IBEP3282

Current Oculomotor Research

Physiological and Psychological Aspects

Current Oculomotor Research
Physiological and Psychological Aspects

Edited by

Wolfgang Becker
University of Ulm
Ulm, Germany

Heiner Deubel
Ludwig-Maximilians University
Munich, Germany

and

Thomas Mergner
University of Freiburg
Freiburg, Germany

Kluwer Academic / Plenum Publishers
New York, Boston, Dordrecht, London, Moscow

Library of Congress Cataloging-in-Publication Data

Current oculomotor research : physiological and psychological
aspects / edited by Wolfgang Becker, Heiner Deubel, and Thomas
Mergner.
    p. cm.
    "Proceedings of the Ninth European Conference on Eye Movements,
held September 23-26, 1997, in Ulm, Germany"--T.p. verso.
    Includes bibliographical references and index.
    ISBN 0-306-46049-1
    1. Eye--Movements--Congresses. 2. Eye--Movement
disorders--Congresses. I. Becker, Wolfgang, Dr. -Ing. II. Deubel,
Heiner. III. European Conference on Eye Movements (9th : 1997 :
Ulm, Germany)
    QP477.5 .C87 1999
    612.8'46--dc21
                                                        98-31568
                                                           CIP

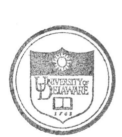

Proceedings of the Ninth European Conference on Eye Movements,
held September 23 – 26, 1997, in Ulm, Germany

ISBN 0-306-46049-1

© 1999 Kluwer Academic / Plenum Publishers, New York
233 Spring Street, New York, N.Y. 10013

10 9 8 7 6 5 4 3 2 1

A C.I.P. record for this book is available from the Library of Congress.

Printed in the United States of America

PREFACE

This volume contains the proceedings of the Ninth European Conference on Eye Movements (ECEM 9), held in Ulm, Germany, on September 23–26, 1997. ECEM 9 continued a series of conferences initiated by Rudolf Groner of Bern, Switzerland, in 1981 which, from its very beginning, has brought together scientists from very diverse fields with a common interest in eye movements. About 40 of the papers presented at ECEM 9 have been selected for presentation in full length while others are rendered in condensed form.

There is a broad spectrum of motives why people have become involved in, and fascinated by, eye movement research. Neuroscientists have been allured by the prospect of understanding anatomical findings, single unit recordings, and the sequels of experimental lesions in terms of the clearly defined system requirements and the well documented behavioural repertoire of the oculomotor system. Others have been attracted by the richness of this repertoire and its dependence on an intricate hierarchy of factors spanning from "simple" reflexes to visual pattern recognition and spatio-temporal prediction. Neurologists, neuro-ophthalmologists and neuro-otologists have long standing experience with eye movements as sensitive indicators of lesions in the brain stem, the midbrain, and the cerebellum. By studying oculomotor malfunctions they have made, and are continuing to make, important contributions to our understanding of oculomotor functions. Engineers, early on, were intrigued by the often machine-like responses of our eyes and tried to analyze the underlying logical structure by means of systems theory. Others are interested in developing ever more sophisticated and reliable eye movement recording systems or look at the way eye movements scan the visual space in order to devise optimum strategies for the presentation and search of visually coded information. Finally, psychologists have discovered eye movements as indicators of cognitive processes and of variations of a subject's attentive state. They are investigating the role of eye movements in reading and are considering their interactions with the uptake of visual information. In doing so, they have come to pose the very same questions about the logical structure of the visuo-oculomotor interface that also preoccupy their colleagues on the neuroscience and engineering side. Characteristically, the originator of ECEM series himself is a psychologist.

Screening the more than 160 mostly excellent presentations given at ECEM 9 and selecting 40 of them for full length presentation was not an easy task. We have tried to identify the most outstanding contributions that would best reflect the broad and interdisciplinary scope of the conference. We are indebted to the conference chairpersons for assisting us herein with their invaluable advice. However, the ultimate responsibility for the final selection is entirely with the editors—it is they who should be blamed for inconsistencies and important papers that have been overlooked.

The conference, and hence this book, could not have been realized without the dedicated help of numerous people. We wish to thank the staff of Sektion Neurophysiologie at the University of Ulm, including T. Boß, V. Diekmann, B. Glinkemann, R. Jürgens, and R. Kühne, for their participation in the organization of the conference, Fray L. Frey for her secretarial help, and W. Krause of Neurologische Klinik at the University of Freiburg for helping to prepare the book.

Finally, we also gratefully acknowledge the financial support of Deutsche Forschungsgemeinschaft and the Faculty of Medicine of the University of Ulm. We also thank the participants who all contributed to an exciting and challenging conference.

The picture on the front cover shows the EYE OF HORUS, a symbol of the god Horus from the mythical world of ancient Egypt (here as artwork of T. Mergner). The symbol was also considered a powerful amulet and was worn to ensure good health. The pharmacist's mark for prescription, ℞, is derived from this symbol. Furthermore, the scheme also represented a fractional quantification system to measure parts of a whole. Each piece of the eye was thought to represent a fraction of the descending geometric series 1/2, 1/4, 1/8, ... 1/64. Its sum equals 63/64, or approximately 1. The eye is also thought to represent the "whole" of sensory inputs, its parts standing for Touch, Taste, Hearing, Thought, Sight and Smell. Following very precise laws related to the fraction values, it represented a kind of "model" for what we call today sensory physiology.

W. Becker, Ulm
H. Deubel, Munich
T. Mergner, Freiburg

CONTENTS

BRAINSTEM ANATOMY OF SACCADES AND OCULAR FOLLOWING

J. A. Büttner-Ennever and A. K. E. Horn

Institute of Anatomy
Ludwig-Maximilian University
Munich, Germany

1. INTRODUCTION

It is convenient to divide eye movements into different types (saccades, vestibular ocular reflexes, optokinetic responses, smooth pursuit and vergence) and to consider the neuroanatomical circuits generating each type as relatively separate. Although it is clear that this is an oversimplification (Büttner and Büttner-Ennever, 1988; Büttner-Ennever and Horn 1997), individual cell groups with a function specific for one particular type of eye movement can be identified in experimental material. With the help of histochemical markers they can be identified in man too. In this report we describe the identification of two cell groups essential for the generation of saccadic eye movements in monkey, their location in man and their differential control from the superior colliculus.

2. DIFFERENT TYPES OF EYE MOVEMENTS

2.1. Saccades

A simple description of the premotor circuits for saccadic eye movements would be as follows: immediate premotor burst neurons in the paramedian pontine reticular formation (PPRF) for horizontal saccades, in the rostral interstitial nucleus of the medial longitudinal fascicle (riMLF) for vertical saccades, activate the eye muscle motoneurons during a saccade. During slow eye movements and fixation the burst neurons are inhibited by omnipause neurons (OPN) in the nucleus raphe interpositus (RIP). Burst neurons and omnipause neurons receive afferents from the superior colliculus (SC), while the frontal eye fields of the cerebral cortex appear only to contact the omnipause neurons (Moschovakis et al. 1996).

Current Oculomotor Research, edited by Becker *et al.*
Plenum Press, New York, 1999.

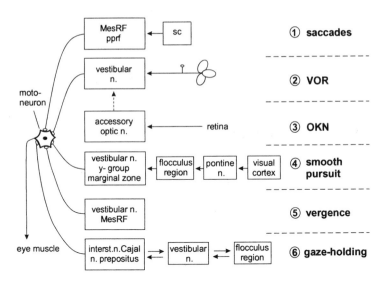

Figure 1. A simplified diagram of the premotor networks subserving 5 different types of eye movements, and gaze-holding. All converge at the level of the motoneuron. Abbreviations: n.= nucleus; MesRF= mesencephalic reticular formation; OKN= optokinetic response; PPRF= paramedian pontine reticular formation; SC= superior colliculus; VOR= vestibulo-ocular reflex.

2.2. The Vestibulo-Ocular Reflex

The vestibulo-ocular reflex is generated by sensory signals from the labyrinthine canals and otoliths, relayed through the vestibular nuclei, where the signals are modulated by the cerebellum, then fed to the extraocular motoneurons in nIII, nIV and nVI via the medial longitudinal fasciculus (MLF) or the brachium conjunctivum (Büttner-Ennever, 1992; Büttner-Ennever 1998).

2.3. The Optokinetic Response

Optokinetic responses (OKN) are elicited by the movement of large visual fields across the retina, which generate responses in the retino-recipient accessory optic terminal nuclei of the mesencephalon: the dorsal, medial, lateral and interstitial terminal nuclei (DTN, MTN, LTN, and ITN). These nuclei along with the nucleus of the optic tract (NOT) in the pretectum, feed the information into the vestibular-oculomotor circuits through which the eye movement response, OKN, is generated (Fuchs and Mustari, 1993; Büttner-Ennever et al. 1996).

2.4. Smooth Pursuit

Smooth pursuit pathways receive retinal information through 2 parallel afferent pathways: a motion-sensitive 'magnocellular pathway', and a form- and colour- sensitive 'parvocellular pathway'. The two inputs supply posterior parietal cortical areas with information concerning object motion in space (the dorsal stream), in contrast to the inferotemporal region more involved in the analysis of form (the ventral stream). Descending projections from the posterior parietal cortex relay in the dorsolateral pontine nuclei (May et al. 1991), which projects to the dorsal and ventral paraflocculus and the caudal vermis of the cerebellum. Cerebellar efferents via the vestibular complex or other relays, reach the oculomotor nuclei to generate smooth pursuit eye movements (Leigh and Zee 1991).

2.5. Vergence

Vergence premotor neurons have been found in the mesencephalic reticular formation dorsal to the oculomotor nucleus and in the pretectum, which provide the vergence command to the oculomotor nuclei (Mays and Gamlin 1995). Recently Chen-Huang and McCrea (1998) have shown that a vergence signal proportional to the viewing distance during horizontal linear acceleration is carried by the ascending tract of Deiters (ATD), to medial rectus motoneurons in nIII. The ascending tract of Deiters originates in the magnocellular division of the medial vestibular nucleus, a region which is arguably part of the lateral vestibular nucleus.

2.6. Gaze-Holding

In addition to these eye movement types perhaps gaze-holding, involving the velocity to position integrator, should be included in the list of eye movement types. Gaze-holding is also subtended by a relatively separate group of neural circuits: the interstitial nucleus of Cajal (iC) for vertical, and the nucleus prepositus hypoglossi (ppH) for horizontal gaze-holding with their reciprocal vestibular and cerebellar connections (Fukushima et al. 1992).

3. LOCATION OF SACCADIC PREMOTOR CELL GROUPS

With transsynaptic tracer and double-labelling experiments we have shown that the horizontal *excitatory burst neurons* (EBNs) form a compact group of neurons in the pontine reticular formation, which can be recognized in the absence of tract tracer labelling on the basis of the following characteristics: 1) their location is in the nucleus reticularis pontis caudalis just beneath the MLF, immediately caudal to locus coeruleus, and rostral to the abducens nucleus: 2) they are medium-sized: and 3) contain the calcium-binding protein parvalbumin (Horn et al., 1995). The region also contains reticulospinal neurons (Robinson et al. 1994).

The *omnipause neurons* (OPNs) are glycinergic, and lie close to the midline between the rootlets of the abducens nerve (Büttner-Ennever et al., 1988; Horn et al., 1994). The OPNs are parvalbumin-positive, and in addition they constitute the majority (70%) of medium-sized neurons with distinctive, horizontally-oriented dendrites, within the nucleus raphe interpositus (RIP). With the help of this experimental information, the homologous cell groups in humans were identified (Horn et al., 1994). In addition we were able to analyse the inputs from different regions of the superior colliculus (SC) to the saccade generator in terms of their termination on EBNs and OPNs cell populations in monkey.

4. SUPERIOR COLLICULUS INPUTS TO THE SACCADE GENERATOR

The superior colliculus is essential for the generation of an orienting resonse to an object of visual or auditory interest (Grantyn et al. 1993). Descending pathways from SC to the saccade generator and reticulospinal cells groups generate the eye and head movements, and have been documented in many studies (Moschovakis, 1996; Moschovakis et al.1996; Olivier et al. 1993). Electrical stimulation and recording studies in the superior colliculus demonstrate a topographical motor map for the saccadic eye movements (Robinson, 1972). Large saccades are represented caudally and small saccades rostrally, and rostrolaterally lies the 'rostral pole of the saccadic motor map', a region described as the fixation zone in behavioural experiments (Munoz and Guitton, 1991; Munoz and Wurtz, 1993; Paré and Guitton, 1994). These physiological studies in cat and monkey report regional specializations in the rostral pole considered to promote 'gaze-fixation'.

4.1. Projections from Superior Colliculus to EBNs and OPNs

We investigated the differential projections to the EBNs and OPNs from the SC 1) rostral pole, 2) small saccade region and 3) large horizontal saccade region (Büttner-Ennever et al. 1997). Injections of ^{3}H-leucine into the rostral pole led to the labelling of fibres in the crossed predorsal bundle (PDB) with thick axon collaterals that terminated around the soma of neurons in nucleus raphe interpositus (RIP), the OPNs. Very little input to other regions, containing EBNs or reticulospinal neurons, was evident. Injections into the small saccade area led to a diffuse projection over the whole dendritic field of contralateral OPNs, which arose from PDB axons of smaller diameter than those from the rostral pole. In addition, labelling of EBNs and other reticulospinal areas was seen. Finally, tracer deposits in the caudal SC regions labelled the PDB, reticulospinal EBN areas, but no terminals over the OPNs in RIP. However we consider it to be significant that the labelled PDB fibres passed through the dendritic fields of the OPNs, because this could provide a point of interaction between SC efferents (e.g. from build-up neurons) and the OPNs, i.e. the saccade generator.

4.2. Discussion

The results fit in some respects with the hypothesis put forward by of Everling et al. (1998), after comparing the pattern of discharge in SC 'fixation neurons' with omnipause cells, in the behaving monkey. The authors proposed, that the OPNs receive 3 different inputs from the SC: 1) a monosynaptic input from the 'fixation neurons': 2) a disynaptic in-

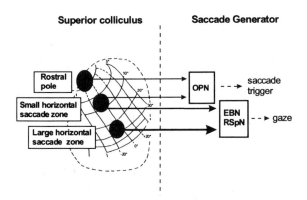

Figure 2. A simplified diagram of the connections between the superior colliculus (SC) and two cell groups of the horizontal saccade generator in the caudal pons: the omnipause neurons (OPN) and the excitatory burst neurons (EBN), which lie intermingled with reticulospinal neurons (RSpN). The shaded areas represent deposits of ^{3}H-leucine at 3 different locations on the saccadic motor map according to Robinson (1972). The arrows indicate the labelled efferent pathways.

hibitory input from the tectal long-lead burst neurons, to trigger a saccade: 3) an input from the build-up neurons to compensate for the decreased input from the 'fixation cells' just before a saccade. First, we demonstrate anatomically the somatic input to OPNs from cells in the rostral pole with thick axon collaterals. Second, we show that there is a diffuse pattern of terminal labelling over the contralateral OPNs and their dendritic area: the function of this is unclear, since details in synaptic connectivity cannot be interpreted from light microscopic data. Finally the interaction between build-up neurons and OPNs could very well be anatomically represented by axo-dendritic contacts between the OPN horizontal dendrites and the descending fibres of the predorsal bundle, which approach so close to the OPN dendritic field.

5. CONCLUSIONS

Relatively separate neural circuits for five different types of eye movements, and gaze-holding, can be distinguished in primates. Omnipause (OPN) and horizontal excitatory burst neuron (EBN) areas of the saccade burst generator can be cytoarchitectonically recognised in both monkey and *man*. Differential inputs to these two cell groups from the different regions of the motor map of the superior colliculus (SC) suggest an anatomical basis for their activation during saccade generation, and for the supression of saccades (fixation) from the rostral pole of the motor map.

ACKNOWLEDGMENT

This work was supported by a grant from the German Research Council: SFB 462/B3.

REFERENCES

Büttner U, and Büttner-Ennever JA (1988) Present concepts of oculomotor organization. Rev Oculomot Res 2: 3–32

Büttner-Ennever JA, Cohen B, Pause M, and Fries W (1988) Raphe nucleus of the pons containing omnipause neurons of the oculomotor system in the monkey, and its homologue in man. J Comp Neurol 267: 307–321

Büttner-Ennever JA (1992) Patterns of connectivity in the vestibular nuclei. Ann N Y Acad Sci 656: 363–378

Büttner-Ennever JA, Cohen B, Horn AKE, Reisine H (1996) Efferent pathways of the nucleus of the optic tract in monkey and their role in eye movements. J Comp Neurol 373: 90–107

Büttner-Ennever JA, Horn AKE, Henn V (1997) Differential projections from rostral and caudal superior colliculus to the horizontal saccadic premotor and omnipause neurons in pons of the primate. Soc Neurosci Abstr 23: 1296

Büttner-Ennever JA, and Horn AKE (1997) Anatomical substrates of oculomotor control. Current Opinion in Neurobiology 7: 872–879

Büttner-Ennever JA (1998) Otolith pathways to brainstem and cerebellum. Ann N Y Acad Sci (in press)

Chen Huang C, and McCrea RA (1998) Viewing distance related sensory processing in the ascending tract of deiters vestibulo-ocular reflex pathway. J Vestib Res 8: 175–184

Everling S, Paré M, Dorris MC, and Munoz DP (1998) Comparison of the discharge characteristics of brain stem omnipause neurons and superior colliculus fixation neurons in monkey: Implications for control of fixation and saccade behavior. J Neurophysiol 79: 511–528

Fuchs AF, Mustari MJ (1993) The optokinetic response in primates and its possible neuronal substrate. In: Miles FA, Wallmann J (eds) Visual motion and its role in the stabilization of gaze. Elsevier, Amsterdam, London, New York, Tokyo, pp 343–369

Fukushima K, Kaneko CRS, and Fuchs AF (1992) The neuronal substrate of integration in the oculomotor system. Prog Neurobiol 39: 609–639

Grantyn A, Olivier E, Kitama T (1993) Tracing premotor brain stem networks of orienting movements. Curr Opin Neurobiol 3: 973–981

Horn AKE, Büttner-Ennever JA, Wahle P, and Reichenberger I (1994) Neurotransmitter profile of saccadic omnipause neurons in nucleus raphe interpositus. J Neurosci 14: 2032–2046

Horn AKE, Büttner-Ennever JA, Suzuki Y, and Henn V (1995) Histological identification of premotor neurons for horizontal saccades in monkey and man by parvalbumin immunostaining. J Comp Neurol 359: 350–363

Leigh RJ, Zee DS (1991) The neurology of eye movements. F.A.Davis Company, Philadelphia,

May JG, Keller EL, and Suzuki DA (1991) Smooth-pursuit eye movement deficits with chemical lesions in the dorsolateral pontine nucleus of the monkey. J Neurophysiol

Mays LE, and Gamlin PD (1995) Neuronal circuitry controlling the near response. Curr Opin Neurobiol 5: 763–768

Moschovakis AK (1996) The superior colliculus and eye movement control. Curr Opin Neurobiol 6: 811–816

Moschovakis AK, Scudder CA, and Highstein SM (1996) The microscopic anatomy and physiology of the mammalian saccadic system. Prog Neurobiol 50: 133

Munoz DP, and Guitton D (1991) Control of Orienting gaze shifts by the tectoreticulospinal System in the had-free cat. II Sustained discharges during motor preparation and fixation. J Neurophysiol 66: 1624–1641

Munoz DP, Wurtz RH (1993) Fixation cells in monkey superior colliculus. II. Reversible activation and deactivation. J Neurophysiol 70: 576–589(Abstract)

Olivier E, Grantyn A, Chat M, and Berthoz A (1993) The Control of Slow Orienting Eye Movements by Tectoreticulospinal Neurons in the Cat - Behavior, Discharge Patterns and Underlying Connections. Exp Brain Res 93: 435–449

Paré M, and Guitton D (1994) The fixation area of the cat superior colliculus: Effects of electrical stimulation and direct connection with brainstem omnipause neurons. Exp Brain Res 101: 109–122

Robinson DA (1972) Eye movements evoked by collicular stimulation in the alert monkey. Vision Res 12: 1795–1808

Robinson FR, Phillips JO, and Fuchs AF (1994) Coordination of gaze shifts in primates: Brainstem inputs to neck and extraocular motoneuron pools. J Comp Neurol 346: 43–62

C-FOS EXPRESSION IN THE OPTOKINETIC NUCLEI OF THE RAT FOLLOWING DIFFERENT VISUAL STIMULUS CONDITIONS

Giampaolo Biral, Renata Ferrari, and Sergio Fonda

Dipartimento di Scienze Biomediche
Università di Modena
Via Campi, 287, 41100 Modena, Italy

1. ABSTRACT

In the present study we characterised by means of the c-Fos method the neuronal populations of the optokinetic nuclei system of the rat activated by different directions of external visual world motion as well as by saccadic exploration of a patterned stationary scene. A major difference was found between the nucleus of the optic tract (NOT) and the nuclei of the accessory optic system (AOS): dorsal terminal (DTN), lateral terminal (LTN) and medial terminal (MTN). c-Fos-positive cells are expressed in the AOS nuclei only after optokinetic stimulation (OKS) according to the direction for which each nucleus is strictly committed: in the DTN after horizontal OKS, in the LTN and MTN after vertical OKS. No segregation of direction-selective cells was observed in the MTN for opposite directions of motion. In the NOT, c-Fos cells became immunoreactive after OKS of any direction, with the greatest expression induced by horizontal OKS in the nucleus contralateral to the eye stimulated nasalward, and even following the presentation of a non-rotating drum. However, the spatial location of the activated neurones is distributed along the nucleus for horizontal OKS and strongly restricted to its rostral region for other stimuli. Given these findings, a larger spectrum of competencies than previously supposed should be attributed to the NOT.

2. INTRODUCTION

The bulk of metabolic and electrophysiological data support the idea that the medial terminal nucleus (MTN), the most prominent of the accessory optic system (AOS) nuclei in rodents and lagomorphes, represents the first relay station along the vertical optokinetic

Current Oculomotor Research, edited by Becker *et al.*
Plenum Press, New York, 1999.

7

pathway (Walley 1967; Simpson et al. 1979; Grasse and Cynader 1982; Biral et al. 1987; Soodak and Simpson 1988; Benassi et al. 1989; Lui et al. 1990; Van der Togt et al. 1993).

In concert with the other AOS nuclei and the pretectal nucleus of the optic tract (NOT), the analogous structure involved in the processing of horizontal optokinetic signals, the MTN contributes to visual stabilisation of the external scene for translatory movements of the animal (Collewijn 1975; Simpson et al. 1979; Cazin et al. 1980; Simpson 1984; Simpson et al. 1988). In addition, these visual nuclei become the complementary counterpart of the vestibular reflex for head rotation in the low frequency range (Collewijn 1981). Consequently, optokinetic nuclei have been regarded as a specialised system committed to detecting self-motion in all directions.

As proved by the great populations of GABAergic cells present in these nuclei, in a large proportion projecting neurones, a consistent reciprocal, inhibitory input connects AOS nuclei, in particular MTN with the DTN and the pretectal NOT (Giolli et al. 1985; Van der Togt et al. 1991; Giolli et al. 1992; Van der Want et al. 1992). The functional properties of the optokinetic nuclei cells, mainly their strict direction selectivity (D.S.), seem to be widely if not exclusively dependent on this extended net of mutual interconnections. In fact, lesions of the NOT alter the range of the direction selectivity of the MTN neurones (Natal and Britto 1987) and lesions of the AOS lead to a disturbed horizontal optokinetic nystagmus (Clement and Magnin 1984). Furthermore, a complete silencing of NOT cells is obtained during electrical stimulation of the MTN (Van der Togt and Schmidt 1994), thus showing that the operational modality of the optokinetic system is founded on preventing other signal elaboration when a specific directional channel is working.

However, some indications suggest that at least a number of the NOT neurones do not fire during optokinetic stimulation (OKS) but their activity appears related to fast moving visual stimuli in whatever direction (Ballas and Hoffmann 1985; Ibbotson and Mark 1994) or associated to eye saccades (Schmidt and Hoffmann 1992; Schweigart and Hoffmann 1992; Ibbotson and Mark 1994; Schmidt 1996; Mustari et al. 1997). This peculiarity has not yet been investigated for the AOS nuclei and specifically for MTN, for which, on the other hand, some conflicting findings question a regional segregation of units in relation to their D.S. (Simpson et al. 1979; Grasse and Cynader 1982; Biral et al. 1987; Benassi et al. 1989; Lui et al. 1990; Van der Togt et al. 1993).

The present study pursues two objectives. First, it tries to provide evidence for a tight commitment of each optokinetic nucleus to a determined direction of motion and, at the same time, to ascertain the existence of neurones unrelated to the retinal slip signal in the MTN and to localise the exact position of such a class of cells in the NOT. Secondly, to determine the degree of segregation of the D.S. units within the MTN. For these purposes we used the c-Fos immunohistochemical procedure because it provides a cellular resolution of activated neurones in all nuclei of the brain and, more importantly, allows the mapping of their position in each nucleus. It is generally accepted that the expression of immediate early genes, such as c-Fos, in post-synaptic neurones following incoming stimulation could represent a neuroanatomical method for studying functional activity (Morgan and Curran 1989).

3. MATERIALS AND METHODS

Twenty Long-Evans rats weighing 240–300 g were used for this study. Two weeks before the actual experiments the animals were anaesthetised (pentobarbital: 40 mg/kg i.p.) and a pair of metal nuts were cemented onto their skull with dental acrylic. The nuts served to fasten a steel screw connected to a rigid support of a small plastic box allowing painless fixation of the head. To reduce the stressful effects of novelty and acute restraint, all animals were handled extensively and underwent a cycle of training sessions in the experimental condition. On the day of the experiment, under brief ether anaesthesia, the rats were housed in their box and placed at the centre of an optokinetic drum (90 cm both in diameter and in height) lined with black and white alternating stripes. Stimulation was started after 1 hour, enough time to recover from anaesthesia.

The animals, all tested in the binocular condition, were divided into 4 groups according to the experimental design: control (still illuminated pattern, 5 rats); horizontal optokinetic stimulation (pattern rotating clockwise around its vertical axis at 4.50°/s, 5 rats); vertical downward optokinetic stimulation (pattern rotating around an horizontal axis at 2°/s, 5 rats) and vertical upward optokinetic stimulation (pattern rotating at 2°/s, 5 rats). In the case of vertical OKS the animals were placed perpendicular to the axis of the drum so that both eyes received the same direction of stimulation. In some preliminary experiments we tested the animals for optokinetic performance to different velocity steps and for spontaneous oculomotor behaviour by means of a magnetic search coil. The speeds used in the present experiment had been shown to elicit the most consistent optokinetic response. Spontaneous eye movements towards the non-rotating illuminated drum were mainly horizontal saccades (4–5/min) of various amplitude occurring in both directions. After 1 hour of stimulation, during which the animals were continuously kept alert by a random noise, they were placed in the dark and allowed to move freely in the cage for an additional 30 minutes.

Subsequently, the rats were deeply anaesthetised with an overdose of pentobarbital and transcardially perfused with 150 ml of 0.1M phosphate buffer solution (PBS) followed by 350 ml of 4% paraformaldehyde in PBS. The brain was removed, postfixed for another two hours in the same fixative at 4°C then transferred in 30% sucrose until it sunk. One out of every two 40 μm section was incubated overnight in the primary antibody raised in sheep against a c-Fos synthetic peptide (CRB, Cambridge, UK, Lot OA-11–823) diluted 1:3000 in PBS-0.3% Triton. After rinsing in PBS the sections were incubated for 2 hours in biotinylated rabbit anti-sheep serum, 1:200 in PBS-Triton. Then they were washed in PBS and placed for 1hr in avidin-biotin-peroxidase complex (Elite-ABC kit Vector Labs). Following two rinses in PBS, the sections were developed in 1 mg/ml diaminobenzidine in PBS with 0.02% hydrogen peroxide, mounted on gelatinized slides and coverslipped. Adjacent sections were stained with cresyl violet.

For better anatomical identification of nuclei, especially for the pretectal nucleus of the optic tract, we referred to the Atlas by Paxinos and Watson (1986) and to our histological sections. For quantitative analyses, c-Fos positive cells were manually counted in duplicate in the areas of interest under the light microscope at 100 X magnification. Therefore, the counts were expressed as total cell number per rat.

The statistical analysis was performed using the Student's t-test (single tail, nonpaired groups).

4. RESULTS

The counts of c-Fos positive cells in the two main nuclei of the optokinetic system, MTN and NOT, for each animal group are given in Table 1.

Table 1. Mean and standard deviation of total number of immunoreactive cells
in the NOT (and DTN) and in the MTN.

Experimental groups	NOT		MTN	
	Left	Right	Left	Right
Non-rotating drum	° 30.33 ± 8.08	§ 22.66 ± 3.51	0.10	0.22
Horizontal OKS	128.00 ± 46.53	& 284.00 ± 30.20	# 2.20 ± 1.30	# 4.21 ± 3.49
Vertical OKS up → down	49.80 ± 28.15	51.80 ± 26.50	70.27 ± 27.15	71.41 ± 32.56
Vertical OKS down → up	59.00 ± 10.79	68.00 ± 14.26	75.00 ± 20.82	88.00 ± 42.16

& Significant difference ($P<0.001$) from left side. § Significant difference ($P<0.01$) from the right NOT in vertical and horizontal optokinetic stimulated groups. ° Significant difference from the left NOT in vertical upward
($P<0.05$) and horizontal ($P<0.01$) optokinetic stimulated groups. # Significant difference ($P<0.01$) from vertical
stimulated groups.
Note that the strongest c-Fos expression in the NOT was found following horizontal OKS: the right NOT was
related to the nasally stimulated eye and the left NOT received a temporalward stimulus. In the MTN the largest
number of c-Fos labelled cells occurs in animals subjected to vertical OKS.

4.1. Non-Rotating drum

No cell expressing c-Fos was found in the MTN and LTN when the animal was facing
the non-rotating illuminated drum. On the other hand, some c-Fos immunoreactivity was
present in the NOT (Fig. 1), almost exclusively confined to its rostral portions. Immunoreactive cells were not encountered in the DTN and neighbouring regions of the NOT.

4.2. Horizontal Stimulation

In the NOT, the number of c-Fos labelled cells increased considerably following
horizontal optokinetic stimulation (Fig. 2). NOT receiving nasalward stimulation showed
a significantly ($P<0.001$) higher number of c-Fos positive cells (284 ± 30.2) than the NOT

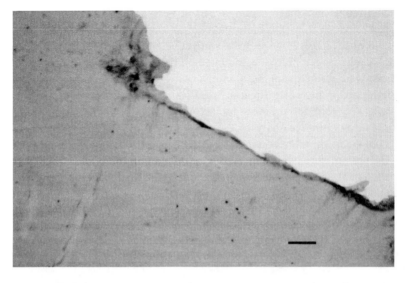

Figure 1. Coronal brain section at the level of pretectal region showing c-Fos expressing cells in the NOT of a rat
facing the immobile illuminated drum. Bar = 0.1 mm.

receiving input from the naso-temporal stimulated eye (128 ± 46.53). The c-Fos induced cells were distributed throughout the NOT and in the DTN, but the majority of cells were concentrated in the rostral regions of the NOT where a population of efferent neurones projecting to the inferior olive has been described (Robertson 1983; Schmidt et al. 1995). As for the MTN and LTN, very few cells were induced to express c-Fos protein by horizontal optokinetic stimulation.

4.3. Vertical Stimulation

A less conspicuous increase of c-Fos than in horizontal OKS induction, but still significantly different from rats facing the non-rotating illuminated drum, was found in the NOT following vertical optokinetic stimulation. With downward stimulation c-Fos expressing cells accounted to 49.8 ± 28.15 and 51.8 ± 26.5 in the left and right NOT, respectively. A similar number of immunoreactive cells were counted in the rat group subjected to upward OKS. In fact, the mean number of neurones was 59 ± 10.79 in the left NOT and 68 ± 14.26 in the right NOT. It was noted that the cells were often grouped in clusters, as shown in Fig. 3, and distributed almost exclusively in the rostral regions of the nucleus.

Following a prolonged vertical optokinetic stimulation all animals showed a consistent appearance of c-Fos immunoreactive cells in the entire MTN along its caudal to rostral extension (Fig. 4). The amount of c–Fos expression was largely independent of the direction of vertical motion. In fact, following downward stimulation the MTN labelled cells were 70.2 ± 27.15 and 71.4 ± 32.5 on the left and right side respectively. Similar values were found for the upward direction: 75 ± 20.82 c-Fos-stained cells were counted in the left and 88 ± 42.16 in the right MTN. As for the distribution of the cells, about 80% were confined to the ventral portion of the nucleus, without differences between the two directions of vertical OKS. A few c-Fos labelled cells appeared in the LTN following ver-

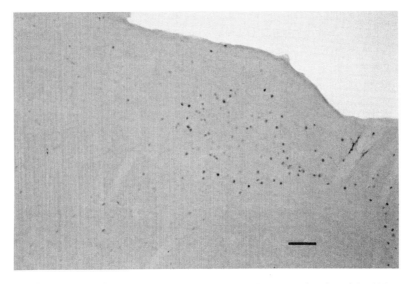

Figure 2. Coronal brain section showing c-Fos immunoreactive cells in the rostral region of the NOT contralateral to the nasalward stimulated eye following the binocular horizontal OKS. Bar = 0.1 mm.

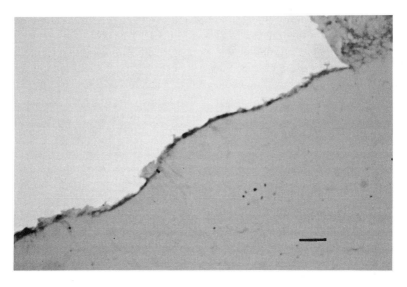

Figure 3. c-Fos labelled cells grouped in a cluster in the rostral region of the NOT from a rat subjected to vertical downward OKS. Bar = 0.1 mm.

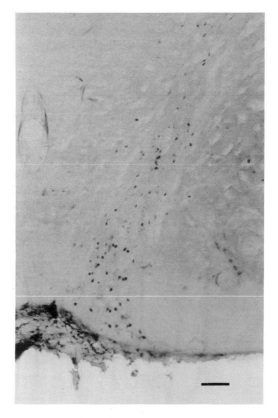

Figure 4. Coronal brain section at the level of MTN of a rat subjected to vertical OKS. The greatest c-Fos expression was concentrated in the ventral region of the nucleus. Bar = 0.1 mm.

tical OKS, but the high variability in the staining level did not allow us to replicate the counting, and so it is not reported in Table 1.

5. DISCUSSION

The c-Fos expression seems to be a valuable marker for assessing the functional performance of the optokinetic brainstem nuclei. In fact, external world motion, in whatever way induced, determines a very strong appearance of c-Fos positive cells in the neuronal structures known to be involved in the first steps of elaboration of retinal slip signals. Furthermore, besides the cellular resolution of the method, the concurrent overview of all nuclei provides compelling evidence of the operations performed by the single nucleus in respect to all others in the context of the same experimental condition.

The present study provides support for a differential characterisation of the optokinetic nuclei. The activation of MTN and LTN, as demonstrated by the appearance of c-Fos expression in a consistent number of their neurones, is limited only to vertical optokinetic stimulation. Neither horizontal motion of the drum nor saccadic scanning of the stationary pattern activated the cells of these nuclei strong enough to express c-Fos protein. Therefore, saccade related neurones have so far not been described in these optokinetic nuclei (and in the DTN). This class of cells appears to be confined to restricted portion of the NOT, as will be discussed below. Absence of immunoreactivity in the vertical committed nuclei following horizontal OKS can be attributed to a strong inhibition by neurones in the NOT and DTN by means of their heavy GABAergic efferents (Giolli et al. 1985; Van der Togt et al. 1991; Giolli et al. 1992; Van der Want et al. 1992). However, analysis of the neuronal responses (Natal and Britto 1988) evidenced a large spectrum of directions, including the horizontal one, for which MTN neurones could fire. Nonetheless, the majority of these neurones display a preference for vertical downward motion with a nasal component, or for the upward direction with a temporal component. c-Fos expression probably depicts a more general behaviour of the output of the neuronal population, while the unit analysis emphasises on the single cell behaviour. In fact, the c-Fos method provides us with an exact insight into the spatial distribution of MTN neurones selectively activated for each vertical direction in a given single rat. Both upward as well as downward vertical motion give overlapping immunoreactive patterns: c-Fos positive neurones are mainly concentrated in the ventral part of the nucleus along its entire rostro-caudal extension.

Recently Van der Togt et al. (1993) described in anaesthetised rats a possible segregation between upward and downward direction selective units, in the dorsal and in the ventral part of MTN, respectively, in relation to the area in which retinal fibers of the two fascicles of the accessory optic tract are distributed. A similar segregation was previously noted by Natal and Britto (1987). On the other hand, previous data from metabolic studies, using the deoxyglucose method in fully awake rats and guinea pigs, provided a clear demonstration that the functional activity, as assessed by labelling uptake, was always independent of drum motion direction and related only to the amount of retinal afferents (Biral et al. 1987; Benassi et al. 1989; Lui et al. 1990). It is possible that this discrepancy is based on methodological difference, in addition to the level of vigilance of the animals. The deoxyglucose as well as the c-Fos method reflect the harmonised activity of an entire population of neurones regardless of the single cell size. Electrophysiological recording might introduce an intrinsic bias, by selecting the largest cells, thereby giving an incomplete and distorted representation of the entire population. The same methodological framework together with species differences could be invoked to explain the inverted direction selectivity obtained in two other mammals (Walley 1967; Simpson et al. 1979; Grasse and Cynader 1982). In conclusion, we claim likely that MTN cells that are driven by the vertical retinal slip signals of different direction are largely intermingled. Furthermore, MTN seems to be exclusively committed to operations of the optokinetic system with a strict competence for external world vertical motion.

As for the NOT, a different and more general role can be inferred from our data. c-Fos positive cells are found, as expected, following horizontal optokinetic stimulation in the NOT and DTN and, more surprisingly, although exclusively in the NOT, even after vertical optokinetic stimulation and in rats facing the stationary drum. The largest number of c-Fos expressing neurones, observed in animals subjected to horizontal OKS, confirms NOT (at least a part of it) and DTN as the first relay station involved in transferring the horizontal retinal slip signal to the appropriate optomotor structures. On the other hand, groups of neurones, mainly or almost exclusively confined to the rostral portions of the NOT, are induced to express c-Fos protein in response to non-specific visual stimuli. We have to exclude that a minor part of the cell population of the NOT might be driven by vertical motion, given the inhibitory pathway arising from the MTN and the fact that its electrical stimulation evokes inhibition of NOT cells (Van der Togt and Schmidt 1994). We have to exclude also that c-Fos expression could arise spontaneously and always with the same pattern in the same region of the nucleus. One possible explanation would consider the NOT a mixed population of cells with a wide spectrum of functional properties, as in fact has been reported in several papers (Schmidt and Hoffmann 1992; Schweigart and Hoffmann 1992; Ibbotson and Mark 1994; Schmidt 1996; Mustari et al. 1997). Besides of retinal slip cells, as the more representative and consistent ones of NOT, another class of neurones have been described in the cat (Ballas and Hoffmann 1985) and in the wallaby (Ibbotson and Mark 1994). These neurones, "jerk" neurones, respond to visual stimuli moving in any direction and at high speed. Furthermore, in a previous report that was largely neglected or misinterpreted (Bon et al. 1977), a class of neurones in the pretectal region, perhaps in the NOT, was described responding in relation to eye saccades even in the dark. Only recently Schmidt (1996) in an in depth reassessment of this problem found a class of neurones, termed saccade neurones, in the pretectum and mainly in the NOT, projecting to the dorsal subdivision of the lateral geniculate nucleus, which responded to saccades in the dark. The c-Fos positive cells which we found following vertical OKS and after spontaneous saccadic exploration evidently belong to subclasses of NOT cells different from retinal slip cells. In agreement with the proposal advanced in a recent review (Büttner-Ennever and Horn 1997) based on a detailed survey of data collected in higher mammals, our results underline the functional heterogeneity of the output NOT cells. At the same time, they suggest that only the more lateral part of the NOT could be considered a close ally of the AOS nuclei in the optokinetic reflex and that this part is integrated in the NOT/DTN complex. Finally, it seems that the complexity of the NOT organisation, as is emerging from recent studies in non-human primates, might represent the consequent evolution of the basic layout present in the rat. On the other hand, consistent similarities have been pointed out between lateral-eyed and frontal-eyed mammals in the anatomical arrangement of NOT efferent pathways (Schmidt et al. 1995).

Further investigations are needed to establish how many classes of specialised neurones inhabit the NOT and to localise each class within this multifaceted nucleus.

ACKNOWLEDGMENTS

This research was supported by EC grant BMH4-CT96-0976 and by grants from the Ministero dell'Universita' e della Ricerca Scientifica e Tecnologica.

REFERENCES

Ballas I, Hoffmann K-P (1985) A correlation between receptive field properties and morphological structures in the pretectum of the cat. J Comp Neurol 238: 417–428

Benassi C, Biral GP, Lui F, Porro CA, Corazza R (1989) The interstitial nucleus of the superior fasciculus, posterior bundle (INSFp) in the guinea pig: another nucleus of the accessory optic system processing the vertical slip signal. Visual Neurosci 2: 377–382

Biral GP, Porro CA, Cavazzuti M, Benassi C, Corazza R (1987) Vertical and horizontal visual whole-field motion differently affect the metabolic activity of the rat medial terminal nucleus. Brain Res 412: 43–53

Bon L, Corazza R, Inchingolo P (1977) Neuronal activity correlated with eye movements in the cat's pretectum. Neurosci Letters 5: 69–73

Büttner-Ennever JA, Horn AKE (1997) Anatomical substrates of oculomotor control. Curr Opin Neurobiol 7: 872–879

Cazin L, Precht W, Lannou J (1980) Firing characteristics of neurons mediating optokinetic responses to rat's vestibular neurons. Pflügers Arch 386:221–230

Clement G, Magnin M (1984) Effects of accessory optic system lesions on vestibulo-ocular and optokinetic reflexes in the cat. Exp Brain Res 55: 49–59

Collewijn H (1975) Direction-selective units in the rabbit's nucleus of the optic tract. Brain Res 100: 489–508

Collewijn H (1981) The oculomotor system of the rabbit and its plasticity. Springer-Verlag, Berlin

Giolli RA, Peterson GM, Ribak CE, McDonald HM, Blanks RHI, Fallon JH (1985) GABAergic neurons comprise a major cell type in rodent visual relay nuclei: An immunocytochemical study of pretectal and accessory optic nuclei. Exp Brain Res 61: 194–203

Giolli RA, Torigoe Y, Clarke RJ, Blanks RHI, Fallon JH (1992) GABAergic and non-GABAergic projections of the accessry optic nuclei, including the visual tegmental relay zone, to the nucleus of the optic tract and dorsal terminal accessory optic nucleus in rat. J Comp Neurol 319:349–358

Grasse KL, Cynader MS (1982) Electrophysiology of medial terminal nucleus of accessory optic system in the cat. J Neurophysiol 48: 490–504

Ibbotson MR, Mark RF (1994) Wide-field nondirectional visual unis in the pretectum: do they suppress ocular following of saccade-induced visual stimulation? J Neurophysiol 72: 1448–1450

Lui F, Biral GP, Benassi C, Ferrari R, Corazza R (1990) Correlation between retinal afferent distribution, neuronal size, and functional activity in the guinea pig medial terminal accessory optic nucleus. Exp Brain Res 81: 77–84

Morgan JI, Curran T (1989) Stimulus-transcription coupling in neurons : role of cellular immediate-early genes. Trends Neurosci 12: 459–462

Mustari MJ, Fuchs AF; Pong M (1997) Response properties of pretectal omnidirectinal pause neurons in the behaving primate. J Neurophysiol 77: 116–125

Natal CL, Britto LRG (1987) The pretectal nucleus of the optic tract modulates the direction selectivity of accessory optic neurons in rats. Brain Res 419: 320–323

Natal CL, Britto LRG (1988) The rat accessory optic system: effects of cortical lesions on the directional selectivity of units within the medial terminal nucleus. Neurosci Letters 91: 154- 159

Paxinos G, Watson C (1986) The rat brain in stereotaxic coordinates. Academic Press, Sidney

Robertson RT (1983) Efferents of the pretectal complex: separate populationsof neuronsproject to lateral thalamus and to inferior olive. Brain Res 258: 91–95

Schmidt M, Hoffman K-P (1992) Physiological characterization of pretectal neurons projecting to the lateral geniculate nucleus in the cat. Eur J Neurosci 4: 318–326

Schmidt M, Schiff D, Bentivoglio M (1995) Independent efferent populations in the nucleus of the optic tract: an anatomical and physiological study in rat and cat. J Comp Neurol 360: 271–285

Schmidt M (1996) Neurons in the cat pretectum that project to the dorsal lateral geniculate nucleus are activated during saccades. J Neurophysiol 76: 2907–2917

Schweigart G, Hoffmann K-P (1992) Pretectal jerk neuron activity during saccadic eye movements and visual stimulation in the cat. Exp Brain Res 91: 273–283

Simpson JI, Soodak RE, Hess R (1979) The accessory optic system and its relation to the vestibulocerebellum. In: Granit R and Pompeiano O (eds) Progress in Brain Research. Reflex control of posture and movement. Elsevier, Amsterdam: pp 715–724

Simpson JI (1984) The accessory optic system. Annu Rev Neurosci 7: 13–44

Simpson JI, Giolli RA, Blanks RHI (1988) The pretectal nuclear complex and the accessory optic system. In: Büttner-Ennever JA (ed) Neuroanatomy of the Oculomotor System. Elsevier, Amsterdam: pp 335–364

Soodak RE, Simpson JI (1988) The accessory optic system of the rabbit. I. Basic visual response properties J Neurophysiol 60: 2037–2054

Van der Togt C, Nunes Cardoso B, Van der Want J (1991) Medial terminal nucleus terminals in the nucleus of the optic tract contain GABA: an electron microscopical study with immunocytochemical double labeling of GABA and PHA-L. J Comp Neurol 312: 231–241

Van der Togt C, Van der Want J, Schmidt M (1993) Segregation of direction selective neurons and synaptic organization of inhibitory intranuclear connections in the medial terminal nucleus of the rat: an electrophysiological and immunoelectron microscopical study. J Comp Neurol 338: 175–192

Van der Togt C, Schmidt M (1994) Inhibition of neuronal activity in the nucleus of the optic tract due to electrical stimulation of the medial terminal nucleus in the rat. Eur J Neurosci 6: 558–564

Van der Want JJL, Nunes Cardoso JJ, Van der Togt C (1992) GABAergic neurons and circuits in the pretectal nuclei and the accessory optic system of mammals. In: Mize RR, Marc R, Sillito A (eds) Progress in Brain Research, vol 90, Elsevier, Amsterdam, pp 283–305

Walley RE (1967) Receptive fields in the accessory optic system of the rabbit. Exp Neurol 17: 27–43

NEURONAL ACTIVITY IN MONKEY SUPERIOR COLLICULUS DURING AN ANTISACCADE TASK

Stefan Everling, Michael C. Dorris, and Douglas P. Munoz

MRC Group in Sensory-Motor Neuroscience
Department of Physiology, Queen's University
Kingston, Ontario K7L 3N6, Canada

1. INTRODUCTION

It well known that the primate superior colliculus (SC) is involved in the generation of visually guided saccadic eye movements (for review see Sparks and Hartwich-Young 1989). Its intermediate layers contain neurons which display motor bursts for saccades within the response field of the neuron. These neurons project directly to preoculomotoneurons in paramedian pontine reticular formation and the rostral interstitial nucleus of the medial longitudinal fasciculus, which provide the input to the extraocular muscle motoneurons (for review see Moschovakis et al. 1996).

The importance of the SC in the generation of saccades is shown by the prolonged latencies, reduced velocities and decreased precision of saccades after lesion or chemical deactivation of the SC (Lee et al. 1988; Schiller et al. 1987; Hikosaka and Wurtz 1985; Wurtz and Goldberg 1972). While the SC is generally considered to be involved in the generation of reflexive saccades, the frontal eye field (FEF) and supplementary eye field (SEF) are considered to be predominately involved in the generation of purposive or voluntary saccades. This hypothesis is supported by the difficulties of patients with frontal cortex lesions (Guitton et al. 1985; Pierrot-Deseilligny et al. 1991) to correctly perform the anti-saccade task (Hallett 1978, Hallett and Adams 1980). This task requires subjects to suppress a saccade to a suddenly appearing visual stimulus and generate a saccade to a mirror symmetric position. Recently, it has also been shown that many neurons in the SEF have a higher saccade-related burst for anti-saccades compared with pro-saccades (Schlag-Rey et al. 1997).

However, the interaction between the frontal oculomotor areas and the SC are unknown for the anti-saccade task. The situation is complicated, because the FEF and SEF project directly and also indirectly via the basal ganglia to the SC. Moreover, both areas also project directly to the preoculomotoneurons in the brain stem. At least three possibilities of neural activity in the SC during anti-saccades would be in accordance with this projection pattern: 1) *Bypass hypothesis*: The signal for the generation of an anti-saccade is

Current Oculomotor Research, edited by Becker *et al.*
Plenum Press, New York, 1999.

generated within the FEF or SEF and then send to the brain stem, whereas the SC generates the movement signal for the pro-saccade. In this case, a strong signal from the FEF or SEF would be needed to overrule the conflicting movement signal to the stimulus arising from the SC. This hypothesis would be in agreement with the finding of a stronger saccade-related motor burst for anti-saccades compared with pro-saccades in the SEF (Schlag-Rey et al. 1997). 2) *Inhibition hypothesis*: The FEF or SEF send the movement signal for the anti-saccade to the brain stem and at the same time inhibit the movement signal for the pro-saccade in the SC. 3) *Serial hypothesis*: The FEF or SEF send the movement signal for the anti-saccade to the SC which relays this command to the brain stem.

The *bypass hypothesis* predicts the inappropriate motor signal for anti-saccades in the SC. The *inhibition hypothesis* predicts that no motor command is generated in the SC during the anti-saccade task, whereas the *serial hypothesis* predicts the occurrence of a saccade-related motor burst on the side ipsilateral to the stimulus in the SC.

The objective of the current study was to distinguish between these three hypotheses by recording from single neurons in the SC in monkeys during the performance of a task with pro-saccade and anti-saccade trials.

2. METHODS

2.1. Experimental Procedures

We recorded single-neuron activity from neurons in the SC of two male rhesus monkeys (*Macaca mulatta*) weighing between 5 and 9 kg. The surgical procedures for preparing the monkeys were described recently (Dorris et al. 1997). The magnetic search coil technique (Fuchs and Robinson 1966) was used for eye movement recording.

A real-time data acquisition system (REX) (Hays et al. 1982) was used for the control of the behavioral paradigm, visual displays, and storage of data. Single neurons were recorded by the use of tungsten microelectrodes (Frederick Haer) with impedances of 1–5 MΩ which were driven through stainless steel guide tubes. The guide tubes were held in position by a delrin grid fixed to the recording cylinders (Crist et al. 1988). During the experiments, monkeys were seated in a primate chair with the head restrained. They faced a tangent screen 86 cm in front of them for which they had an unobstructed view of 70° x 70°, i.e. ± 35° of center. Red and green light emitting diodes (LEDs, 0.3 cd/m^2) were back projected onto the screen to produce visual stimuli. During the intertrial intervals, the screen was illuminated diffusely (1.0 cd/m^2) to prevent the animals from becoming dark-adapted.

2.2. Behavioral Paradigm

The monkeys were trained to perform saccades during randomly interleaved pro-saccade and anti-saccade trials. A trial started with the appearance of either a central green fixation point (FP) which signalled an anti-saccade trial or a red FP which signalled a pro-saccade trial. The animals were required to look at it and maintain steady fixation for 700–900 ms. On one half of the trials the FP was extinguished for 200 ms (gap period) before stimulus presentation. On the remainder of trials the FP remained illuminated during the whole trial. An eccentric red stimulus was then pseudorandomly projected with equal probability either into the response field of the neuron or at the mirror position opposite to the horizontal and vertical meridian. A liquid reward was given to the monkey if it made a saccade within 500 ms to the correct position and maintained fixation there for at least 200 ms. Trials with reaction times below 80 ms were excluded as anticipations and trials with reaction times above 500 ms were excluded as no response trials. After the experimental session the monkeys received water until satiation, after which they were returned to their home cage. Records were kept of the weight and health status of the monkeys and additional water and fruit was provided as needed.

2.3. Data Collection and Analysis

Single-neuron discharges were sampled at 1 kHz after passing through a window discriminator that produced a pulse for each spike that met both amplitude and time constraints. Horizontal and vertical eye position signals were digitized at 500 Hz and stored on a hard disk. The off-line analysis was performed on a SUN Sparc 2 Workstation with the use of a computer program that identified and marked the onset and termination of each saccade using velocity and acceleration threshold criteria (Waitzman et al. 1991). Each trial was visually inspected by the experimenter and identified failures were corrected if necessary.

To evaluate the relation between neuron discharge and stimulus appearance or saccade onset, we produced rasters and constructed average peristimulus and perisaccade histograms with a binwidth of 10 ms from these spike rasters.

2.4. Neuron Identification

We describe here the activities of three classes of neurons in the SC, which were classified according to the following criteria:

Visual neurons. To be classified as a visual neuron, a neuron had to be located 0 to 1.5 mm below the dorsal surface of the SC and had to discharge for the presentation of a visual stimulus into the neuron's response field, but not for saccadic eye movements.

Buildup neurons. To be classified as a buildup neuron, a neuron had to be located 1 to 3 mm below the dorsal surface of the SC and display: 1) long-lead pretarget activity during the end of the gap epoch (Dorris et al. 1997; Munoz and Wurtz 1995) that was significantly greater than during the visual fixation epoch (t-test, $p<0.05$); and 2) saccade-related activity above 100 spikes/s for pro-saccades into the neuron's response field.

Burst neurons. To be classified as a burst neuron, a neuron had to be located 1 to 3 mm below the dorsal surface of the SC and to display 1) no increase in discharge during the gap period and; and 2) saccade-related activity above 100 spikes/s for pro-saccades into the neuron's response field.

3. RESULTS

Figure 1 shows the activity of a visual neuron located in the superficial layers, a burst neuron in the intermediate layers, and a buildup neuron in the intermediate layers aligned on stimulus presentation on gap pro-saccade trials. Buildup neurons had a low-frequency increase in discharge during the gap period (Fig. 1, left and right panel, bottom). All three types of neurons displayed a burst of action potentials around 80 ms in response to the presentation of the visual stimulus into their response field, which is always on the side contralateral to the stimulus (left panel). The neurons do not show any increase in discharge for stimulus presentations at the mirror location on the ipsilateral side. The sac-

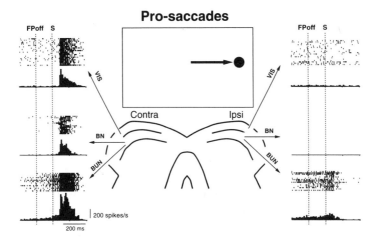

Figure 1. Activity of neurons in the superficial and intermediate layers of the superior colliculus during pro-saccade trials aligned on the onset of the visual stimulus. In the rasters, each tickmark represents one actionpotential, and each line represents the discharge on one trial. Below each raster is a histogram showing the discharge summed over trials (binwidth 10 ms). BN, burst neuron. BUN, buildup neuron. VIS, visual neuron.

cade-related burst neuron and buildup neuron in the intermediate layers of the SC then show a motor burst time-locked to the start of the saccade to the stimulus (Fig. 2, left panel, middle and bottom).

The discharge pattern of the same SC neurons is shown in the gap anti-saccade condition in Fig. 3 aligned on the presentation of the stimulus and in Fig. 4 aligned on the onset of the correct anti-saccades. The stimulus conditions were identical to those in the gap pro-saccade condition, except that the monkeys were instructed by the color of the initial FP to generate an anti-saccade. Visual neurons in the superficial layers displayed a burst of

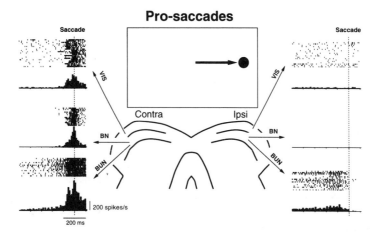

Figure 2. Activity of neurons in the superficial and intermediate layers of the superior colliculus during pro-saccade trials aligned on the onset of saccadic eye movements. In the rasters, each tickmark represents one actionpotential, and each line represents the discharge on one trial. Below each raster is a histogram showing the discharge summed over trials (binwidth 10 ms). BN, burst neuron. BUN, buildup neuron. VIS, visual neuron.

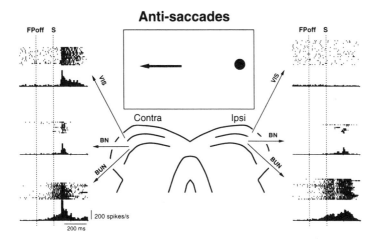

Figure 3. Activity of neurons in the superficial and intermediate layers of the superior colliculus during anti-saccade trials aligned on the onset of the visual stimulus. In the rasters, each tickmark represents one actionpotential, and each line represents the discharge on one trial. Below each raster is a histogram showing the discharge summed over trials (binwidth 10 ms). BN, burst neuron. BUN, buildup neuron. VIS, visual neuron.

action potentials in response to the presentation of the visual stimulus into their response field on the side contralateral to the stimulus (Fig. 3, left panel, top). We did not observe an increase in discharge in visual neurons on the side ipsilateral to the stimulus, i.e., when the monkey generated an anti-saccade to this location (Fig. 3, right panel, top). Burst neurons in the intermediate layers of the SC with visual responses also discharged in response to the presentation of the stimulus into their response field on anti-saccade trials (Fig. 3, left panel, middle). In contrast to visual neurons, burst neurons showed a later discharge when the stimulus was presented on the side ipsilateral to neuron's response field (Fig. 3,

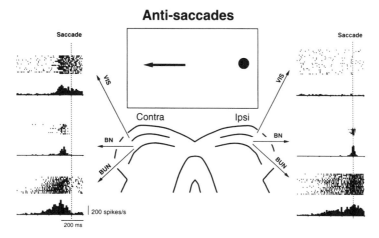

Figure 4. Activity of neurons in the superficial and intermediate layers of the superior colliculus during anti-saccade trials aligned on the onset of saccadic eye movements. In the rasters, each tickmark represents one actionpotential, and each line represents the discharge on one trial. Below each raster is a histogram showing the discharge summed over trials (binwidth 10 ms). BN, burst neuron. BUN, buildup neuron. VIS, visual neuron.

right panel, middle). This discharge was time-locked to the onset of the anti-saccades (Fig. 4, right panel, middle). Buildup neurons displayed a low-frequency discharge during the gap period on anti-saccade trials (Fig. 3, left and right panel, bottom), similar to pro-saccade trials. Like the burst neuron, the buildup neuron also discharged for stimulus presentations into its response field (Fig. 3, left panel, bottom) and it displayed a motor burst when the stimulus was presented on the ipsilateral side (Fig. 4, right panel, bottom). A comparison of the saccade-related discharges of the burst neuron and the buildup neuron between the pro-saccade condition (Fig. 2, left panel, middle and bottom) and the anti-saccade condition (Fig. 4, right panel, middle and bottom) shows that although saccade-related neurons in the SC discharge a motor burst for anti-saccades, the amplitudes of these motor bursts are considerably lower than the burst amplitude for pro-saccades with the same amplitudes.

4. DISCUSSION

We have provided evidence for the serial hypothesis in anti-saccade generation outlined in the introduction. Our findings show that SC neurons display a visual response for stimulus presentations into their response field, regardless of whether the monkeys generated pro-saccades to the stimulus or anti-saccades to the opposite side. Furthermore, saccade-related neurons in the intermediate layers of the SC display saccade-related discharges for anti-saccades into their response field. The latter finding contradicts the bypass hypothesis which predicted a saccade-related discharge for stimulus presentations into the neuron's response field. The finding also contradicts the inhibition hypothesis which predicted no saccade-related motor burst for anti-saccades.

The strong cortical projections to the SC directly and indirectly via the basal ganglia (for review see Wurtz and Goldberg 1989) suggest that cortical inputs are responsible for the suppression of neural activity on the side contralateral to the stimulus in the SC after the visual response and for the increase of neural activity on the ipsilateral side which is required to drive the anti-saccade. A clear function of the frontal cortex in the inhibition of reflexive pro-saccades is shown by the known difficulties of patients with frontal lobe lesions or neurological or psychiatric diseases which affect the frontal lobe to suppress reflexive saccades in the anti-saccade task (for review see Everling and Fischer 1998). Therefore, it may be assumed that the input from the FEF or SEF is necessary to suppress the neural activity in the contralateral SC. It is less clear, where the necessary spatial transformation for the anti-saccades is performed. One candidate would be the SEF where visual-and-eye movement neurons encode the stimulus location and the direction of the impending saccade (Schlag-Rey et al. 1997). Another candidate would be parietal cortex which is known to be involved in spatial transformation processes (for review see Andersen et al. 1997). Indeed, an event-related potential study with humans has shown a shift of a negative potential in the parietal cortex from the contralateral to the ipsilateral side prior to anti-saccade generation (Everling et al. 1998). The poor spatial resolution of event-related potentials, however, makes it hard to localize the cortical areas involved in this transformation. Single-cell recordings in the lateral intraparietal (LIP) area have provided no evidence for a participation of LIP in the computation of the vector for the anti-saccade (Gottlieb and Goldberg 1997). The vast majority of LIP neurons only display visual bursts for the direction of the visual stimulus but do not discharge for the antisaccade.

In this respect, SC neurons resemble SEF neurons in that they discharge for the location of the stimulus and for the direction of the saccade. However, we found lower saccadic motor bursts for anti-saccades compared with pro-saccades. The opposite result was obtained in the SEF (Schlag-Rey et al. 1997). It is currently unknown, why SC neurons display weak saccade-related discharges for anti-saccades despite increased discharges in the SEF.

We conclude from our results that the SC in primates is not merely involved in the generation of reflexive visually-guided saccades, but also in the generation of voluntary anti-saccades.

REFERENCES

Andersen RA, Snyder LH, Bradley DC, Hing J (1989) Multimodal representation of space in the posterior parietal cortex and its use in planning movements. Ann Rev Neurosci 20: 303–330

Christ CF, Yamasaki DSG, Komatsu H, Wurtz RH (1988) A grid system and microsyringe for single cell recordings. J Neurosci Methods 26: 117–122

Dorris MC, Paré M, Munoz DP (1997) Neuronal activity in monkey superior colliculus related to the initiation of saccadic eye movements. J Neurosci 17: 8566–8579

Everling S, Fischer B (1998) The antisaccade: A review of basic research and clinical studies. Neuropsychologia (In Press)

Everling S, Spantekow A, Krappmann P, Flohr H (1998) Event-related potentials associated with correct and incorrect responses in a cued gap antisaccade task. Exp Brain Res 118: 27–34

Fuchs AF, Robinson DA (1966) A method for measuring horizontal and vertical eye movements chronically in the monkey. J Appl Physiol 21: 1068–1070

Gottlieb J, Goldberg ME (1997) Encoding of stimulus and saccade direction in rhesus monkey lateral intraparietal area (LIP). Soc Neurosci Abstr 23: 14.9

Guitton D, Buchtel HA, Douglas RM (1985) Frontal lobe lesions in man cause difficulties in suppressing reflexive glances and in generating goal-directed saccades. Exp Brain Res 58: 455–472

Hallett PE (1978) Primary and secondary saccades to goals defined by instructions. Vision Res 18: 1279–1296

Hallett PE, Adams BD (1980) The predictability of saccadic latencies in a novel voluntary oculomotor task. Vision Res 20: 329–339

Hays AV, Richmond BJ, Optican LM (1982) A UNIX-based multiple process system for real-time data acquisition and control, W ESCON Conf. Proc. 2: 1–10

Hikosaka O, Wurtz RH (1985) Modification of saccadic eye movements by GABA-related substances. I. Effect of muscimol and bicuculline in monkey superior colliculus. J Neurophysiol 53: 266–291

Lee C, Rohrer W, Sparks DL (1988) Population coding of saccadic eye movements by neurons in the superior colliculus. Nature 332: 357–360

Munoz DP, Wurtz RH (1995) Saccade-related activity in monkey superior colliculus. I. Characteristics of burst and buildup cells. J Neurophysiol 73: 2313–2333

Moschovakis AK, Scudder CA, Highstein SM (1996) The microscopic anatomy and physiology of the mammalian saccadic system. Proc Neurobiol 50: 133–254

Pierrot-Deseilligny CP, Rivaud S, Gaymard B, Agid Y (1991) Cortical control of reflexive visually-guided saccades. Brain 114: 1472–1485

Schiller PH, Sandel JH, Maunsell JHR (1987) The effect of frontal eye field and superior colliculus lesions on saccadic latencies in the rhesus monkey. J Neurophysiol 57: 1033–1049

Schlag-Rey M, Amador N, Sanchez H, Schlag J (1997) Antisaccade performance predicted by neuronal activity in the supplementary eye field. Nature 390: 398–401

Sparks DL, Hartwich-Young R (1989) The deep layers of the superior colliculus. In Wurtz RH, Goldberg ME (eds.) The neurobiology of saccadic eye movements. Amsterdam, Elsevier.

Waitzman DM, Ma TP, Optican LM, Wurtz RH (1991) Superior colliculus neurons mediate the dynamic characteristics of saccades. J Neurophysiol 66: 1716–1737

Wurtz, RH, Goldberg ME (1972) Activity of superior colliculus neurons in behaving monkey, IV. Effects of lesions on eye movements. J Neurophysiol 35: 575–586

Wurtz RH, Goldberg ME (1989) The neurobiology of saccadic eye movements. Amsterdam, Elsevier.

4

SPACE AND SALIENCE IN PARIETAL CORTEX

Keith D. Powell,[1] Carol L. Colby,[2] Jacqueline Gottlieb,[1] Makoto Kusunoki,[1,3] and Michael E. Goldberg[1,4]

[1]Laboratory of Sensorimotor Research
National Eye Institute
Bethesda, Maryland 20892-4435
[2]Department of Neuroscience and Center for the Neural Basis of Cognition
University of Pittsburgh
Pittsburgh, Pennsylvania 15260
[3]Department of Physiology
Nihon University School of Medicine
Tokyo 173, Japan
[4]Department of Neurology
Georgetown University School of Medicine
Washington, DC 20007

1. INTRODUCTION

The parietal cortex has long been thought to participate in the neural mechanisms underlying visual attention, spatial perception, and eye movements (Critchley 1953). This review will begin by describing the attentional and spatial aspects of saccadic performance in a patient with a frontoparietal deficit, and then show how single neuron activity in one particular area, the lateral intraparietal area (LIP) renders the clinical deficits understandable in neurophysiological terms.

2. OCULOMOTOR DEFICITS IN A PATIENT WITH FRONTOPARIETAL DAMAGE

A patient sustained an intracerebral hemorrhage from a ruptured aneurysm that bled into the overlying cerebral cortex (Duhamel et al. 1992). She had significant damage to the right parietal and frontal lobes. Fourteen years later, at the time of study, she had a mild left hemiparesis, mild left visual and somatosensory neglect and a left inferior quadrantanopsia that spared the central 6° of the visual field. With the head in a fixed position,

Current Oculomotor Research, edited by Becker *et al.*
Plenum Press, New York, 1999.

she had a directional deficit for saccades between targets presented 5° to the left and to the right in a random walk: leftward saccades were hypometric and had a longer latency than rightward ones. These deficits did not vary with the starting position of the eye: the same spatial location acquired by an accurate rightward saccade would only be approached by a hypometric leftward saccade.

Her most unexpected deficit lay in her performance of the double step task (Figure 1). This task, first described by Hallett and Lightstone (1976), has been used to demonstrate that the saccadic system can perform in a spatially accurate fashion even when there is a mismatch between the spatial location of the target and its location on the retina. In this task, the subject looks at a fixation point (Figure 1, top panel). The fixation point goes out and two lights are flashed sequentially in the visual periphery. The subject makes successive saccades from the fixation point to the first target and then from the first to the second target. Programming the first saccade is easy, because the vector of the saccade necessary to acquire the target is identical to the vector from the fixation point to the retinal location of the stimulus. A simple retinal strategy can drive accurate saccades in this

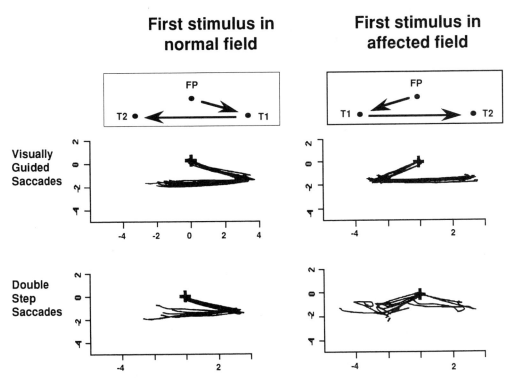

Figure 1. Sequential saccades in a patient with a right frontoparietal lesion. The cartoons (top row) show the arrangement of stimuli and saccade directions for the experiments in the columns beneath. The middle and bottom rows show eye position plotted in horizontal and vertical coordinates. This reproduces the spatial pattern of the eye movements. The subject begins by looking at the fixation point (FP), and makes saccades to T1 and T2 in response to sequential flashes. In the left column the stimulus flashes first in the ipsilesional, normal left visual field, and then in the contralateral, affected visual field. In the right column the stimulus flashes first in the contralesional, affected visual field and then in the ipsilesional, normal visual field. The middle row shows eye movements in the visually guided task, in which the stimuli remain illuminated long enough (500ms each) so that each sequential saccade is visually guided. The bottom row shows eye movement in the true double-step case, with the T1 flashing for 100ms and T2 for 80 ms. Adapted from Duhamel et al., 1992b.

case. However, once the subject fixates the spatial location of the first target, this equivalence no longer exists for the second target. If the subject used a retinal strategy, she would make a downward and rightward saccade, equivalent to the retinal vector of the stimulus when it appeared. Normal subjects can compensate for the first saccade, and make accurate saccades to the spatial location of the second target.

In the patient described above, saccadic accuracy was measured in two tasks, successive visually guided saccade (slow double step) and true double step. First, in the slow version of the double step task, the patient was instructed to make sequential saccades to the two targets in the order in which they appeared (Fig. 1, middle). Each target stayed on for 500 ms, so both saccades were visually guided, and the retinal and saccade vectors were identical. Leftward saccades followed by rightward saccades were just as accurate as the reverse order, although all leftward saccades were somewhat inaccurate, as was predicted from the random walk experiment.

The double step task proved more difficult for the patient (Figure 1, bottom row). When the target stepped first into the good field (bottom left panel) the patient made an accurate first saccade, and then a second saccade which was slightly more inaccurate than the simple visually guided saccades. The most profound deficit appeared only when the first stimulus appeared in the affected field. For some saccades, the patient ignored the stimulus in the affected field entirely, and made a saccade directly to the second stimulus presented in the normal field. When she did make the first saccade into the affected field, she was unable to generate a subsequent saccade to the location of the second target (bottom right panel).

This finding is somewhat unexpected: the patient often failed on saccades in the good direction, to targets that appeared in the good field. Nevertheless, she clearly did not have a general spatial deficit for either field or a memory deficit. On trials in which she neglected the first target (in the affected field) and went directly to the second target (in the good field) she acquired the second target accurately. Her specific deficit was an inability to calculate the change in target position relative to eye position. She could not compensate for the first saccade when it was in the direction of the affected field. Although this was only a single case report, the phenomenon has been replicated in a large number of patients and was exhibited by patients whose lesion included only the right posterior parietal cortex and not in patients with damage limited to frontal cortex (Heide et al. 1995) .

These observations demonstrate three different roles for the parietal cortex in visuospatial behavior. The first role is related to the generation of saccades: the patient's saccades to visual targets were inaccurate and had longer reaction times. The second role is attentional: given the rapid presentation of stimuli in the affected and normal fields, on a certain number of trials she neglected the stimulus in the affected field. The third role is in spatially accurate behavior: although the patient demonstrated knowledge of the spatial location of the target, on some trials she did not compensate for a saccade in the affected direction. The remainder of this paper will discuss activity in one particular region of the posterior parietal cortex, the lateral intraparietal area, where activity of single neurons is consistent with all three functions - oculomotor, attentional, and spatial- that were illustrated in this case report.

3. THE LATERAL INTRAPARIETAL AREA

The lateral intraparietal area was first described anatomically. It lies in the posterior bank of the intraparietal sulcus and is one of several areas that receives a visual projection from the parieto-occipital area (Colby et al. 1988). It has projections to and from the frontal eye field, and to the intermediate layers of the superior colliculus (Andersen et al. 1985; Lynch et al. 1985; Schall et al. 1995; Stanton et al. 1995). These connections are appropriate for transmitting spatial information to the oculomotor system. LIP also has projections to visual areas such as V4, TE, and TEO (Baizer et al. 1991; Webster et al. 1994) which are known to have activity dependent upon spatial attention (Moran and Desimone 1985), but are not known to be involved in the generation of saccadic eye movements. It also projects to the parahippocampal gyrus (Suzuki and Amaral, 1994) which is critical in spatial memory. A signal that is related to visuospatial attention is useful for all of the projection targets of LIP.

4. BEHAVIORAL MODULATION OF VISUAL RESPONSES IN LIP

Nearly all LIP neurons respond to the appearance of a visual stimulus in the receptive field in a simple fixation task (Robinson et al. 1978), in which a monkey looks at a spot of light and a behaviorally irrelevant stimulus appears in the receptive field of the neuron. These responses can be behaviorally modulated: when the monkey must respond in some way to the stimulus about a third of the neurons respond at a significantly higher frequency to its appearance (Bushnell et al. 1981; Colby et al. 1996). This enhanced response in LIP is not dependent upon what the monkey will do with the stimulus as long as the monkey attends to it. The amount of enhancement is similar whether the (the delayed saccade task) or a task in which the monkey releases a lever in response to a dimming of the stimulus (the peripheral attention task). This is strikingly different from the enhancement of visual responses in the monkey frontal eye field and superior colliculus, where enhancement only occurs when the stimulus in the receptive field is the target for a saccade (Goldberg and Bushnell 1981; Goldberg and Wurtz 1972). Because of this dramatic difference between LIP and the more clearly oculomotor frontal eye field and superior colliculus, it was postulated that enhancement in LIP reflects visuospatial attention (Colby et al. 1996; Goldberg et al. 1990).

All of the standard tasks (fixation, delayed saccade, and peripheral attention) probe the visual activity of a neuron with the use of a stimulus flashed in the receptive field. A flashed stimulus presents a problem that has been ignored by investigators who, since the dawn of behavioral neurophysiology, have used it to describe the 'visual' responses of neurons (Robinson et al. 1978; Wurtz 1969). Psychological analysis indicates that an abrupt onset captures attention (Yantis and Jonides 1984). When a stimulus flashes in the visual field of a monkey, it may itself capture attention, regardless of the wishes of the investigator. This raises the possibility that activity evoked by a suddenly appearing stimulus is primarily an attentional response rather than a purely visual one.

To distinguish between neural activity associated with attention, and that associated with the arrival of a stimulus in the visual receptive of a neuron, we developed a new task, the stable array task (Gottlieb et al. 1998). In this task, the monkey sees a stable array of symbols back-projected by a computer-controlled video projector onto tangent screen in front of him. The symbols do not change at all during the experiment, but remain constantly illuminated and immobile. The advantage of these stimuli is that as the monkey makes saccades across the array, the eye movements bring the stimuli into and out of the receptive fields. However, unlike the flashed stimuli used in most tasks, these stimuli are new only to the receptive field, and not to the visual environment as a whole. When the monkey makes a saccade that brings a stable, non-novel stimulus into the receptive field of a neuron in LIP, the activity evoked by the stimulus is marginal. In contrast, in the fixation task, the same stimulus evokes a strong response when it suddenly appears in the receptive field (Figure 2). Control tasks indicate that the different responses in these two cases are not due to visual factors, such as the motion of the stimulus across the retina during the saccade or the presence of other stimuli outside the receptive field. In the control task, one member of the array (the one that will be in the receptive field) appears immediately before the saccade. In this case, the neurons respond as if the stimulus had flashed in the receptive field (Figure 2).

This result suggests that a large portion of the 'visual' activity evoked in a passive fixation task is in fact due to the salience of the abrupt appearance of the stimulus, and not to the actual photons arriving in the receptive field. This is in contrast to striate cortex, where neurons respond at high frequencies to stimuli brought into their receptive fields by a saccade (Livingstone et al. 1996). The LIP response resembles the activity of visual neurons in the monkey frontal eye field. These FEF neurons respond to flashed stimuli but do not respond when a monkey explores a complex visual environment, unless the monkey is going to make a saccade to an object in the receptive field (Burman and Segraves 1994).

The stable array experiment shows that previous LIP studies significantly underestimate the amount of enhancement. If we consider the baseline visual response of neurons to be that elicited when a saccade brings a stable target into the receptive field, then

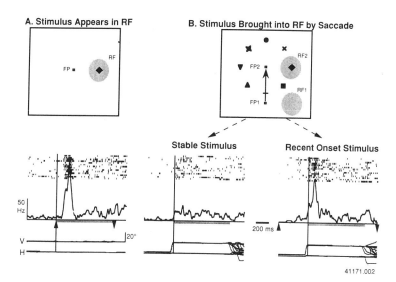

Figure 2. Effect of recent onset on neuronal response. A. Response to the onset of a diamond-shaped stimulus flashed in the receptive field. The cartoon above illustrates the spatial relationship of the fixation point (FP), the stimulus (diamond) and an estimate of receptive field (RF). Raster and spike density plots, synchronized on the appearance of the stimulus, are below the cartoon. The eye position traces from each trial illustrated in the raster diagram are superimposed on the vertical (V) and horizontal (H) eye position traces. Stimulus appears at the up-triangle and disappears at the down triangle. B. Responses when the stimulus is brought into the receptive field by a saccade. The cartoon above illustrates the array of symbols, which remain stably on the tangent screen in front of the monkey. The trial begins when the monkey fixates FP1. At that time the receptive field lies outside the array. The monkey makes a saccade from FP1 to FP2, which moves the receptive field onto the diamond-shaped stimulus. When the diamond is stable, its arrival in the receptive field is accompanied by a weak response of the neuron that begins at the end of the saccade (Stable stimulus). When the diamond stimulus flashes immediately before the saccade (Recent onset stimulus), the cell discharges almost as intensely as in the flashed stimulus case. Reproduced with permission from Gottlieb et al., 1998.

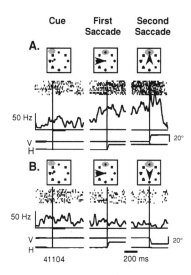

Figure 3. Responses of a neuron during the stable target task. The cartoon above each diagram illustrates the task. The monkey fixates the small square that is located so that the receptive field is outside the array. A cue that matches a member of the array (the circle) briefly appears near the fixation point. The fixation point steps to the center of the array and the monkey makes a saccade to it. The fixation point then disappears and the monkey makes a second saccade to the member of the array that matches the cue. A. The cue matches the stimulus in the receptive field and the monkey makes a saccade to the stable stimulus in the receptive field. B. The cue matches a stimulus outside the receptive field, and the monkey makes a saccade to a stimulus not in the receptive field. The first saccade brings the stimulus into the receptive field in both cases. Adapted from Gottlieb et al., 1998.

roughly 75% of LIP neurons exhibit enhancement, and the average increase in activity is more than double. In studies comparing the modulation of on-responses by task relevance, the amount of enhancement was about 50%, and this only occurred in a third of neurons (Bushnell et al. 1981; Colby et al. 1996).

Although stable objects in the environment are irrelevant to behavior most of the time, they can be made important. For example, you usually ignore the clock on the wall, unless you want to know the time. Then you direct your attention to it, even though it is not new. Attention can be directed to a stable object by requiring the monkey to use that stimulus for some sort of behavior. The stable target task (Figure 3) accomplishes this by cueing the monkey to make a saccade to a stable target that itself never changes during the experiment. The monkey first fixates outside the array, and a cue that matches a member of the array appears briefly at a fixed location in the visual field. Then the monkey makes a saccade to the center of the array, which brings one member of the array into the receptive field. Finally, the monkey makes a second saccade to the stable symbol that matched the cue. Trials in which the cue matches each of the eight symbols are randomly intermixed. When the cue matches the symbol in the receptive field, the cell begins to discharge around the time of the first saccade. When the cue does not match the symbol in the receptive field, the cell does not discharge. The simplest interpretation of these data is that the stimulus in the receptive field has become salient by virtue of the match, and the neural response reflects the representation of a salient stimulus. Making the stimulus behaviorally relevant has enhanced the response, just as its sudden appearance enhanced the response.

5. RELATIONSHIP OF LIP ACTIVITY TO SACCADE PLANNING

Another interpretation is that this activity is related specifically to planning the second saccade. In order to test whether activity in LIP is related to motor planning, we performed a learned-saccade variant of the stable target task. This task dissociates activity evoked by a saccade target from activity related to planning the saccade. In this version of the task, the symbols remain on the screen as in the stable target task. The monkey fixates

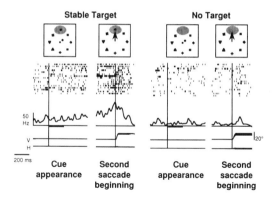

Figure 4. Dependence of activity on the presence of a saccade target (Same neuron as in Figure 3.) Stable target: the monkey fixates in the center of the array, and a cue appears outside the receptive field matching the stimulus in the receptive field. When the fixation point disappears, the monkey makes a saccade to the target. Unlike the previous experiment, where saccade direction is randomized, in this experiment the saccade direction is always into the receptive field. Rasters are shown synchronized on the cue appearance (left) and the beginning of the saccade to the target (right). In the next block of trials, the symbol in the receptive field is removed from the array, and the monkey makes a saccade to the empty spatial location in the receptive field. Rasters are again shown synchronized on the cue appearance (left) and the beginning of the saccade (right). Reproduced with permission from Gottlieb et al., 1998.

in the center of the array, the cue appears outside the receptive field, and the monkey makes a saccade to the stimulus in the receptive field when the fixation point disappears. After a block of trials, that symbol is removed, and the monkey makes the saccade to the spatial location of the now-vanished symbol. The symbol never appears again for the entire block of trials. For most neurons, the activity falls significantly (Figure 4, same neuron as Figure 3) even though the monkey plans and executes the same saccade. Clearly, activity in the stable target task cannot be attributed to the monkey's intention to make the saccade. Maximal activity in the majority of LIP neurons requires a stimulus. That stimulus need not be new, but it must be salient.

Further evidence that activity in LIP reflects salience rather than a motor plan comes from experiments in which the stimulus evoking the response cannot be construed as a saccade target. In the stable target task described above, the cue that dictated the saccade was outside the receptive field. It is also possible to place the cue in the receptive field. In this case, the neuron responds to the cue regardless of the saccade that the monkey will make (Figure 5). This experiment shows that paying attention to information in the receptive field drives the neuron no matter what direction of saccade the monkey is planning.

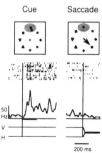

Figure 5. Response to cue that signals a saccade elsewhere. The monkey performs a stable target task like Figure 3, but the cue is in the receptive field and the saccade is made to a stable target outside the receptive field. Rasters synchronized on cue (left) and saccade (right). Reproduced with permission from Gottlieb et al., 1998.

Because flashed stimuli are themselves salient, we studied the effect of saccade planning on the response to a flashed stimulus. In this experiment, the monkey performed a memory-guided delayed saccade task. The saccade target could be inside or outside the receptive field. Five hundred ms after the saccade target disappeared, and roughly 300 ms before the fixation point disappeared, signaling the monkey to make the saccade to the remembered target location, an identical stimulus appeared as a distractor. The distractor could also appear inside or outside of the receptive field. Not only did LIP neurons respond to the stimulus despite the ongoing planning of a saccade elsewhere, the response to the distractor inside the receptive field was greater when the monkey was planning a saccade elsewhere than when it was planning the saccade to the receptive field (Figure 5). This result is reminiscent of those obtained by Steinmetz et al. in Area 7a (1994) and Robinson et al. in LIP (1995). A stimulus flashing in an area to which attention has already been shifted evokes a lesser response than it does when attention is elsewhere. However, we emphasize that even this diminished response is greater than that evoked when a saccade brings a stable stimulus into the receptive field, and so must represent an enhanced response to a salient or attended object.

We conclude that the function of LIP is the representation of attended or salient spatial locations. The hallmark of neuronal activity in LIP is that, like spatial perception itself, it is not tied to any particular modality. Neurons in LIP respond to salient visual stimuli, but they also respond to attended auditory stimuli (Stricanne et al. 1996), respond weakly before saccades without visual targets, and respond even in anticipation of the appearance of a salient target (Colby et al. 1996). For the reasons outlined above, their activity cannot be linked to the planning of any particular movement. Rather, LIP represents attended objects and their locations, and damage to it may cause the neglect described in patients and monkeys with parietal lesions (Critchley 1953; Duhamel et al. 1992; Lynch and McLaren 1989). The next critical problem is to understand the reference frame in which LIP represents attended space.

6. SPATIAL REPRESENTATION IN LIP

Because humans and monkeys perform the double-step task in a spatially accurate manner, one would expect that neurons in the oculomotor system that describe the distance and direction (i.e. the vector) of saccades or saccade targets would also describe those vectors in a spatially accurate fashion. This is precisely the result found in the superior colliculus (Mays and Sparks 1980), in LIP (Barash et al. 1991; Goldberg et al. 1990), and in the frontal eye field (Goldberg and Bruce 1990). If the monkey has to make a saccade of a particular direction and amplitude, neurons discharge in association with that saccade regardless of the retinal location of the stimulus.

7. PERISACCADIC REMAPPING

The double-step task is a laboratory curiosity, but it illustrates a more general problem that the brain must solve . The latency of frontal and parietal visual neurons is at least 60 ms (Bushnell et al. 1981; Goldberg and Bushnell 1981). Without a mechanism that compensates for saccades, every time we move our eyes the information in the brain is inaccurate for the purposes of localization for at least 60 ms after the saccade. If we assume that humans ordinarily make three saccades a second during visual exploration, then the

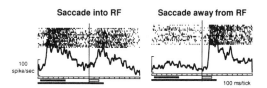

Figure 6. Effect of saccade planning on the response to a task-irrelevant stimulus. The monkey plans a saccade either into (left) or away from (right) the receptive field. Traces show stimulus appearance, distractor appearance, and fixation point appearance. Rasters synchronized on distractor appearance.

cortical representation of the visual world would be inaccurate for the purpose of spatial localization at least 180 ms out of every second, or, roughly twenty percent of the time! Such an inaccuracy in spatial localization, and by inference for spatial behavior, would have very adverse consequences for survival.

Every time a monkey makes a saccade, there is a remapping of the visual world into the coordinates of the new center of gaze. This is demonstrated in the experiment illustrated in Figure 7. The cell shown responds when a stimulus is in the receptive field. It does not respond to the same stimulus in the same spatial location when the monkey is fixating a different place and has therefore moved the retinal receptive field away from the stimulus. There is one circumstance, though, in which it will respond to a stimulus that is

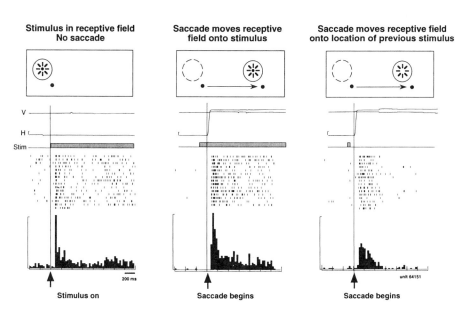

Figure 7. Remapping of visual activity in area LIP. Diagrams show the arrangement of the fixation point, receptive field, stimulus location and saccade. Left: In the fixation task, the neuron responds to the onset of a stimulus in the receptive field. Middle: The same neuron responds when a saccade moves the receptive field onto the location of a recent stimulus. Right: Response after a saccade moves the receptive field onto a previously stimulated location. The stimulus is flashed on for only 50 ms and is extinguished before the saccade begins. The neuron is responding to the remapped memory trace of the previous stimulus. Control experiments (not shown) indicate that neither the stimulus alone nor the saccade alone can drive the neuron. Adapted from Duhamel et al., 1992a.

not in its retinotopic receptive field. When the monkey makes a saccade that brings the spatial location of a recently flashed stimulus into the retinotopic receptive field of the neuron, the cell responds even if the stimulus never actually entered the retinal receptive field. The response is not merely a postsaccadic response to the saccade: there is no post-saccadic activity if the monkey makes a similar saccade that does not move the spatial location of a recently flashed stimulus into the receptive field. Rather, the response reflects a remapped memory trace of the previous stimulus event. These remapped visual responses in LIP and its projection areas may be responsible for the ability of humans and monkeys to perform in a spatially accurate manner across saccades. The inability of patients with parietal deficits such as the one described above can be explained by a lack of this mechanism.

8. CONCLUSIONS

The results describe above support the conclusion that LIP is important in the neural processes underlying visuospatial attention. It selects salient objects from the environment, and transmits this information to its projection targets. Visual areas in the temporal and occipital lobes to which LIP projects can use this information for their own attentional processing. The superior colliculus and frontal eye field can use this information for the generation of saccades, but LIP activity itself is independent of saccade planning or motor intention: LIP neurons respond to stimuli that direct saccades elsewhere, and respond to distractors that cannot be the targets for saccades. It discharges weakly before purposive saccades made without stimuli, even when the saccades go to the spatial location of the neurons' receptive fields. Finally, LIP has a remapping mechanism that enables it to respond to stimuli in spatial locations that enter the receptive field by virtue of a saccade. Patients whose lesions include LIP would, on the basis of these neuronal properties, be expected to have deficits in the selection of targets for saccades, in visuospatial attention, and in the maintenance of spatially accurate behavior across saccades.

REFERENCES

Andersen RA, Asanuma C, Cowan M (1985) Callosal and prefrontal associational projecting cell populations in area 7a of the macaque monkey: a study using retrogradely transported fluorescent dyes. J. Comp. Neurol. 232:443–455.

Baizer JS, Ungerleider LG, Desimoner R (1991) Organization of visual inputs to the inferior temporal and posterior parietal cortex in macaques. J. Neurosci. 11:168–190.

Barash S, Bracewell RM, Fogassi L, Gnadt, JW, Andersen RA (1991) Saccade-related activity in the lateral intraparietal area. II. Spatial properties. J. Neurophysiol. 66:1109–1124.

Burman DD, Segraves MA (1994) Primate frontal eye field activity during natural scanning eye movements. J. Neurophysiol. 71:1266–1271.

Bushnell MC, Goldberg ME, Robinson DL (1981) Behavioral enhancement of visual responses in monkey cerebral cortex: I. Modulation in posterior parietal cortex related to selective visual attention. J. Neurophysiol. 46:755–772.

Colby CL Duhamel J-R, Goldberg, ME (1996) Visual, presaccadic and cognitive activation of single neurons in monkey lateral intraparietal area. J. Neurophysiol. 76:2841–2852.

Colby CL, Gattass R, Olson CR, Gross CG (1988) Topographic organization of cortical afferents to extrastriate visual area PO in the macaque: a dual tracer study. J. Comp. Neurol. 269:392–413.

Critchley M (1953) The Parietal Lobes. London: Edward Arnold.

Duhamel J-R, Goldberg ME, FitzGibbon EJ, Sirigu A, Grafman J (1992) Saccadic dysmetria in a patient with a right frontoparietal lesion: the importance of corollary discharge for accurate spatial behavior. Brain 115:1387–1402.

Goldberg ME, Bruce CJ (1990) Primate frontal eye fields. III. Maintenance of a spatially accurate saccade signal. J. Neurophysiol. 64:489–508.

Goldberg ME, Bushnell M C (1981) Behavioral enhancement of visual responses in monkey cerebral cortex. II. Modulation in frontal eye fields specifically related to saccades. J. Neurophysiol. 46:773–787.

Goldberg ME, Colby CL, Duhamel J-R (1990) The representation of visuomotor space in the parietal lobe of the monkey. Cold Spring Harbor Symp. Quant. Biol. 55:729–739.

Goldberg ME, Wurtz RH (1972) Activity of superior colliculus in behaving monkeys. II. Effect of attention on neuronal responses. J. Neurophysiol. 35:560–574.

Gottlieb JP, Kusunoki M, Goldberg ME (1998) The representation of visual salience in monkey parietal cortex. Nature 391:481–4.

Hallett PE, Lightstone AD (1976) Saccadic eye movements to flashed targets. Vision Res. 16:107–114.

Heide W, Blankenburg M, Zimmermann E, Kompf D (1995) Cortical control of double-step saccades: implications for spatial orientation. Ann Neurol 38:739–48.

Livingstone MS, Freeman DC, Hubel, DH (1996) Visual responses in V1 of freely viewing monkeys. Cold Spring Harb Symp Quant Biol 61:27–37.

Lynch JC, Graybiel AM, Lobeck, LJ (1985) The differential projection of two cytoarchitectonic subregions of the inferior parietal lobule of macaque upon the deep layers of the superior colliculus. J. Comp. Neurol. 235:241–254.

Lynch JC, McLaren JW (1989) Deficits of visual attention and saccadic eye movements after lesions of parieto-occipital cortex in monkeys. J. Neurophysiol. 61:74–90.

Mays LE, Sparks L (1980) Dissociation of visual and saccade-related responses in superior colliculus neurons. J. Neurophysiol. 43:207–232.

Moran J, Desimone R (1985) Selective attention gates visual processing in extrastriate cortex. Science 229:782–784.

Robinson DL, Bowman EM, Kertzman C (1995) Covert orienting of attention in macaques. II. Contributions of parietal cortex. J. Neurophysiol. 74:698–712.

Robinson DL, Goldberg ME, Stanton, GB () Parietal association cortex in the primate: Sensory mechanisms and behavioral modulations. J. Neurophysiol. 41:910–932, 1978.

Schall JD, Morel A, King DJ, Bullier, J () Topography of visual cortex connections with frontal eye field in macaque: Convergence and segregation of processing streams. J. Neurosci. 15:4464–4487, 1995.

Stanton GB, Bruce CJ, Goldberg, ME () Topography of projections to posterior cortical areas from the macaque frontal eye fields. J. Comp. Neurol. 353:291–305, 1995.

Steinmetz MA, Connor CE, Constantinidis C, McLaughlin JR () Covert attention suppresses neuronal responses in area 7a of the posterior parietal cortex. J. Neurophysiol. 72:1020–1023, 1994.

Stricanne B, Andersen RA, Mazzoni P (1996) Eye-centered, head-centered, and intermediate coding of remembered sound locations in area LIP. J. Neurophysiol. 76:2071–2076.

Suzuki WA, Amaral DG (1994) Perirhinal and parahippocampal cortices of the macaque monkey: cortical afferents. J Comp Neurol, 350, 497–533.

Webster MJ, Bachevalier J, Ungerleider LG (1994) Connections of inferior temporal areas TEO and TE with parietal and frontal cortex in macaque monkeys. Cereb. Cortex 4:470–483.

Wurtz RH (1969) Visual receptive fields of striate cortex neurons in awake monkeys. J. Neurophysiol. 32:727–742.

Yantis S, Jonides J (1984) Abrupt visual onsets and selective attention: evidence from visual search. J Exp Psychol Hum Percept Perform 10:601–21.

5

PARIETAL NEURONS ARE ACTIVATED BY SMOOTH PURSUIT OF *IMAGINARY* TARGETS

U. J. Ilg, J. A. Rommel, and P. Thier

Sektion für Visuelle Sensomotorik
Neurologische Universitätsklinik
D-72076 Tübingen, Germany

1. INTRODUCTION

The interpretation of the function of the primate posterior parietal cortex has been influenced for many years by conflicting interpretations of the response properties of posterior parietal cortex neurons, leading to very different and even exclusive interpretations of parietal lobe functions. In the 1970s, neuroscientists began to study the properties of neurons recorded from area 7 of primate posterior parietal cortex using paradigms which required monkeys to direct either their eyes or their hands to visual targets in extrapersonal space (Hyvärinen and Poranen 1974; Mountcastle et al. 1975). Since many of the neurons studied were active in conjunction with distinct oculomotor behaviors such as fixation, saccades, or smooth pursuit, or alternatively in conjunction with visually directed hand movements, Mountcastle et al. (1975) suggested that the neuronal activation reflected commands for the execution of movements to objects in extrapersonal space. Not much later, Robinson and coworkers arrived at a very different interpretation of eye or hand movement related single unit responses (Robinson et al. 1978). Instead of interpreting posterior parietal cortex as a command device programming movements directed to targets in extrapersonal space, they suggested, alternatively, that the posterior parietal cortex of monkeys should be understood as a sensory structure extracting relevant information by focusing spatial attention to relevant sensory stimuli.

Today, these exclusive views, localizing the functional role of the posterior parietal cortex on opposite sides of the sensory vs. motor dividing line, are no longer tenable. Rather than being either sensory or motor in the strict sense, recent work on visually guided saccades has suggested that parietal neurons involved in these types of visually guided behavior are better described as elements of networks underlying intermediate stages of the sensory-to-motor transformations leading to these behaviors (for review see Andersen et al. 1997). While this view is gaining ground, attempts to extend it to smooth pursuit eye movements, the other type of visually guided eye movements, whose parietal implementation was suggested by the early studies of Mountcastle and coworkers (1975),

Current Oculomotor Research, edited by Becker *et al.*
Plenum Press, New York, 1999.

37

have faced especially strong resistance. This is a direct consequence of the influence of models of smooth pursuit eye movements, which from a computational point of view have successfully reduced cortical contributions to smooth pursuit to the extraction of the relevant sensory information such as retinal image motion. In contrast, the actual sensory-to-motor transformation was proposed to be mediated by subcortical structures such as the cerebellum (Lisberger et al. 1987).

The alternative possibility that parietal smooth pursuit-related single units are actually part of a network underlying the sensory-to-motor transformation, rather than being mere sensory error detectors, has proven to be hard to test. The reason is that smooth pursuit eye movements are much more sensory driven than saccades or reaching hand movements. This makes it impossible to disentangle the influence of retinal and nonretinal factors on the discharge of smooth pursuit-related parietal neurons by simply separating the presentation of the visual target and the motor response required in time, a standard strategy in the study of saccade- and reaching-related single-unit activity. Nevertheless, recent work on smooth pursuit-related single-unit activity has come up with ways to demonstrate the involvement of nonretinal smooth pursuit-related signals. This paper discusses these techniques and their limitations, which have prompted us to use a new approach based on the presentation of *imaginary* targets guiding smooth pursuit eye movements. Our results with this new technique support the view that parietal cortex contributions to smooth pursuit cannot be reduced to the extraction of retinal error signals.

2. NONRETINAL SIGNALS AFFECT THE ACTIVITY OF SMOOTH PURSUIT-RELATED PARIETOOCCIPITAL NEURONS

In the 1980s, both electrophysiological observations and the study of the effects of experimental lesions suggested that two parietooccipital areas are involved in the generation of smooth pursuit eye movements (Dürsteler and Wurtz 1988; Komatsu and Wurtz 1988; Erickson and Dow 1989). Both areas are located within the superior temporal sulcus (STS) of rhesus monkeys, the middle temporal area (area MT) on the posterior bank of the sulcus and the middle superior temporal area (area MST) confined to the anterior bank and the fundus, the latter marking the caudal end of the posterior parietal cortex. In both areas, single units were found which were activated by smooth pursuit eye movements.

Newsome and colleagues (1988) set out to reveal the nature of the pursuit-related activity found in the STS of rhesus monkeys by trying to separate the retinal and eye movement-related factors involved. The first step taken towards this end was to rule out the possible impact of the visual background, whose image is shifted passively across the retina by the pursuit eye movement. This was achieved by presenting the target in an otherwise totally dark environment and by avoiding dark adaptation, possibly rendering remaining low contrast contours visible by switching background lights on in the intertrial intervals. While these choices were able to eliminate the influence of self-induced background image motion on the discharge of a single unit under study, they, of course, did not interfere with the other retinal stimulus involved, the target itself. Even during steady state pursuit, well after the onset of target movement, eye velocity does not necessarily match the velocity of the visual target. The resulting residual retinal motion of the target image, however, might activate a motion-sensitive mechanism, giving rise to the discharge of pursuit-related STS neurons.

In order to test whether this was the case, Newsome et al. (1988) adopted two paradigms, which had in common that they tried to temporarily remove target-induced retinal image motion while smooth pursuit continued. The first paradigm was based on the assumption that steady state smooth pursuit is carried on even in the absence of a visible target, provided the target is taken away only briefly. This was achieved in their study by simply switching the target off for 150 ms (*blink paradigm*). The second approach (*stabilization paradigm*) was less radical. Rather than turning the target off completely, they tried to eliminate residual target image slip during steady state pursuit by temporarily clamping the target image to the retina by electronic means, thus compensating for the insufficiencies of the pursuit system. The rationale underlying these two paradigms was as follows: If the activation of a pursuit-related STS neuron during on-going pursuit was not affected by the removal of target image slip *(=target gap)* by either technique it obviously could not have a retinal cause and the persisting activation necessarily had to reflect the impact of a nonretinal pursuit-related input.

When Newsome et al. (1988) applied the blink and the stabilization paradigm to pursuit-related neurons in the representation of the foveal parts of the visual field in MT, they found that none of them continued firing during the target gap. In other words, the activation of these neurons by smooth pursuit resulted from retinal image motion. In contrast, when these authors explored area MST on the anterior bank of the STS, they found many neurons in both the dorsal and lateral parts of this area whose activation was not affected by the target gap, a finding corroborated by later work (Thier and Erickson 1992). Under different circumstances, the same neurons could be shown to be sensitive to retinal image motion. Their ability to respond to smooth pursuit even in the absence of retinal image slip suggested that these neurons were driven by two pursuit-related signals, namely, target image motion and a nonretinal signal related to eye velocity. While the sensitivity to target image motion would enable these neurons to contribute to the initiation of smooth pursuit eye movement, their sensitivity to eye velocity would allow them to maintain smooth pursuit even in the absence of significant image slip, a property with profound ecological significance. Absence of retinal image motion is by no means a laboratory artifact, resulting from the usage of the blink paradigm. Rather, under natural conditions, the object of interest will often be hidden temporarily by non-attended objects such as trees or bushes falling in the line of sight.

3. TARGET BLINKS OR STABILIZATION IMPAIR SMOOTH PURSUIT

The interpretation of the experiments with target gaps presented in the preceding paragraph was based on the assumption that smooth pursuit is not affected by the disappearance of the target or the stabilization of its image on the retina. If, however, the disappearance of retinal image slip affected smooth pursuit, any concomitant change in neuronal activation could either result from the elimination of retinal image motion or, alternatively, from the change in eye velocity. Consequently, the conclusion that a drop in discharge rate during the gap reflected removal of retinal stimulation and the absence of nonretinal input would no longer be legitimate. The complementary conclusion would also become less straightforward. If the firing rate of a neuron depended on a nonretinal signal related to the smooth pursuit eye movement in the absence of retinal stimulation, why should it remain unaffected if eye velocity changed. Actually, we had convinced ourselves earlier (unpublished observations) that the smooth pursuit eye velocity of monkeys almost always drops if the target image is stabilized by electronic means.

Several years ago Becker and Fuchs (1985) reported that human smooth pursuit eye velocity drops if the target is turned off for periods of time similar to the ones prevailing in the experiments by Newsome et al. (1988) and Thier and Erickson (1992). Our own experiments demonstrate that monkeys, similarly to humans, show a drop of their smooth pursuit eye velocity if the target is turned off briefly. One might have expected that monkeys, usually highly overtrained, might be less susceptible to target gaps than humans. However, our results show that even overtrained monkeys are not able to bridge the target gap without significant loss in smooth pursuit eye velocity, thereby complicating the interpretation of the responses of pursuit-related single units for the reasons outlined before. When the target disappeared unpredictably for 300 ms during steady state pursuit of a target moving at 10°/s on a homogeneous background, mean eye velocity of our human subjects (n=11) dropped to 55% of the eye velocity prevailing before the disappearance of the target, while mean eye velocity of the monkey subjects (n=2) dropped somewhat less to only 63% of the pre-gap velocity.

This already small difference between monkeys and humans was further reduced when the demands on the pursuit system were increased by introducing a structured, stationary background on which the target moved. In this case, both monkeys and humans were even less able to bridge target gaps and the performance of monkeys and humans became almost identical (mean eye velocity during the gap of humans 40% and of monkeys 44% of pre-gap velocity). We recorded close to one hundred pursuit-related single units from the superior temporal sulcus (STS) of three monkeys which showed a discharge rate not affected by the gap, although, as mentioned before, the drop in eye velocity was in the order of 1/3 (homogeneous background during single-unit recordings). Obviously, the discharge of such neurons cannot be the neuronal replica of eye velocity assumed by previous work. However, although not offering a true replica of eye velocity, such neurons might still offer a coarse representation of eye velocity. For instance, they might already exhibit response saturation at the velocities prevailing in the gap period (which were in the order of 5°/s). In this case, we would not expect to see much of an effect of the change of velocity induced by the target gap.

Actually, there is evidence that pursuit-related MST neurons are indeed characterized by response saturation at target velocities around 10°/s (Ilg et al. 1998). However, these considerations, plausible as they may be, cannot rule out a radically different explanation for the persistence of discharge despite changes in eye velocity, namely, a neuronal memory of the (para-)foveal image slip prevailing before the introduction of the target gap. In an attempt to critically test this possibility, we sought a way to evoke smooth pursuit eye movements without presenting foveal image slip in the first place, thus avoiding the charging of a putative image slip memory element. If the activation of pursuit-related MST neurons depended on foveal image slip, either presented in *real*-time or memorized, these neurons should be shut down in the case of pursuit without foveal stimulation. Our experiments with *imaginary* targets sparing the fovea show that this is not the case, lending new support to the notion that pursuit-related MST neurons depend on nonretinal information.

4. *IMAGINARY* FIGURES AS TARGETS FOR SMOOTH PURSUIT

Human subjects are able to track a wide variety of moving objects whose location and velocity cannot be directly derived from perifoveal retinal information. Examples are the lower corner of a moving diamond whose lower part is hidden by a stationary foreground or the invisible hub of a spinning wheel (Steinbach 1976). The common denominator of this class of pursuit targets is the fact that they are hidden parts of objects readily completed by our visual system using top-down knowledge of the shape of the object. However, even if we do not complete a meaningful object from sparse retinal cues, we are

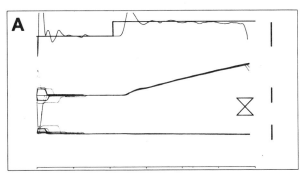

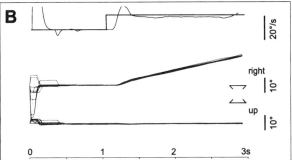

Figure 1. Typical examples of smooth pursuit eye movements guided by the *real* (**A**) and *imaginary* (**B**) target moving at 8°/s rightwards, respectively. The horizontal and vertical eye position traces of single trials (n=20) are shown. In addition, the mean eye velocity and target velocity are displayed. Note the similarity of eye movements guided by the *real* and *imaginary* target.

able to evoke and maintain high-gain smooth pursuit eye movements. An example investigated in detail by Wyatt et al. (1994) is the imagined midpoint between two dots, presented extrafoveally and moving in synchrony. Such figures have in common that they lack any foveal information, thereby allowing us to critically test the hypothesis of a neuronal memory of foveal image slip in area MST. In order to use this approach, we first had to clarify whether monkeys are able to pursue such an *imaginary* target as well. Initially, we trained rhesus monkeys to track the center of an hourglass-like figure (size 20° times 20°) given by the intersection of the two diagonals defining the hourglass. After a monkey had learned to track the center, we removed the central 12°x12° of the hourglass centered on the intersection, while continuously asking the monkey to keep his line of sight on the now invisible center. Finally, the monkeys learned to use the *imaginary* target to initiate and maintain smooth pursuit eye movements (see figure 1).

One might object at this point that our monkeys simply learned to stay away evenly from the four line ends delimiting the void center of the hourglass rather than perceiving and fixating an imagined intersection of the two diagonals. The important difference between these two interpretations obviously is that the first one assumes that smooth pursuit would be generated by the direct conversion of information derived from extrafoveal retinal cues without any need for a filling in of hidden object parts by top-down processes. However, this objection is irrelevant for the single-unit experiment we had in mind, whose only requirement was the absence of foveal retinal information.

5. SINGLE UNIT ACTIVITY RECORDED FROM AREA MT AND MST DURING PURSUIT OF *REAL* AND *IMAGINARY* TARGETS

Monkey area MT is characterized by a high percentage of neurons responding in a directionally selective manner to visual motion (Dubner and Zeki 1971; Zeki 1974). MT

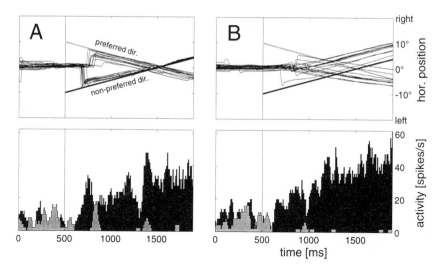

Figure 2. Smooth pursuit eye movements and pursuit-related activity of a typical neuron recorded from area MST. The horizontal eye and target position of single trials (n=10) as well as the neuronal activity are shown. In **A**, the monkey tracked the *real* target moving in the preferred rightward (black) and non-preferred leftward direction (gray), respectively. In **B**, the monkey tracked the *imaginary* target moving in the preferred and non-preferred direction, respectively. Note that the activity observed during pursuit of the *imaginary* target was quite similar to the activity observed during pursuit of the *real* target.

neurons with (para-)foveal receptive fields are typically activated by smooth pursuit eye movements. *Imaginary targets* like the ones discussed in the preceding section allow us to demonstrate that the pursuit-related responses indeed result from visual stimulation of the receptive field center. The purely retinal nature of the pursuit-related response obtained from many area MT neurons is demonstrated by the fact that no significant response was obtained when the monkey pursued the *imaginary* target whose central void region was much larger than the receptive field center of this cell. These MT-neurons also stopped discharging when the conventional dot target was blinked out temporarily. These observations fully support the view that the absence of activation during the target gap first noted by Newsome and colleagues (1988) is indeed a consequence of the exclusively retinal nature of pursuit-related responses of MT neurons and not a result of the inevitable drop in eye velocity during the gap. In contrast, our recordings from neurons located in area MST revealed that some neurons responded equally during pursuit of the *real* as well as during pursuit of the *imaginary* target, a typical example of such a response is shown in figure 2.

Most of these neurons responding similarly during tracking of the *real* and *imaginary* target also showed resistance to the blinking of the target during steady state pursuit although the eye velocity dropped in this condition. We are well aware that receptive fields of MST neurons are typically larger than those of MT neurons at comparable eccentricities. To test if the response to pursuit of the *imaginary* target was not simply the consequence of stimulation of the peripheral parts of large receptive fields, we moved the same stimulus used as target for pursuit while the monkey was asked to keep stationary fixation. In case of moving the *real* figure across the stationary fixation point, a clear passive visual response to the onset of the figure as well as a directionally selective response to the figure crossing the fovea could be observed (see figure 3A). But as the size of the blanked area was increased (see figure 3B to D), this initial visual response gradually de-

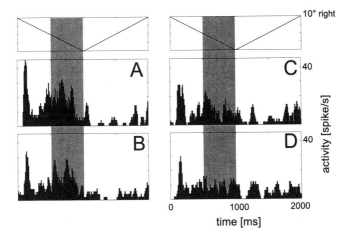

Figure 3. Passive visual stimulation. During fixation of a stationary target, the *real* target moved leftward at 20°/s (preferred direction) starting at 10° right and subsequently rightward for 1s each (**A**). In **B**, the central area of 4° was blanked, in **C** 8°, and in **D** 12° identical as during tracking of the *imaginary* target shown in figure 2. The gray box shows when the stimulus crossed the fovea and moved into the contralateral visual field. Note that the directionally selective visual response disappeared from **A** to **D**.

clined and the directionally selective responses disappeared completely. This lack in response demonstrates the extra-retinal nature of the pursuit-related activity observed during tracking of the *imaginary* target.

In total, we recorded 74 pursuit-related neurons which were activated similarly by pursuit of both *imaginary* and *real* targets from three monkeys. In two monkeys, the reconstruction of the recordings sites of these neurons were verified to be located within area MST. In the third monkey, still used in experiments, the affiliation of these neurons to area MST is based on electrophysiological criteria.

In conclusion, our findings with *imaginary* targets fully support the view that area MST, unlike area MT, is a cortical area which integrates nonretinal information related to smooth pursuit eye movements useful for maintaining smooth pursuit even in the absence of foveal retinal information. This extraretinal signal is available only to a subset of pursuit-related neurons, being absent from MT and also from a substantial number of pursuit-related neurons in MST.

ACKNOWLEDGMENTS

This work was supported by grants from the Deutsche Forschungsgemeinschaft.

REFERENCES

Andersen RA, Snyder LH, Bradley DC, Xing J (1997) Multimodal representation of space in the posterior parietal cortex and its use in planning movements. Annu Rev Neurosci 20: 303–330

Becker W, Fuchs AF (1985) Prediction in the oculomotor system: smooth pursuit during transient disappearance of a visual target. Exp Brain Res 57:562–575

Dubner R, Zeki SM (1971) Response properties and receptive fields of cells in an anatomically defined region in the superior temporal sulcus in the monkey. Brain Res 35:528–532

Dürsteler MR, Wurtz RH (1988) Pursuit and optokinetic deficits following chemical lesions of cortical areas MT and MST. J Neurophysiol 60:940–965

Erickson RG, Dow B (1989) Foveal tracking cells in the superior temporal sulcus of the macaque monkey. Exp Brain Res 78:113–131

Hyvärinen J, Poranen A (1974) Function of the parietal association area 7 as revealed from cellular discharges in alert monkeys. Brain 97:673–692

Ilg UJ, Rommel J, Thier P (1998) Visual tracking (VT) neurons in monkey area MST exhibit similar speed tuning for visual motion and eye velocity. ENA Forum Berlin

Komatsu H, Wurtz RH (1988) Relation of cortical areas MT and MST to pursuit eye movements. I. Localization and visual properties of neurons. J Neurophysiol 60:580–603

Lisberger SG, Morris EJ, Tychsen L (1987) Visual motion processing and sensory-motor integration for smooth pursuit eye movements. Annu Rev Neurosci 10:97–129

Mountcastle VB, Lynch JC, Georgopoulos A, Sakata H, Acuna C (1975) Posterior parietal association cortex of the monkey: command functions for operations within extrapersonal space. J Neurophysiol 38:871–908

Newsome WT, Wurtz RH, Komatsu H (1988) Relation of cortical area MT and MST to pursuit eye movements. II. Differentiation of retinal from extraretinal inputs.
J Neurophysiol 60:604–620

Robinson DL, Goldberg ME, Stanton GB (1978) Parietal association cortex in the primate: sensory mechanisms and behavioral modulations. J Neurophysiol 41:910–932

Steinbach MJ (1976) Pursuing the perceptual rather than the retinal stimulus. Vision Res 16:1371–1376

Thier P, Erickson RG (1992) Responses of visual-tracking neurons from cortical area MST-l to visual, eye, and head motion. Eur J Neurosci 4:539–553

Wyatt HJ, Pola J, Fortune B, Posner M (1994) Smooth pursuit eye movements with imaginary targets defined by extrafoveal cues. Vision Res 34:803–820

Zeki SM (1974) Functional organization of a visual area in the posterior bank of the superior temporal sulcus of the rhesus monkey. J Physiol (Lond) 236:549–573

6

PROPERTIES OF SACCADES DURING OPTOKINETIC RESPONSES TO RADIAL OPTIC FLOW IN MONKEYS

Markus Lappe, Martin Pekel, and Klaus-Peter Hoffmann

Dept. Zoology and Neurobiology
Ruhr University
D-44780 Bochum, Germany

1. ABSTRACT

Optokinetic eye movements stabilize vision in response to large-field visual motion. We have studied oculomotor behavior of rhesus monkeys that viewed large optic flow stimuli. These stimuli present radial motion that is normally experienced during forward self-movement. In previous work (Lappe et al., 1998) we have described that such radial optic flow stimuli also elicit optokinetic responses in the form of slow eye movements which stabilize the moving visual image on the fovea and parafovea. Here we describe the properties of saccades during unrestrained viewing of radial optic flow. We show that the saccades do not share the reflectory nature of the slow phases but rather support an active exploration of the visual scene.

2. INTRODUCTION

During natural locomotor behavior our eyes continuously experience global visual motion. This motion is called the optic flow. Reflectory vestibulo-ocular and optokinetic eye movements will attempt to stabilize vision during movements of the head. In the case of head rotation, an opposite movement of the eyes can almost completely cancel the visual motion and stabilize the full retinal image. This is not possible for translations of the head. Especially during forward translation, the optic flow has a radial structure in which different directions of motion are present in different parts of the visual field. Hence, eye movements can only stabilize part of the retinal image.

We have recorded spontaneous optokinetic eye movements of three macaque monkeys during unconstrained viewing of optic flow stimuli that simulated forward transla-

Current Oculomotor Research, edited by Becker *et al.*
Plenum Press, New York, 1999.

tion. The typical oculomotor behavior in this situation consists of regularly alternating slow phases and saccades at a frequency of about 2Hz. In a previous paper (Lappe et al., 1998) we have analysed the properties of the slow phases. Eye movements in the slow phases follow the direction of motion that is present at the fovea and parafovea. Thus, the slow phases stabilize the retinal image in a small parafoveal region only. Many of the characteristics of the slow phases can be explained by properties of the optokinetic system. In this paper we will investigate the properties of the saccades.

When an optokinetic nystagmus is elicited by a large-field unidirectional motion stimulus, slow phases and saccades are very stereotypic. First, a saccade is made against the direction of the stimulus motion. Then a slow eye movement follows the stimulus motion in order to stabilize the retinal image. After the eye has moved a certain distance, another saccade against the stimulus motion occurs which re-positions the eye and compensates for positional change during the slow phase. Saccades in this situation serve two functions (Carpenter, 1988). The first is to orient gaze towards the direction from which the stimulus motion originates. The second is to reset eye position after the slow phase tracking movement. However, during visual scanning of radial optic flow, each saccade changes the direction and speed of retinal motion on the fovea. After the saccade, the slow phase eye movement has to adapt to these changes (Lappe et al., 1998) Thus, saccades in this situation also influence tracking performance. Moreover, during forward locomotion a constant monitoring of the environment and of possible obstacles in the direction of heading is required, which might necessitate ocular scanning of the visual scene. Thus, saccades in this situation might serve different purposes than merely the resetting of eye position.

3. METHODS

Eye movement were recorded in three awake male rhesus monkeys (Macaca mulatta). Under general anesthesia and sterile conditions a head-holder and two scleral search-coils were chronically implanted. For the experiments, the monkey was seated in a primate chair with its head fixed. Horizontal and vertical position of one eye were registered by an Eye Position Meter 3020 (SKALAR) and recorded to a PC with a sampling rate of 500 Hz. Each experimental trial lasted 15 or 20 seconds during which spontaneous and unrestrained eye movements were recorded. Several trials were performed on each recording day. Monkeys weight was monitored daily and supplementary fruit and water was supplied. All experiments were in accord with published guidelines on the use of animal research (European Communities Council Directive 86/609/ECC).

The optic flow stimuli consisted of full-field (90x90deg) computer generated sequences that were back projected onto a tangent screen, 47 cm in front of the monkey. They simulated forward or backward self-motion with respect to a large number of random dots. The distribution of dots in space simulated four different virtual environments (Fig. 1). In successive trials simulated observer speed and direction was randomly varied. Observer speeds of 1, 2, or 3m/s were used. Different simulated directions of observer movement gave different horizontal positions of the focus of expansion (-20, -10, 0, +10, +20deg).

In the recorded data, saccades were separated from slow phases by a velocity level criterion, typically set at 25deg/s. Beginning and end of saccades were determined as the first and last data points which cross the criterion level, respectively. In addition, a minimum duration of 12ms between the start and end points was required.

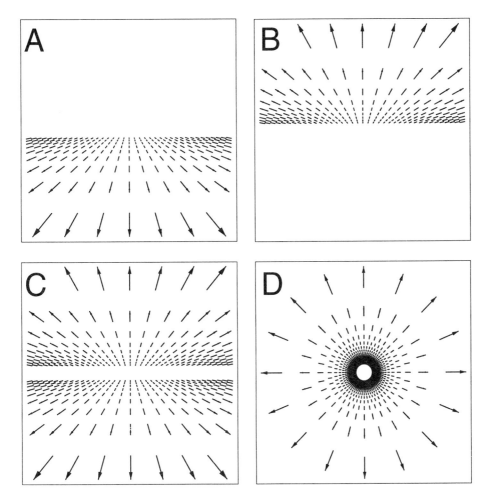

Figure 1. Illustration of the optic flow stimuli. The simulated movement of an observer in different virtual environments. The first consisted of a horizontal ground plane 0.37m below eye level (A). This plane contained lit dots that moved on the screen according to the simulated observer motion. The ground plane stimulus could be inverted such that the observer moved below a ceiling (B), or two planes could be presented, one below and one above the observer (C). A fourth environment consisted of a simulated tunnel, 0.72m in diameter (D).

4. RESULTS

A typical scan path during viewing of an expanding ground plane stimulus is shown in Fig. 2A. Most of the time gaze is slightly below the horizon. Accordingly most saccades are in a horizontal direction. Saccades frequently cross the center of the stimulus. Each crossing reverses the direction of the flow that is projected onto the fovea before and after the saccade. Between saccades, optokinetic slow phase eye movements occur that follow the direction of motion on the fovea. Examples are shown in Fig. 2B, which presents the horizontal eye position as a function of time. In periods between saccades, the eye performed slow motions toward the center. These occurred because the stimulus consisted of a radial visual contraction that simulated backward motion of the monkey. Detailed analy-

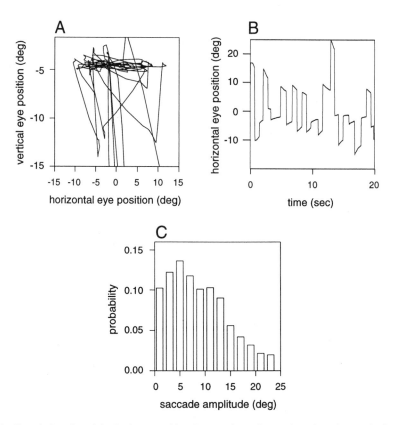

Figure 2. A: Cumulative plot of the (x,y) eye position (scan path) as the monkey viewed an optic flow stimulus such as Fig. 1A for 20 seconds. B: Example trace of the horizontal eye position over time. In this example, the stimulus was a contraction pattern simulating backward motion of the monkey. One can clearly distinguish saccades from optokinetic slow phase eye movements. C: Distribution of saccade amplitudes (Data from all animals and stimulus conditions collapsed).

sis of the relationship between the slow phase eye movements and the optic flow stimulus revealed that direction and speed of the eye movements are linked to the foveal and parafoveal motion (see Lappe et al. 1998). Direction very closely followed the direction of the motion on the fovea. Eye speed roughly matched the average motion within the parafoveal summation area of the optokinetic system.

To describe the saccadic behavior during optic flow stimulation we first looked at the distribution of saccade amplitudes and directions in relation to the parameters of the stimulus. Saccadic amplitude varied in a wide range (Fig. 2C). However, median amplitude, median duration, and median maximum velocity of saccades were not systematically affected by simulated observer speed or placement of the focus of expansion. The distribution of saccade directions, on the other hand, showed a clear relation to the visual environment (Fig. 3). For half-field stimuli, ground plane and ceiling, the distribution of saccade directions had clear peaks at 0 and 180deg, or rightward and leftward directions, respectively (Fig. 3A,B). This changed when full field stimuli were presented (Fig. 3C,D). In the case of the two plane stimulus, the distribution of saccade directions had four shallower peaks, which correspond to 0, 90, 180 and 270deg. This suggests that the animal now shifted gaze also between the upper and lower stimulus fields in addition to horizontal

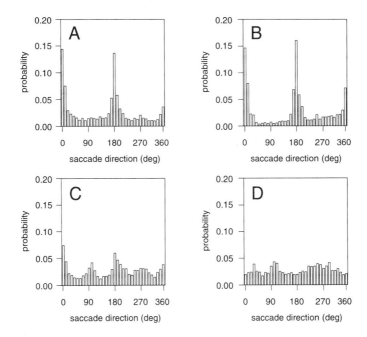

Figure 3. Distribution of saccade directions for four different environments (see Fig. 1). In ground plane (A) and ceiling (B) conditions horizontal saccades are the most frequent. This is consistent with the observation that gaze in these conditions is mostly directed towards the horizon. For the double plane (C) and tunnel (D) environments saccade directions are more equally distributed.

saccades along the two horizons. For the tunnel stimulus, which is completely radial-symmetric no clear preference of any saccade direction was observed. The median temporal separation of successive saccades also depended on the simulated visual environment. Median intersaccadic interval was 415ms for half-field stimuli and 320ms for full-field stimuli.

The properties of the saccades therefore show a clear relation to the visual environment. This would be expected from typical visual scanning behavior (Yarbus, 1967). However, the slow phase eye movements between the saccades have many characteristics that link them to the optokinetic system (Lappe et al., 1998). Therefore, we wondered whether saccades during optic flow stimulation also show properties related to optokinetic quick phases.

In the regular optokinetic nystagmus evoked by full-field unidirectional motion, saccades are directed against the motion of the stimulus and against the eye movement direction during the slow phase. We examined whether such a relationship also exists for optokinetic responses to radial motion. We compared saccade directions to the direction of the slow phase eye movement that preceded the saccade and computed the angular difference between the two. Fig. 4 shows this angular difference as a function of saccadic amplitude in scatter plots that contain data from all animals for the ground plane stimuli. For a radial flow pattern with a centered focus of expansion, saccade directions showed no correlation with the direction of the preceding slow phase eye movements (Fig. 4A). However, when the focus of expansion was 20deg eccentric on the screen the proportion of saccades in a direction opposite to the direction of the preceding slow phase increased (Fig. 4B). Evaluation of the number of saccades that were directed leftward or rightward

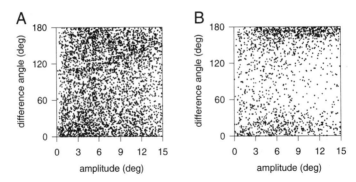

Figure 4. Distributions of saccadic amplitudes and directions relative to the direction of the preceding slow phase eye movement for central (A) and 20deg eccentric (B) positions of the focus of expansion. Each dot represents a single saccade. Typical optokinetic quick phases would appear in the upper part of the plots because their direction would be 180deg apart from the direction of the slow phase.

also showed a dependence on the location of the focus of expansion. For eccentric locations, about twice as many saccades were directed towards the focus of expansion than away from it. For contraction stimuli, this ratio was reversed. When the focus was eccentric, differences between expansion and contraction also occurred in the distribution of eye positions. Median eye position was shifted towards the focus position for expansion, but in the opposite direction, i.e. away from the focus position, in the case of contraction. This behavior might be linked to the shift of the 'Schlagfeld' of the optokinetic nystagmus (Lappe et al., 1998).

Optokinetic slow phases continuously change eye position. Part of the function of saccades must therefore lie in the compensation for this continuous eye drift. We quantified the proportion of saccadic amplitude that was necessary for the compensation of positional changes during slow phase eye movements. This was done by calculating the ratio between the sum of all slow phase amplitudes and the sum of all saccade amplitudes. The results are shown in Fig. 5. The percentage of saccades needed for compensation is lowest for a centered radial expansion. With increasing observer velocity or with increasing eccentricity of the focus of expansion on the screen the ratio increases. However, for expanding optic flow, which is the typical motion pattern during forward locomotion, less than 20% of saccadic amplitudes are required to compensate for slow phase eye movements. More than 80% of saccadic amplitudes is used for active exploration of the environment.

5. DISCUSSION

The oculomotor behavior of monkeys that view radial optic flow stimuli consists of slow optokinetic tracking movements and quick saccadic changes of gaze direction. During slow phases the eye movement follows the motion in that part of the optic flow stimulus that falls on the fovea and parafovea. These slow phase eye movements are strongly correlated to stimulus motion. This is true for both eye movement direction and speed (Lappe et al., 1998). In contrast, most properties of the saccades did not depend on the stimulus motion. This was true for amplitude, duration, velocity, and to a large degree also

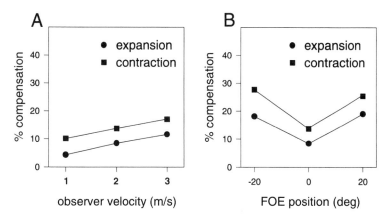

Figure 5. Proportion of saccadic amplitudes that was necessary to compensate for the positional drift of the eyes during the slow phase between two successive saccades. In A only data from stimuli with central focus of expansion were used. B contains only data from a single observer speed (2m/s).

for direction of saccades. Instead, saccade parameters depended strongly on the structure of the visual scene. The distribution of saccade directions and saccade frequency was different for half-field and for full-field stimuli. This is consistent with an ocular scanning behavior that relates to the content of the visual scene. Such ocular scanning occurs during inspection of static images (Yarbus, 1967; Burman & Segraves, 1994) but also in moving scenes during self-motion (Land, 1992; Land & Lee, 1994). Indeed, a dependence of saccade frequency on the size of the visual stimulus was also observed in humans during driving in a car (Osaka, 1991).

With fully radial optic flow stimuli, centered expansion or contraction, little support was found for the opposing hypothesis that saccades in this situation are linked with the optokinetic eye movements during the slow phases. Saccade direction was not correlated with the direction of the preceding slow phase eye movement. Saccadic amplitudes on average exceeded the distance required to compensate for the eye drift during slow phases by a factor of 4. However, this behavior changed when the focus of expansion was eccentric on the screen. In this case, saccades were more often directed against the direction of the preceding slow phase and the ratio between saccadic amplitude and the amplitude of the slow phases decreased. These observations are consistent with a greater optokinetic potential of the stimulus in this situation, which also leads to a higher gain of the slow phase eye movements (Lappe et al., 1998). As the focus of expansion becomes eccentric the stimulus motion on the screen becomes more homogeneous and more like a typical optokinetic stimulus. Saccadic properties in this case gradually change towards those observed in an optokinetic nystagmus.

While slow phase eye movements of monkeys during unrestrained viewing of radial optic flow show many properties of the optokinetic system, saccades in this situation are used to a large degree for an active exploration of the moving scene. This is unlike the stereotypic reflectory behavior of saccadic quick phases during optokinetic nystagmus. Thus, slow phases and saccades in this situation are likely generated by different oculomotor processes. The basic neuronal circuit that drives optokinetic eye movements consists mainly of subcortical structures (Hoffmann, 1986). However, lesions of the frontal eye field in rats have shown systematic effects on the saccades, but not the slow phases, of the optokinetic nystagmus (Bähring et al., 1994). Saccades in optokinetic nystagmus serve to compensate for eye drifts during the slow phases and to orient gaze towards the origin of the motion. Lesions of the frontal eye field in rats selectively impaired the orientation but not the compensation. This suggests that the frontal eye field contributes to saccadic behavior also during optokinetic nystagmus, specifically in the orientation of gaze towards novel parts of the stimulus. Such a contribution might also underlie the generation of saccades during the ocular scanning of radial optic flow.

REFERENCES

Bähring R, Meier RK, Dieringer N (1994) Unilateral ablation of the frontal eye field of the rat affects the beating field of ocular nystagmus. Exp Brain Res 98:391–400.

Burman DD, Segraves MA (1994) Primate frontal eye field activity during natural scanning eye movements. J Neurophysiol 71:1266–1271.

Carpenter RHS (1988) Movement Of The Eyes. Pion, London.

Hoffmann KP (1986) Visual inputs relevant for the optokinetic nystagmus in mammals. In Freund HJ, Büttner U, Cohen B, Noth J (Eds.) Progress in Brain Research. Elsevier.

Land MF (1992) Predictable eye-head coordination during driving. Nature 359:318–320.

Land MF, Lee DN (1994) Where we look when we steer. Nature 369:742–744.

Lappe M, Pekel M, Hoffmann KP (1998) Optokinetic eye movements elicited by radial optic flow in the macaque monkey. J Neurophysiol 79:1461–1480.

Osaka N (1991) Effects of window size and eccentricity upon eye fixation and reaction time in negotiation of curves. In Gale AG, Freeman MH, Haslegrave CM, Smith P, Taylor SP (Eds.) Vision in Vehicles III. Elsevier.

Yarbus AL (1967) Eye Movements And Vision. Plenum, New York.

7

ERRONEOUS PROSACCADES IN A GAP-ANTISACCADE-TASK

Production, Correction, and Recognition

Burkhart Fischer,[*] Stefan Gezeck, and Annette Mokler

Brain Research Unit
Hansastr. 9
79104 Freiburg, Germany

1. ABSTRACT

In an antisaccade-task subjects are required to look to the side opposite of a suddenly presented stimulus so that the voluntary and the reflexive components operate in opposite directions. In this study the gap-antisaccade- and the overlap-prosaccade-task were used to investigate the number of erroneous prosaccades in the antisaccade-task, their reaction times, and their correction times in relation to the number of express saccades a same subject produced in the overlap-prosaccade-task. Out of 234 subjects 126 were selected who produced more than 20 % errors. Among the data sets we differentiated between a "fast" group with many express saccades and a "slow" group with only a few express saccades in the overlap-prosaccade-task. Both groups showed differences in the reaction and correction time of their errors. In a second experiment we wanted to know whether the subjects (N=38) recognized their errors and whether a recognized sequence of an erroneous prosaccade and the corrective saccade is different from an unrecognized sequence. The results indicate that for each subject one has to differentiate between the disability to suppress reflex-like saccades due to an insufficient fixational control or due to a weak voluntary control or the disability to generate voluntary saccades. The erroneous prosaccades and their corrections escape the conscious perception in many cases despite large (4°+8°) and long lasting (>100 ms) changes of the retinal image. It is discussed that the perceptual spatial frame transforms differently prior to voluntary as compared to involuntary saccades.

---

[*] www.brain.uni-freiburg.de/fischer

Current Oculomotor Research, edited by Becker *et al.*
Plenum Press, New York, 1999.

2. INTRODUCTION

Most of the time the direction of gaze is stabilized due to a fixation mechanism which inhibits the saccade system (Munoz and Wurtz, 1993 a,b). Saccades can be generated reflexively or voluntarily using a cortical-tectal pathway or a frontal pathway (Schiller et al. 1987). In a gap condition (fixation point offset precedes stimulus onset by a temporal gap) the fixation process is largely disengaged and the reflex pathway is most sensitive favouring express saccades (Fischer and Ramsperger, 1984; Fischer and Boch, 1983). By contrast, during overlap conditions long latency (regular) saccades are favoured depending on the strength of inhibition of the saccade system (Mayfrank et al. 1986). In an antisaccade-task subjects are required to look to the side opposite of a suddenly presented stimulus (Hallett, 1978) and therefore the voluntary and the reflexive components operate in opposite directions. Even normally developed adult subjects produce 10–15 % errors on average if the gap-antisaccade-task is used (Fischer and Weber, 1992). Many children at age 10 years are still unable to perform the gap-antisaccade-task producing an average of 60 % errors (Fischer et al. 1997). The number of errors is increased by a factor of 2 or 3 if the side to which the antisaccade has to be made is validly indicated by a short cue presented 100 ms before stimulus onset (Fischer and Weber, 1996). The question arises why these errors occur. Does the error rate reflect a certain status of the optomotor system, which is reflected also in the subject's saccadic performance in other tasks?

In this study, both the gap-antisaccade- and the overlap-prosaccade-task were used to investigate the number and the reaction times of the erroneous prosaccades and their corrections obtained in the gap-antisaccade-task in relation to the number of express saccades a subject produced in the overlap-prosaccade-task. The idea was that a relatively weak fixation system would lead to relatively many express saccades in the overlap-prosaccade-task and at the same time to excessive numbers of erroneous prosaccades in the gap-antisaccade-task (Cavegn and Biscaldi, 1996). On the other hand, high numbers of errors due to a weak voluntary control are also expected despite a normal fixation system. This differentiation of reasons for excessive numbers of errors may have impacts on the clinical significance as pointed out earlier (O'Driscoll et al. 1995) and reviewed in a recent article (Everling and Fischer, 1998).

We also wanted to know whether the subjects recognized their errors and whether a recognized sequence of an erroneous prosaccade and the corrective saccade is different from an unrecognized sequence.

The results show that indeed subjects with many express saccades in the overlap-prosaccade-task produce and correct their errors differently as compared to subjects with only few express saccades. Also, it turns out that about 50% of the errors escape the subjects' conscious perception.

3. METHODS

3.1. Eye Movement Recording and Calibration

Eye movements were recorded by infrared light techniques with a temporal resolution of 1ms and a spatial resolution of 0.1 °. Reaction times were determined for all correct prosaccades in the overlap-prosaccade-task. Reaction and correction times were measured for all erroneous prosaccades in the gap-antisaccade-task.

3.2. Stimulus Presentation

The visual stimuli, a central red fixation point (Fp, $0.1°$ x $0.1°$) and white target stimuli (St, $0.2°$x$0.2°$) on a $20°$x $15°$ green background, were generated by a personal computer and presented on a RGB colour monitor using a high resolution graphic interface (mirograph 510). Target onset time was synchronized to the screen (frame rate 83 Hz), taking into account also the constant time delay between the synchronization pulse and the horizontal level at which the stimuli were presented. The luminance of all stimuli was well above perceptual threshold. Viewing distance was 57 cm.

3.3. Data Analysis

The time from stimulus onset to the beginning of the first saccade is called the reaction time (SRT), the time from the end of an erroneous prosaccade in the antisaccade-task to the beginning of the second corrective saccade, which brings the eyes onto the opposite side, i. e. the intersaccadic interval, is called the correction time (CRT). Thus the secondary corrective saccade is opposite in sign and larger as the primary saccade. Erroneous saccades which are not corrected in the second saccade within 600 ms are considered as uncorrected. Sacccades with a reaction time below 80 ms were considered as anticipations and were analysed seperately. Further details of variable definition have been published elsewhere (Fischer et al. 1997)

3.4. Experiment 1

3.4.1. Subjects. In this study 234 subjects between the age of 8 and 70 years participated. Each subject contributed 2 sessions of 200 trials, 100 to each side in random order. From these 126 were selected by the criterion of making more than 20% errors in the antisaccade-task. They were all healthy in the sense that they were not under medical treatment. They were all volunteers paid for their participation in two sessions of 10 minutes each. Subjects were classified into age groups of increasing bin width: age below 11, 11–13, 13–16, 16–20, 20 -25, 25–31, 31–38, 38–46, 46–55, 55–75. This was necessary because some of the variables considered in this study clearly depend on age (Fischer et al. 1997).

3.4.2. The Tasks. In the prosaccade-task subjects were required to look to the stimulus when it was presented, in the antisaccade-task they were instructed to make a saccade in the direction opposite to the stimulus. The antisaccade-task was used together with a gap paradigm and the prosaccade-task was used with the overlap paradigm. The stimuli were presented always randomly $4°$ to the right or left of the fixation point. The fixation point was presented for 1000 ms on gap trials and for 2000 ms on overlap trials. The stimulus was presented 1200 ms after fixation point onset for 800 ms. The inter-trial interval was 1000 ms throughout. Each experimental session consisted of a block of 200 trials, 100 for each side of stimulus presentation.

3.5. Experiment 2

3.5.1. Subjects. In the second experiment we used 38 naive and trained subjects. They were older than 20 years. Each subject contributed at least 1 session consisting of 400 trials. Ninetythree data sets were analysed.

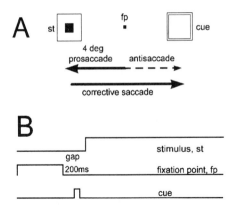

Figure 1. A, Spatial and B, temporal stimulus arrangements in experiment 2 together with the directions of three saccades: a prosaccade to the left, a corrective saccade of double size to the right following a prosaccade, and an antisaccade to the right (broken line). A central fixation point, which remained on for 1s from the beginning of each trial, is flanked at both sides in a distance of 4 deg by the outlines of a 2°x2° box. The box on the side to which the next saccade had to be made briefly (40 ms) lit up 100 ms after fixation point offset. Another 100 ms later a stimulus was presented at the side opposite to that cue, in that box which had not lit up. The subjects were instructed to generate a saccade to the side opposite of this stimulus (antisaccade). Therefore, on each trial, a temporal gap of 200 ms existed between fixation point offset and stimulus onset. The side was selected randomly between 4° to the right or left.

3.5.2. The Tasks. To increase the error rate we used the gap condition together with a peripheral cue presented 100 ms before stimulus onset for 40 ms as indicated in Fig. 1 (Fischer and Weber, 1996). The cue, a frame of 2°x2° around both 4° positions, was presented randomly at 4° to the right or left but always at the side to which the saccade was to be made. The subjects were asked to press a key at the end of every trial in which they recognized an error. We determined the error rate, the percentage of unrecognized errors, the size, the reaction (SRT), and the correction times (CRT) from the error trials. For comparison we asked the subjects to repeat the session with the instruction to generate a saccade to the stimulus on purpose followed by the antisaccade as quickly as possible. In this pro- antisaccade-task (PA condition) the sequence of saccades is the same as on trials when the subjects make and correct an error. The difference is that in the PA case the sequence is made voluntarily while in the antisaccade-task it occurs involuntarily and against the subjects own intention. We determined the time between the end of the first prosaccade and the following antisaccade (PAT), which is equivalent to the CRT.

4. RESULTS

The general observation in both experiments confirmed the earlier results: most subjects irrespective of their age and state of training produced some errors in the gap-antisaccade-task (Weber and Fischer, 1991). The error rate was increased by the introduction of the valid cue presented at the side to which the next antisaccade had to be directed (Fischer and Weber, 1996). Children and certain adults produced reasonable numbers of express saccades in the overlap-prosacccade-condition (Fischer et al. 1997).

Table 1. Mean reaction time and correction time
of erroneous prosaccades, the percentage
of the errors that are corrected in the second
saccade, and the percentage of errors for
the two groups A and B.

	SRT - err (ms)	CRT - err (ms)	Corrections (%)	Errors (%)
Group A	142	142	85	35
Group B	165	164	75	48

Therefore, it was possible to investigate the question whether the production of the errors and their corrections are related to the phenomenon of express saccades and whether or not the corrections depend on the subjects conscious experience.

4.1. Experiment 1

Data sets of the 126 subjects with more than 20% errors were divided into two groups: group A contains N=83 sets. In this group the express saccade rates in the overlap-prosaccade-task were higher than error rate minus 20% in the antisaccade-task. Group B contains 127 sets. Here express saccade rates are small. The analysis shows that the two groups differ in several aspects as shown in table 1.

The fast group A exhibits a short mean reaction time of their errors, corrects them after short intersaccadic intervals, corrects the errors more often, and produces less errors as compared with group B. All diffenrences between the mean values reached significance.

To test several hypotheses we looked at the scatterplots of the different variables separately for two age groups: teenies and adults versus children (below age 13 y). Fig. 2 shows 4 pairs of such plots together with the questions and answers at the right side. In this case the data of all subjects were used. The answer to the question whether many errors occur because of fast reaction times is "no": a speed - accuracy trade off effect cannot be seen in this data. Also fast errors are not corrected any faster than slow errors. Teenies and adults produce fewer errors and correct them more often than children do. In the children data, but not in the adult data, one sees a clear correlation: the more errors a subject produces the more remain uncorrected. Finally, there is no correlation between correction time and number of corrections.

In conclusion from the first experiment we have seen that the behaviour of a subject in the overlap-prosaccade-task is reflected in the performance of the gap-antisaccade-task. On the other hand, the number of errors and their corrections show little correlations of the type one could have expected from earlier studies on reaction time, errors and corrections.

4.2. Experiment 2

When a vaild cue is added to the gap-antisaccade-task, error rates increased from about 12% to 19% on average varying between 0.3% and 60% depending on the subject and the side of stimulation. The percentage of unrecognized errors was 50±25% on average. The reaction times of the errors range from 80 to 170 ms with a strong express saccade mode around 100 ms. Both types of errors had the same mean SRT of 123 ms and

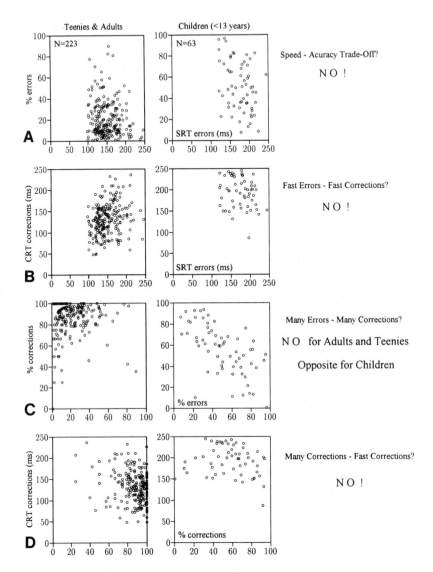

Figure 2. Scatterplots of the different variables of the antisaccade-task shown separately for subjects older than 13 years (left) versus children younger than 13 years (right). At the right the questions we asked and the corresponding answers are shown. A, the percentage of errors in the antisaccade-task as a function of the mean reaction time of these errors. Thus the answer to the question whether many errors occur because of fast reaction times is "no": a speed - accuracy trade off effect cannot be seen in this data. B, the mean correction time for errors as a function of the mean reaction time of these errors: Fast errors are not corrected any faster than slow errors. C, the percentage of corrected errors (100%= all errors corrected) as a function of the percentage of these errors (100%= each trial an error): Teenies and adults produce fewer errors and correct them more often than children do. In the children data, but not in the adult data, one sees a clear correlation: the more errors a subject produces the more remain uncorrected. D, the correction time as a function of the percentage of corrected errors: There is no correlation between correction time and number of corrections.

131 ms, respectively. The unrecognized errors were .4° on average smaller than the recognized errors and they were corrected 50 ms faster (95 ms vs 145 ms) than the recognized errors.

These results are illustrated in Fig. 3. One sees the essential overlap of the distributions indicating that from a single trial one cannot tell whether the error was recognized or not even if one takes into account all 3 variables analysed here. Quite clearly the distribution of the correction times of the unperceived errors contain a fast mode with a peak around 50 ms, which is rather weak in the distribution of the correction times of the recognized errors.

To further look at the difference between involuntary saccades, i. e. the errors and their corrections, and voluntary saccades, we repeated the gap experiment with the instruction to generate on every trial a sequence of a prosaccade to the stimulus and then as quickly as possible a saccade to the opposite side. Thus the sequence of the two saccades would be the same as on an error trial.

The bottom histogram of Fig. 3 shows the distribution of the time the subjects spent at the stimulus, i. e. the time they needed to start the next saccade to the opposite side after having made a voluntary saccade to the stimulus. This intersaccadic interval is drastically longer (222 ms) than the one following an involuntary saccade (95 ms and 145 ms).

The distribution of the correction times of the unrecognized errors shows a seperate mode of very fast corrections, which can not be visually guided. This mode is missing in the recognized errors as well as in the distribution of the intersaccadic interval in the voluntary sequence. A correlation analysis shows, that the very fast corrections (<63 ms) form a distinct population. In these cases of very fast corrections under 63 ms the correction time (CRT) shows a strong positive correlation with the amplitude (AMP) of the error (r=0.27 for 1105 cases of unperceived and r=0.21 for 269 cases of recognized errors) and with the amplitude of the corrective saccade (r=0.42 and 0.44) (Fig. 4) and a strong negative correlation with the saccadic reaction time (SRT) of the error (r=-0.25 and -0.23) (Fig.5). All these correlations are highly significant: The faster such an immediatly corrected error (CRT<63ms) is corrected the smaller is its size and consequently the size of the corrective saccade. The later such an error is produced, the quicker it is corrected. Anticipated saccades, which happen to be prosaccades, are not corrected very quickly (see left of the line in Fig. 5).

From this experiment we can conclude that involuntary saccades are generated and corrected differently and that their relevance for conscious perception is different as well.

5. DISCUSSION

These results indicate that for each subject one has to differentiate between the ability to suppress reflex-like saccades due to a sufficiently strong fixation system and the ability to produce voluntary saccades. If the inhibition of the saccade system by fixation is too weak (as indicated by the relatively large number of express saccades in the prosaccade-task) saccades may occur in response to any stimulus onset irrespective of the subjects voluntary decision. In this case, however, the subject will correct the error in most cases after reasonably short times. This indicates that the subject despite the primary error is very able to generate saccades to the side oppposite to the stimulation. If on the other hand the inhibition is strong enough (as indicated by the relative absence of express saccades and correspondingly long reaction times) the subject may still generate too many saccades to the stimulus. These errors will have longer reaction times, they will be left un-

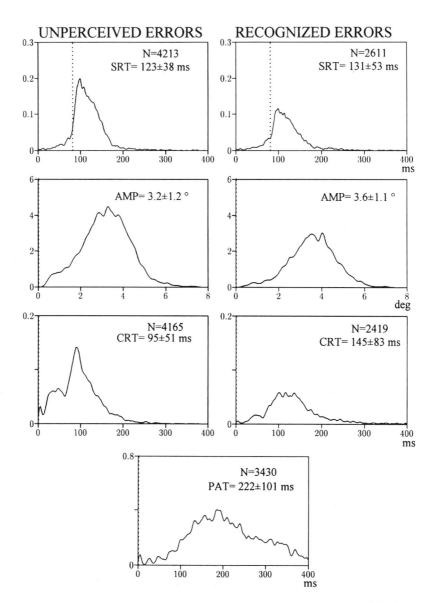

Figure 3. Distributions of the reaction times of the first prosaccades (SRT), the sizes of the first prosaccades (AMP) and the correction times of the corrective saccades (CRT). At the left side the data from the unperceived error trials are depicted (no button press), at the right side the data from the recognized error trials. Anticipated saccades with a SRT below 80 ms (indicated by the broken line in the upper panels) were excluded from this analysis. The bottom distribution shows the intersaccadic interval between the first voluntary prosaccade and the following saccade to the opposite side (PAT condition, see text).

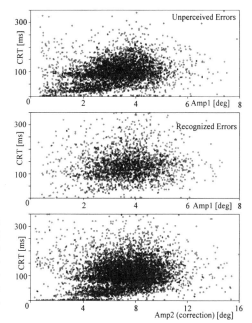

Figure 4. Scatterplots of the correction time (CRT) versus the amplitude (Amp1) of the unperceived prosaccade (top), versus the amplitude (Amp1) of the recognized prosacade (middle) and versus the amplitude (Amp2) of the corrective saccade following an unperceived or a recognized erroneous prosaccade (bottom). Note that the corrections are about twice as large as the prosaccades.

corrected and if corrected the intersaccadic interval will be relatively long. This dual aspect of saccade control makes sense in view of fixation being mediated by a parietal-tectal system (Munoz and Wurtz, 1993 a,b) and voluntary saccade initiation relying largely on an intact frontal system (Guitton et al. 1985). Both systems are also differentiated by their development with age (Fischer et al. 1997): while the number of express saccades changes very little after age 10 years, the variables from the antisaccade-task undergo drastic changes until age 18 y. The clinical findings from the antisaccade-task supporting the idea of two different possible reasons for high error rates are summarized elsewhere (Everling and Fischer, 1998).

The fact that a large proportion of the errors escape the subjects' conscious perception is most surprising from the viewpoint of the physiology of the visual system. Why is

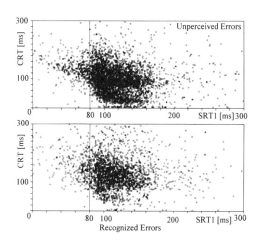

Figure 5. Scatterplots of the correction time (CRT) versus the saccadic reaction time (SRT) of the unperceived prosaccades (top) and of the recognized prosacade (bottom). Left of the line there are anticipated saccades with an SRT<80ms.

it that the relatively large ($4°+8°$) and long lasting (50–150 ms) changes of the retinal image when the stimulus rests on or close to the fovea are not consciously perceived? Conscious perception of location corresponds to what the subject expected to see. This study adds further evidence to a series of studies (Matin and Matin, 1969; Matin et al. 1970; Morrone et al. 1997), which show that in the temporal neighbourhood of saccades perceptual space (concerning both temporal and spatial aspects) is distorted, so that the correct identification of stimulus-location is not possible. To maintain stability of the visual world across saccades despite this temporal breakdown of perceptual space, the visual system has to make use of other information, such as information about intended movements. If extraretinal information of only intended eye movements would be used for the reconstruction of perceptual space (Duhamel et al. 1992; Andersen, 1995; Andersen et al. 1997), the prosaccades, because of being unintended, would have greater chances to escape conscious perception. Thus, our perception is "as if we were doing what we wanted to do".

To prevent the prosaccade an inhibitory action is needed. If this inhibition comes too late or is too weak, a prosaccade can occur which is then followed by an antisaccade. This could be called a "race model", because both saccades are considered as being generated in parallel with one winning the race. The presaccadic activity observed in the frontal cortex allows to predict whether the monkey makes a pro- or an antisaccade during the later course of a trial (Schlag-Rey et al. 1998). This seems to support this notion. If the same sequence of eye movements is made on purpose (PA condition) the subject becomes unable to generate the second saccade following the first as quickly as in case of involuntary errors. Probably only saccades, which can be planned in parallel can follow each other with such a short intersaccadic interval. That means, that intended and unintended saccades seem to have different brain sites of generation. In contrast, the voluntary saccades have to pass both the same bottleneck, which they only can pass sequentially. Neither anticipated saccades are corrected very quickly (Fig.5). It seems that the perceptual spatial frame transforms differently prior to voluntary as compared to involuntary saccades. A similar observation can be made when looking at large saccades falling short of the target (undershoots). These are corrected by a second saccade, which remains unconscious and may be considered as an involuntary reflex. While the motor response takes the mismatch into account, this is not consciously perceived. As soon as there is a temporal gap (introduced artificially) between the landing of the first saccade and the appearance of the final goal the subjects perceive this mismatch very clearly (Deubel et al. 1996). They have to generate another voluntary saccade to reach the final destination.

Another observation may also relate to the present finding: subjects report directions of gaze shift long before saccades (Deubel 1998). These saccades were also voluntary saccades.

As a speculative conclusion from these new and intriguing findings we propose that involuntary reflexes are prepared differently as compared to voluntary saccades: they may constitute a group of "attentionless" saccades which therefore escape the subjects' conscious perception in most cases. It remains open though, why only part of he errors remained unconscious.

ACKNOWLEDGMENTS

This work was supported by the Deutsche Forschungsgemeinschaft (DFG FI 227).

REFERENCES

Andersen R (1995) Encoding of intention and spatial location in the posterior parietal cortex. Cerebral cortex 5: 457–469

Andersen RA, Snyder LH, Bradley DC, Xing J (1997) Multimodal representation of space in the posterior parietal cortex and its use in planning movements. Annual Review of Neuroscience 20: 303–330

Cavegn D, Biscaldi M (1996) Fixation and saccade control in an express-saccade maker. Exp Brain Res 109: 101–116

Deubel H, Schneider WX, Bridgeman B (1996) Postsaccadic target blanking prevents saccadic suppression of image displacement. Vision Res 36, 985–996

Deubel H (1998) Die Rolle der visuellen Aufmerksamkeit bei der Selektion von Blickbewegungszielen. Beiträge zur ersten Tübinger Wahrnehmungskonferenz. Knirschverlag Kirchenstellinsfurt 37

Duhamel JR, Colby C, Goldberg ME (1992) The updating of the representation of visual space in parietal cortex by intended eye movements. Science 255: 90–92

Everling S, Fischer B (1998) The antisaccade: a review of basic research and clinical studies. Neuropsychologia (in press)

Fischer B, Biscaldi M, Gezeck S (1997) On the development of voluntary and reflexive components in saccade generation. Brain Res 754:285–297

Fischer B, Boch R (1983) Saccadic eye movements after extremely short reaction times in the monkey. Brain-Res 260: 21–26

Fischer B, Gezeck S, Hartnegg K (1997) The analysis of saccadic eye movements from gap and overlap paradigms. Brain Research Protocols 2: 47–52

Fischer B, Ramsperger E (1984) Human express saccades: extremely short reaction times of goal directed eye movements. Exp Brain Res 57: 191–195

Fischer B, Weber H (1992) Characteristics of "anti" saccades in man. Exp Brain Res 89: 415–424

Fischer B, Weber H (1996) Effects of procues on error rate and reaction times of antisaccades in human subjects. Exp Brain Res 109: 507–512

Guitton D, Buchtel HA, Douglas RM (1985) Frontal lobe lesions in man cause difficulties in suppressing reflexive glances and in generating goal-directed saccades. Exp Brain Res 58: 455–472

Hallett P (1978) Primary and secondary saccades to goals defined by instructions. Vision Res 18: 1279–1296

Matin L, Matin E (1969) Visual perception of direction when voluntary saccades occur. I.Relation of visual direction of a fixation target extinguished before a saccade to a flash presented during the saccade. Perception & Psychophysics 5: 65–80

Matin L, Matin E, Pola J (1970) Visual perception of direction when voluntary saccades occur: II.Relation of visual direction of a fixation target extinguished before a saccade to a subsequent test flash presented before the saccade. Perception & Psychophysics 8: 9–14

Mayfrank L, Mobashery M, Kimmig H, and Fischer B (1986) The role of fixation and visual attention in the occurrence of express saccades in man. European Archives of Psychiatry & Neurological Sciences 235: 269–275

Morrone CM, Ross J, Burr DC (1997) Apparent Position of Visual Targets during Real and Simulated Saccadic Eye Movements. The Journal of Neuroscience 17: 7941–7953

Munoz DP, Wurtz RH (1993,a) Fixation cells in monkey superior colliculus. I. Characteristics of cell discharge. J Neurophysiol 70: 559–575

Munoz DP, Wurtz RH (1993,b) Fixation cells in monkey superior colliculus. II. Reversible activation and deactivation. J Neurophysiol 70: 576–589

O'Driscoll GA, Alpert NM, Matthysse SW, Levy DL, Rauch SL, and Holzman PS (1995) Functional neuroanatomy of antisaccade eye movements investigated with positron emission tomography. Proc Natl Acad Sci USA 92: 925–929

Schiller PH, Sandell JH, Maunsell JH (1987) The effect of frontal eye field and superior colliculus lesions on saccadic latencies in the rhesus monkey. J Neurophysiol 57: 1033–1049

Schlag-Rey M, Amador N, Sanchez H, Schlag J (1998) Antisaccade performance predicted by neuronal activity in the supplementary eye field. Nature 390: 398–401

8

THE SUBJECTIVE DIRECTION OF GAZE SHIFTS LONG BEFORE THE SACCADE

Heiner Deubel,[1] David E. Irwin,[2] and Werner X. Schneider[1]

[1]Institute of Psychology
Ludwig-Maximilians-University
Munich, Germany
[2]University of Illinois
Urbana-Champaign

1. ABSTRACT

Subjects in eye movement experiments sometimes report that they have moved their eyes to some location before their eyes have actually moved (Deubel and Schneider, 1996). We investigated this by presenting a brief test stimulus at various points in time after directing subjects to make a saccadic eye movement to a peripheral cue. The subjects had to report where they were looking when the test stimulus was presented. We found that visual stimuli presented at the saccade target location as early as 250 ms before saccade onset were reported as occurring after the saccade. In a second experiment subjects performed, intentionally, a saccade to a static cue. Also under this condition, subjects reported to look at the future saccade target location long before the saccade actually occurred. The data show that subjects are unaware of the time when they make even a large saccade, and that they have no explicit knowledge of the retinal position of stimuli. Rather, they mistake movements of visual attention for movements of the eyes.

2. INTRODUCTION

People are able to maintain an assigned gaze direction in total darkness for periods as long as two minutes, and they can return their eyes accurately to an assigned direction in the dark following a randomly-chosen pattern of large saccades (Skavenski and Steinman, 1970). Clearly this would not be possible if people had no (implicit or explicit) knowledge about where their eyes were pointed. In the light, knowing what one is looking at seems an even more trivial task; fixated objects appear clear and in the center of our

Current Oculomotor Research, edited by Becker *et al.*
Plenum Press, New York, 1999.

65

visual space. Despite this, in previous research we have observed that subjects sometimes report anecdotally that they have moved their eyes to a location when in fact their eyes are still fixating somewhere else (Deubel and Schneider, 1996). This finding suggests that people don't always know where their eyes are pointing, at least not while preparing a saccadic eye movement. We investigated this in two experiments reported here.

3. METHODS

The stimuli were presented under computer control on a color monitor (CONRAC 7550 C21) at a frame rate of 100 Hz (KONTRAST 8000 TIGA graphics board); eye movements were measured with an SRI Generation 5.5 dual-Purkinje eyetracker sampling at 400 Hz. Screen background luminance was set to 3 cd/m^2; the luminance of the stimuli was 30 cd/m^2.

Six paid subjects completed six sessions of 192 trials each during the experiment. Trials in which the subject saccaded in the wrong direction and those with saccade latencies shorter than 120 ms or longer than 600 ms were discarded; this eliminated less than 4% of all trials. Subjects were naive with respect to the object of the study, but they were experienced in eye movement tasks. Each subject showed the same pattern of results.

In Experiment 1 the subject began each trial by fixating a central cross (see Figure 1a). After a delay the central fixation disappeared and a saccade cue was presented, 6 deg in the periphery, to the left or to the right of fixation. A test stimulus consisting of an open circle appeared for 20 ms in the visual field with a temporal asynchrony that varied randomly between -50 ms and 450 ms. The circle could appear either in the screen center, at the position of the saccade cue or at a position opposite to the saccade cue (the example given in Figure 1a is for the "circle opposite" case). Depending on the timing of test appearence, the eyes would have moved or not when the circle was presented; the subject's task was to indicate by pressing one of two buttons whether his or her gaze had been on

a)

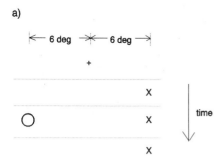

b)

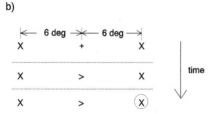

Figure 1. Schematic illustration of the procedure used in Experiment 1 (Figure a) and Experiment 2 (Figure b).

the central fixation point or on the saccade target at the time when the test stimulus occurred.

In Experiment 1, the saccade is triggered by the appearence of a periperal cue. In order to evaluate whether possible effects were not simply due to the subject confusing saccade cue and test stimulus onsets, we performed a second experiment (Experiment 2) in which the saccade was made purely intentionally, without an external cue. For this purpose, the subjects were trained before the experiment to make a (delayed) saccade approximately 1 s after a central visual cue. In the experiment, a central fixation was initially displayed together with two static crosses, 6 deg in the periphery (see Figure 1b). After some delay, a central arrow was displayed indicating the saccade target. The subjects were now told that they should try to move their eyes to the indicated saccade target 1 sec after the arrow cue appeared. As in the previous experiment, the subjects had to judge whether a brief visual test stimulus appeared before or after their gaze shifted. Again the test stimulus consisted of a circle that could apprear either on the screen center, on the indicated saccade target position, or opposite to that position.

4. RESULTS

The results of Experiment 1 are shown in Figure 2. Mean saccade latency in Experiment 1 was 231 ± 71 ms (SD) and was constant across conditions. Figure 2a plots test stimulus / saccade asynchrony on the abscissa; negative values mean that the test appeared before the saccade onset, and positive values mean the test appeared after the saccade onset. The hatched area indicates approximate saccade duration. The percentage of responses in which subjects said they were looking at the saccade target location when the test was presented is on the ordinate. The data are shown separately for the cases when the test stimulus was shown in the center (filled circles), on the side of the saccade cue (open circles), and on the opposite side (open triangles). Figure 2b replots the same data, here as a function of the time between saccade cue onset and test stimulus onset.

The results show that perception of gaze position was approximately veridical when the test was presented at the central fixation point (Figure2, filled circles); the 50% point (the point of subjective synchrony) is close to a stimulus/saccade asynchrony of 0 (see Figure 2a). This means that when the test appears at the center subjects were able to veridically report the time of occurrence with respect to the time of their saccade, though with relatively low temporal resolution. In contrast, when the test circle appeared at the saccade target location (open circles), subjects reported they were fixating the saccade target location long before their actual saccade. The point of subjective synchrony was approximately 300 ms before the saccade in this case. A smaller amount of perceived asynchrony was found for the contralateral position as well (open triangles). Figure 2b shows the same experimental data, but now given as a function of the delay between saccade cue and test stimulus. These data suggest that, at least for the condition where the test circle appears at the target location of the future saccade, the subjective gaze shift follows the presentation of the saccade target almost without delay; it seems that as soon as the saccade cue is presented, subjects already believe they are "on target".

In the first experiment the saccades were stimulus-induced; that is, they were made in immediate response to a saccade cue. To rule out the possibility that our results were due to subjects confusing the onset of the saccade cue for the saccade itself, in Experiment 2 we examined whether a perceived asynchrony between stimulus flash and saccade would be found for voluntary (self-triggered) saccades.

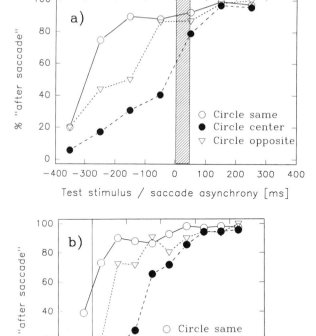

Figure 2. Results of Experiment 1. a) Stimulus/saccade asynchrony is plotted on the abscissa; negative values mean that the test appeared before the saccade onset, and positive values mean the test appeared after the saccade onset. The hatched area indicates approximate saccade duration. The percentage of responses in which subjects said they were looking at the saccade target location when the test was presented is on the ordinate. b) Same data, now plotted as a function of the temporal interval between saccade cue and test circle presentation.

The results are shown in Figure 3, in the same manner as for Experiment 1. It can be seen that also for intentional saccades, subjects considerably misjudge their gaze position before saccades. The points of subjective synchrony were found at -45 ms, -145 ms, and -102 ms for the test circle appearing at the center, the cue location, and the opposite side, respectively.

5. DISCUSSION

The results demonstrate that the perceived direction of gaze shifts a long time before the eyes move. This is true for both stimulus-induced and voluntary saccades. These results show that people don't always know what they are looking at with foveal gaze, or at least, when they are looking where. Apparently, they have no explicit knowledge about their (orbital) eye position. Further, they are unable to gain explicit knowledge about the position at which objects appear on their retinae - otherwise, they would have noticed when the stimulus was presented in their visual periphery. Finally, subjects seem not to notice the occurrence of even large saccadic eye movements. However, because visual attention is known to shift to the location of an intended saccadic eye movement before the eyes move (Deubel and Schneider, 1996; Hoffman and Subramaniam, 1995; Kowler et al., 1995; Shepherd et al., 1986; Schneider and Deubel, 1995), we believe that our results are due to subjects mistaking shifts of visual attention for shifts of the eyes—when that hap-

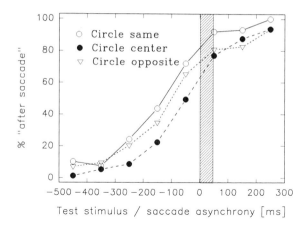

Figure 3. Results of Experiment 2.

pens, the subjective direction of gaze does not correspond to objective eye position. Visual attention moves to the saccade target location before the eyes move, making that location the new center of perceived visual space.

Our results are analogous to physiological findings that the receptive fields of individual neurons in parietal cortex in monkeys shift to new positions in space shortly before a saccade (Duhamel et al., 1992). It has been suggested that parietal cortex might be able to generate a continuously accurate representation of visual space by anticipating the retinal consequences of eye movements in this way. In a similar fashion, we find that the perceived direction of gaze shifts prior to an eye movement, at least for some positions in the visual field. Our results suggest that a global remapping of space does not occur, however; rather, it appears to be primarily the saccade target location that is affected. This agrees with recent evidence showing that information at the saccade target location is critical for linking the contents of successive eye fixations so that one perceives a stable and continuous visual world across eye movements (Deubel et al., 1996; Irwin et al., 1994; McConkie and Currie, 1996).

ACKNOWLEDGMENT

This research was supported by the Deutsche Forschungsgemeinschaft, SFB 462 "Sensomotorik".

REFERENCES

Deubel H, Schneider WX (1996) Saccade target selection and object recognition: Evidence for a common attentional mechanism. Vision Res 36: 1827–1837

Deubel H, Schneider W X, Bridgeman B (1996) Post-saccadic target blanking prevents saccadic suppression of image displacement. Vision Res 36: 985–996

Duhamel J, Colby C, Goldberg ME (1992) The updating of the representation of visual space in parietal cortex by intended eye movements. Science 27: 227–240

Hoffman JE, Subramaniam B (1995) The role of visual attention in saccadic eye movements. Percept Psychophys 57: 787–795

Irwin DE, McConkie G, Carlson-Radvansky L, Currie C (1994) A localist evaluation solution for visual stability across saccades. Behav Brain Sci 17: 265–266

Kowler E, Anderson E, Dosher B, Blaser E (1995) The role of attention in the programming of saccades. Vision Res 35: 1897–1916

McConkie G, Currie C (1996) Visual stability across saccades while viewing complex pictures. J Exp Psychol:HPP 22: 563–581

Schneider WX, Deubel H (1995) Visual attention and saccadic eye movements: Evidence for obligatory and selective spatial coupling. In: Findlay JM, Kentridge RW, Walker R (eds) Eye movement research: mechanisms, processes and applications. Elsevier, Amsterdam, pp 317–324

Shepherd M, Findlay JM, Hockey RJ (1986) The relationship between eye movements and spatial attention. Q J Exp Psychol 38A: 475–491

Skavenski AA, Steinman RM (1970) Control of eye position in the dark. Vision Res 10: 193–203

DOES VISUAL BACKGROUND INFORMATION INFLUENCE SACCADIC ADAPTATION?

J. Ditterich, T. Eggert, and A. Straube

Center for Sensorimotor Research
Dept. of Neurology, Klinikum Grosshadern
Ludwig-Maximilians-University
Marchioninistr. 23, D-81377 Munich, Germany

1. INTRODUCTION

It is well-known that the saccadic system shows an adaptive behavior (e.g. McLaughlin 1967; Deubel et al. 1986). Whenever a large systematic postsaccadic fixation error occurs, an adaptive modification in the system takes place. An elegant paradigm to study this phenomenon experimentally is based on the fact that changes in the visual world during a saccade are hardly detected (e.g. Bridgeman et al. 1975). Shifting the saccade target during visually guided saccades creates an artificial error. As a consequence, the eye does not land on the target, a corrective saccade is elicited and the additional target shift is gradually anticipated by the system by adapting the amplitude of the primary saccade. The visual processing underlying the signal which drives the adaptive process is still not completely understood.

Deubel (1991) was able to show that systematically shifting a pseudonoise pattern of vertical bars during saccades can also elicit saccadic adaptation. An inversion (black turned into white and vice versa) in a limited area served as saccade target. During the reflexive saccade caused by the transient the whole pattern was shifted. Even though the inverted region was not detectable perceptionally, corrective saccades and an adaptive behavior were observed.

We will present a similar experiment where we were able to induce saccadic adaptation by shifting a large random dot pattern intrasaccadically.

These experiments suggest that the information leading to a corrective saccade came from a matching process relying on visual information extracted from an area with a minimum extent of approximately 2 deg. This estimation is based on the structure of the patterns used in these experiments.

How could the shift of the pattern be detected in order to drive the adaptation? One possible explanation is that the system creates a prediction about the expected visual information after the saccade and compares it with the actual visual information. A possible

Current Oculomotor Research, edited by Becker *et al.*
Plenum Press, New York, 1999.

71

neuronal substrate for such a mechanism would be the area LIP. Duhamel et al. (1992) were able to show that neurons in this area have retinocentric receptive fields and carry visual and visual memory signals. The most interesting aspect is that the receptive fields are shifted prior to a saccade in such a way that a neuron codes the same part of a visual scene immediately prior to and after a saccade.

If such a mechanism is the source of the error signal, presenting a stable structured visual background during adaptation experiments should influence the subject's gain adaptation or corrective saccades, since it creates a discrepancy between the information provided by the target and that provided by the visual background. Deubel (1994) reported no significant influence of presenting a stable background during the adaptation procedure on the saccadic gain in the adapted state.

We asked whether a visual background alters the adaptation dynamics and whether the adaptation process is influenced by shifting the background together with the target in the same or opposite direction during the primary saccade.

2. METHODS

We measured the horizontal movements of both eyes using an infrared reflection device (IRIS, Skalar) with a resolution better than 0.5 deg. The position signal was digitized with a sampling rate of 1 kHz. A nonlinear polynomial calibration (3rd order) based on fixation data was applied off-line. For providing the eye position on-line a linear calibration was used.

The visual stimuli were presented on a computer screen (40x30 cm). The viewing distance was 60 cm, thus the screen covered a visual field of 37x28 deg. We used a graphical resolution of 1280x1024 pixels and a frame rate of 60 Hz. A hardware overlay feature allowed us to shift background and target independently from each other.

Our subjects were seated in a darkened room. They placed their head on a chin rest and were instructed not to move their head. The subjects were told to fixate a target appearing in the periphery as fast and as accurately as possible. When a saccade was detected (eye velocity > 100 deg/s), the target was shifted in the opposite direction by 25% of the target step size.

Due to the frame rate of 60 Hz used by our graphic device a maximum of 25 ms (1.5 cycles) can pass between the command to shift the target and the effect on the screen. The time between the occurrence of an eye movement velocity greater than 100 deg/s and the command to shift the target was less than 5 ms yielding an overall maximum delay of 30 ms. From a post hoc analysis it can be inferred that in about 93% of the trials the shift must have taken place during the saccade.

In the off-line analysis saccades were detected automatically using a velocity criterion (v > 100 deg/s). Start and end of a saccade were defined by an algorithm which starts at the peak velocity and searches for the first drop of the velocity below 10% of the peak in both directions. The saccade amplitude was computed as the difference in eye position between end and start. The gain of the primary saccade was defined as the quotient of the amplitude of the primary saccade and the size of the initial target step. All time courses shown here are smoothed using a running median filter with a width of 49 points.

For the time series analysis we filtered the data using a running median filter with a width of 25 points. The width was reduced appropriately at the beginning and the end of the time series with a minimum of 9 points. We extracted the first sample available, then the next one with a minimum distance of 25 points and so on, ensuring that all these samples were calculated from different data points. These samples served as the input for all forthcoming analyses. A single test was always performed on the data from all subjects. A repeated measures ANOVA was used to decide if the gain showed a significant development over time. The question if there was a significant difference in the development over time between two conditions was answered by performing a repeated measures ANOVA on the difference data calculated for each subject. In order to perform a parametric analysis of the adaptation dynamics we subtracted the individual mean from the data and fitted either a linear or an exponential function using a least square fit with the constraint that the sum of the function values at the sample positions had to be zero. What we call time constant in the case of the exponential function is the number of trials necessary for the gain to decrease by 63% of the total gain change. The decision if the descriptive model was sufficient to explain the time variability of the data was based on a repeated measures ANOVA performed on the residual error testing if time is still a significant factor. If this would be the case the hypothesis that the descriptive model can explain the time variability in the data had to be rejected. Estimated parameters were compared using a t test.

3. EXPERIMENTS AND RESULTS

3.1. Experiment (1): Adaptation Induced by Shifting a Random Dot Pattern Intrasaccadically

The random dot pattern used in this experiment consisted of roughly 300 white filled ellipses with the length of both axes taken randomly from the interval 0.25–1 cm on a black background.

The ellipses lying within a virtual circle with a diameter of 4.8 deg were slightly brighter than the others and indicated where the subjects had to fixate ("fixation spot"). Suddenly their brightness changed to the normal value and at the same time the ellipses lying within another virtual circle with the same diameter somewhere in the periphery were shifted in random directions with random amplitudes (maximum: 7 mm; see Fig. 1). Thus, the subjects were able to detect a transient in the periphery which served as the saccade target but they were not able to tell where the shift had taken place when looking at the pattern after the displacement. We requested only horizontal saccades. When a saccade

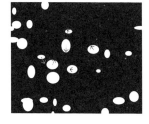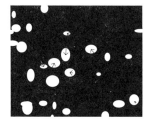

Before transient　　　　　　　　　　　　After transient

Figure 1. Illustration of the stimulus used in Experiment (1). The images show the same small portion of the screen before and after presenting the peripheral motion transient defining the target position. The arrows were not presented on the screen. They only indicate which of the ellipses changed place.

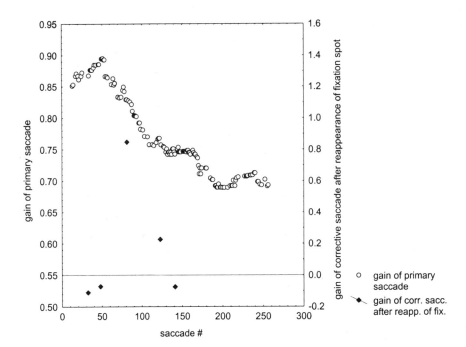

Figure 2. Example of a gain time course observed in the experiment with the intrasaccadic shift of a random dot pattern together with the corrective saccades observed after the reappearance of the fixation spot. Notice that these are not the corrective saccades caused by the intrasaccadic shift of the pattern. In analogy to the definition of the gain of primary saccades we defined the gain of these saccades as the quotient of the saccade amplitude and the size of the initial target step.

was detected the whole pattern was shifted in the direction opposite to the one of the requested saccade by 25% of the requested saccade size. 600 ms later the fixation spot reappeared where the subject was looking at at the moment. Seven subjects took part in this experiment.

A significant gain decrease over time was observed in this experiment. The critical point is, of course, that the reappearance of the fixation spot, determined by measuring the eye position on-line, must not cause a systematic retinal error, for then one could argue that the retinal error of the fixation spot or the corrective saccades to the fixation spot possibly drove the adaptation. Figure 2 shows an example of a gain time course observed in such an experiment together with the saccades, which occurred after highlighting the fixation spot. Since there were not many corrective saccades, and since backward and onward corrections were equally distributed, the gain adaptation must have been caused by the intrasaccadic shift of the random dot pattern.

3.2. Experiment (2): Influence of Presenting a Stable Visual Background on the Adaptation Process

A small white cross subtending a visual angle of 0.3 deg served as target. It was presented on a black horizontal bar with a vertical width of 0.5 deg in all experimental conditions to make sure that the target was easily detectable. This target made random steps with a minimum size of 5 deg and a maximum size of 20 deg in both horizontal directions.

There were five different experimental conditions. A cyclic change in the order of the experiments was applied for the 5 subjects:

a. In the control condition there was no visual background. Only the target was presented.
b. The first structured background was a random dot pattern consisting of roughly 125 randomly distributed red ellipses covering the whole screen with both diameters taken from the interval 0.25–1 cm (about 10% of the pixels were red).
c. The second structured background used consisted of four geometrical objects (filled squares and circles with different colors and a size of 2.5 cm; about 2% of the pixels were not black).
d. The third background was a colored photo covering the whole screen.
e. To evaluate the influence of the luminance we additionally used an unstructured red background.

In contrast to the target, which was shifted during the saccades, all the backgrounds remained stable on the screen.

A significant gain decrease over time was observed under all conditions. The time course could be explained by exponential descriptive models for all conditions. The only significant differences between the control condition without a background and the experimental conditions with a stable background were found in the condition with an unstructured background, where the tests indicated a significant difference in the gain time course

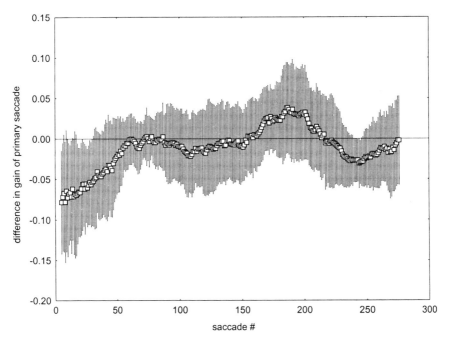

Figure 3. Gain difference when presenting a stable unstructured background compared to the control condition (no background) in the double step paradigm. The negative values observed at the beginning indicate an immediate gain reduction caused by the brighter background.

and in the estimated gain change. Figure 3 presents the time development of the difference in the gain between the condition with a stable unstructured background and the control condition. These differences were calculated separately for each subject. The plot shows the mean value and the standard deviation for each point in time.

The plot shows that the presentation of a stable unstructured background caused an immediate gain drop. Similar observations could be made for all types of backgrounds. There was always a quick gain reduction effect which reached its maximum after at the most, 20 saccades.

This means, of course, that the adaptation process was confronted with altered starting conditions. But did the presentation of a stable background influence the adaptation dynamics? If we consider the estimated time constant a measure of the adaptation dynamics, we have to state that presenting a stable background did not significantly influence the adaptation process.

3.3. Experiment (3): Control Experiment: Influence of an Unstructured Background in a Single Step Paradigm

The only difference between this experiment and the control condition and the condition with the unstructured red background in the last experiment was that the intrasaccadic back step was missing. Seven subjects took part in this experiment.

The immediate gain reduction effect observed when presenting an unstructured background in the double step paradigm was also found in the control experiment with a single step paradigm. Presenting the background led to a significant difference in the gain time course and in the estimated slopes obtained from linear descriptive models, which were sufficient to explain the time variance of the data. Interestingly, a significant gain decrease over time was observed in the case of the single step paradigm in otherwise complete darkness. Figure 4 shows the average time course of the individual gain differences between the condition with an unstructured background and the condition without a background.

3.4. Experiment (4): Influence of Shifting a Background Intrasaccadically on the Adaptation Process

In this experiment we combined the foveal target from Experiment (2) with the random dot pattern from Experiment (1). There were three different conditions:

a. The background remained stable on the screen.
b. The background was shifted together with the target during the primary saccade with the same amplitude in the same direction (opposite to the target step).
c. The background was shifted together with the target during the primary saccade with the same amplitude but in the opposite direction (same direction as the target step).

Ten subjects took part in this experiment.

The gain development over time was significant under all three conditions. Exponential descriptive models were suitable to explain the time variance of the data. The differences between the condition with a stable background (random dot pattern) and the conditions with an intrasaccadic displacement of the background were far from being significant.

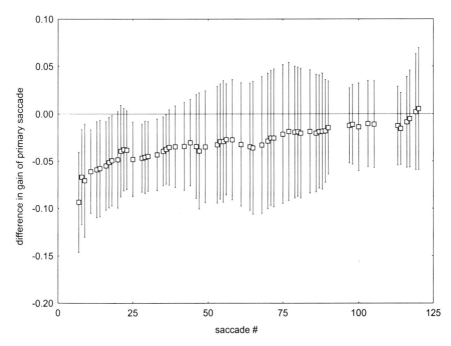

Figure 4. Gain difference when presenting an unstructured background compared to no background in the single step paradigm. Notice the different time scale compared to Fig. 3.

Table 1 summarizes the results obtained from the different experimental conditions. Table 2 shows the results obtained from the comparisons between different conditions.

4. DISCUSSION

In accordance with Deubel's (1991) findings we were able to show that shifting a large random pattern intrasaccadically can induce saccadic adaptation. This again supports the idea that there must be some kind of pattern matching algorithm which is able to detect intrasaccadic displacements by comparing the postsaccadic visual information with a prediction based on the presaccadic visual information. Since there were no single objects in these patterns which could be re-identified to accomplish this, we have to postulate a low-level process operating on presumably the complete visual information taken from a larger visual field. The result of such a correlation mechanism would then be used to program a corrective saccade or to drive saccadic adaptation.

If such a mechanism would be the only one to detect intrasaccadic target displacements which induce an adaptation phenomenon, one would predict that presenting a structured stable visual background in addition to the jumping target in a double step paradigm should interfere with the adaptation process, since there is a mismatch between the displacement information provided by the target and the one provided by the background. Again in agreement with Deubel's (1994) results, we were able to show that the presentation of a stable background in addition to a small foveal target does not influence the adaptation process irrespective of the background type. The fact that the adaptation

Table 1. Significance levels for a gain development over time and the results obtained from the parameter estimations based on a linear or exponential descriptive model. The calculation procedures underlying these results are explained in the Methods section

Experiment	Condition	Sign. f. developm. over time	Lin. mod.: est. slope	St. dev. of est. slope	Sign. f. LIN. mod. not being sufficient	Exp. mod.: est. gain change	St. dev. of est. gain change	Est. time constant	St. dev. of est. time constant	Sign. f. EXP. mod. not being sufficient
1		**0.03**	-3.4E-4	8.3E-5	0.82					
2	no BG	**<0.001**				-0.17	0.02	33	10	0.43
2	RDP	**<0.001**				-0.11	0.02	32	10	0.65
2	geom. obj.	**<0.001**				-0.15	0.03	31	11	0.31
2	photo	**<0.001**				-0.15	0.02	38	12	0.52
2	unstruct. BG	**0.04**				-0.08	0.03	30	22	0.21
3	no BG	**0.03**	-6.0E-4	2.2E-4	0.21					
3	unstruct. BG	**1.0**	3.5E-6	1.8E-4	0.98					
4	stable	**<0.001**				-0.14	0.03	34	10	0.70
4	back step	**<0.001**				-0.13	0.03	42	16	0.96
4	onward step	**<0.001**				-0.12	0.02	44	14	0.83

Bold numbers indicate statistical significance

Table 2. Significance levels for differences in the gain time course or estimated parameter. The calculation procedures underlying these results are again explained in the Methods section*

Experiment	First condition	Second condition	Sign. f. diff. in development over time	Sign. f. diff. in est. slope	Sign. f. diff. in est. gain change	Sign. f. diff. in est. time constant
2	no BG	RDP	0.46		0.07	0.95
2	no BG	geom. obj.	0.14		0.66	0.91
2	no BG	photo	0.12		0.54	0.73
2	no BG	unstruct. BG	**0.04**		**0.01**	0.90
3	no BG	unstruct. BG	**0.02**	**0.04**		
4	stable BG	back step	0.53		0.88	0.67
4	stable BG	onward step	0.66		0.65	0.58
4	back step	onward step	0.90		0.80	0.95

Bold numbers indicate statistical significance.

dynamics, expressed in terms of the estimated time constant obtained from an exponential descriptive model, is not altered contrasts with our hypothesis. Thus, the postulated correlation mechanism operating on the complete visual information taken from a larger part of the visual field could not have been used in these experiments to detect the intrasaccadic target shift.

Presenting a background always led to a quick, immediate decrease in the gain of the primary saccade. Since this effect was maximal when presenting an unstructured background and since it could also be observed in a control experiment with a single step paradigm, this phenomenon cannot be based on structural background information and it has nothing to do with the double step paradigm. It seems as if the target selection process or the saccade programming would be influenced by the background luminance. At the moment we have no explanation for this phenomenon.

Displacing a random dot pattern in the background during the primary saccade made to a small jumping foveal target did not influence the adaptation process, either. Thus, the only information used by the adaptive system in these experiments was the intrasaccadic target displacement. The background even did not serve as a visual reference when evaluating the target shift.

Combined, we propose that either the postulated low-level correlation mechanism is not the only one which can be used by the system responsible for saccadic adaptation for detecting intrasaccadic displacements or that there is some kind of selection process which made sure that this low-level correlation mechanism worked only on the visual target information in our experiments with the small foveal target. A possible mechanism which comes to mind, which would be compatible with the first suggestion, would be a high-level process operating on an abstract representation of objects and their position in space.

However, the displacement detection could still be based on a low-level correlation mechanism, if one postulates more flexibility regarding this process. A possible explanation for the findings compatible with the second proposal would be that it is not the complete visual information which is used. In other words, the system could be able to carry out a selective search for the target based on its characteristic features. This would imply the possibility of suppressing irrelevant visual information when visually matching the saccade target.

Another possible explanation would be that only information from a smaller region could have been used in the experiments with the small foveal target. The part of the visual system dealing with object recognition operates only on a spatially selected portion of the visual information available. The selection is carried out by an attentional mechanism. Since the size of the attention focus is supposed to be variable (e.g. Eriksen and St. James 1986), we can assume that it was small in Experiments (2) and (4) due to the clearly defined small target and larger in Experiment (1) due to the presented pattern. Probably only visual information taken from within the attention focus is used for our purpose. This could have prevented an interaction with the background in the experiments with the small foveal target.

REFERENCES

Bridgeman B, Hendry D, Stark L (1975) Failure to detect displacement of the visual world during saccadic eye movements. Vision Res 15:719–722

Deubel H, Wolf W, Hauske G (1986) Adaptive gain control of saccadic eye movements. Human Neurobiol 5:245–253

Deubel H (1991) Adaptive Control of Saccade Metrics. In: Obrecht G, Stark LW (ed) Presbyopia Research. Plenum Press, New York, pp 93–100

Deubel H (1994) Is saccadic adaptation context-specific? In: Findlay JM, Kentridge RW, Walker R (ed) Eye Movement Research: Mechanisms, Processes and Applications. Elsevier Science.

Duhamel J-R, Colby CL, Goldberg ME (1992) The Updating of the Representation of Visual Space in Parietal Cortex by Intended Eye Movements. Science 255:90–92

Eriksen CW, St. James JD (1986) Visual attention within and around the field of focal attention: A zoom lens model. Percept Psychophys 40:225–240

McLaughlin SC (1967) Parametric adjustment in saccadic eye movements. Percept Psychophys 2:359–362

EFFECTS OF TARGET SIZE AND BRIGHTNESS AND FIXATION POINT SIZE ON HUMAN VISUALLY-GUIDED VOLUNTARY SACCADES

Yoshinobu Ebisawa

Faculty of Engineering
Shizuoka University
Hamamatsu, Japan

1. INTRODUCTION

The peak velocity of saccades elicited by a visual target is known to be higher than that of saccades elicited by an invisible target (Smit et al. 1987; Smit and Van Gisbergen 1989). Other factors that may influence human saccades, however, are not well known. Therefore, the present study examines the relationship between saccades and the stimuli by which they are generated. This examination consisted of simultaneously presenting a fixation point and a saccade target directly in front of subjects. The subjects produced saccades from the fixation point to the target. Separate experiments were conducted in which the size and luminance of the target as well as the size of the fixation point were varied independently. This paper shows that the amplitude and peak velocity of the saccade vary according to the stimulus.

2. METHODS

The present study examined four male university students having normal vision and oculomotor functions. Three experiments were conducted in which the heads of the subjects were immobilized using a dental bite. These experiments were conducted in complete darkness. Visual stimuli were produced using a 15-inch non-interlaced computer display (frame rate: 72.1 Hz) that was placed 50 cm in front of the subject. All visual stimuli were white circles. The luminance of the display background was 0.15 cd/m^2. Visual stimuli were viewed by the right eye only. Horizontal positions of the viewing eye were recorded at a rate of 500 Hz using an infrared limbus reflection system (bandwidth: 70 Hz). The recorded data were then subjected to computer analysis. In each experiment, a small target (0.2 deg, 20 cd/m^2) was presented in the center of the monitor at the beginning of each trial. Each subject was instructed to fix his eye on the target and, after target fixation, to click a computer

Current Oculomotor Research, edited by Becker *et al.*
Plenum Press, New York, 1999.

mouse, causing the target to be extinguished and a buzzer warning to sound for 500 ms. Immediately after the buzzer warning, the small target was replaced by the fixation point (FP), which simultaneously appeared in the center of the monitor with the saccade target (ST), which was presented randomly either 4 deg or 8 deg to the right of the FP. The subject was instructed to continue FP fixation for one second (as judged by the subject) after the appearance of the ST and to then make a single saccadic movement to the ST. If a saccade occurred within one second after the appearance of the ST, the trial was immediately stopped, and the subject was again presented with a buzzer warning. The following three experiments were conducted in the order in which they are presented.

Experiment 1. The ST diameter was chosen randomly from 0.2, 0.4, 0.8, 1.6, and 3.2 deg for each trial. The ST luminance was 20 cd/m^2. The diameter and luminance of the FP were 0.2 deg and 20 cd/m^2, respectively.

Experiment 2. The ST luminance was chosen randomly from 4, 20, and 120 cd/m^2 for each trial. The ST diameter was 0.8 deg. The diameter and luminance of the FP were 0.2 deg and 20 cd/m^2, respectively.

Experiment 3. The FP diameter was chosen randomly from 0.2, 0.8, and 3.2 deg for each trial. The FP luminance was 20 cd/m^2. The diameter and luminance of the ST were 0.8 deg and 20 cd/m^2, respectively.

To quantify the peak velocities of saccades having different amplitudes, the following normalization was executed (Smit et al., 1987). For each experiment and for each subject, all data for all ST diameters, all ST luminance, or all FP diameters representing the relationship between the amplitude (A) and peak velocity (V) was fitted using the following formula:

$$V(A)=V_0(1-\exp(-A_0 01A))\tag{1}$$

where V_0 and A_0 are constants. The normalized peak velocity for each saccade, V_{ni}, was calculated using the following formula:

$$V_{ni}=V_i/V(A_i)\tag{2}$$

where V_i and A_i are the peak velocity and amplitude of the corresponding saccade, respectively. Thus the normalized peak velocities are independent of saccade amplitude.

3. RESULTS

Figures 1a-c show the saccadic gain (saccadic amplitude / target eccentricity) for the stimulus conditions of experiments 1, 2, and 3, respectively. The symbols and bars indicate the mean and standard deviation, respectively. In the figures, the Mean column shows the average of the means of the four subjects for each FP. The results of experiment 1 show that saccadic gain has a tendency to decrease as ST diameter increases and tends to reach a maximum for ST diameter=0.4-deg. Averaging all subjects, the saccadic gain for ST diameter=3.2-deg was 8.88% less than that for ST diameter=0.4-deg. The results of experiment 2 show that saccadic gain was lowest for the brightest ST (120 cd/m^2) when compared to the darker STs (4 and 20 cd/m^2), between which there was no difference. The gain for ST luminance=120-cd/m^2 was 5.23% smaller than that for ST luminance=4-cd/m^2. The results of experiment 3 show that the largest FP produced the smallest gain. The gain for FP diameter=3.2-deg was 17.32% smaller than that for FP diameter=0.2-deg.

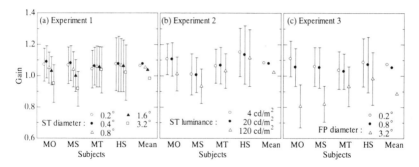

Figure 1. Saccadic gain.

Figures 2a-c show the normalized peak velocities obtained in experiments 1, 2, and 3, respectively. The results of experiment 1 show that for all subjects the normalized peak velocity (NPV) tends to decrease as the ST diameter increases. Averaging all subjects, the NPV ratio for ST diameter=3.2-deg was 6.72% less than that for ST diameter=0.2-deg. The results of experiment 2 show that NPV decreased for the brightest ST (120 cd/m^2) when compared to the darker ones. The average decrease in the NPV ratio from ST luminance=4-cd/m^2 to ST luminance=120-cd/m^2 was 2.39%. The results of experiment 3 show that for all subjects the NPV decreased significantly for the largest FP compared to the smaller FPs. The NPV ratio decreased an average of 10.29% from FP diameter=0.2-deg to FP diameter=3.2-deg.

4. DISCUSSION

In all experiments in the present study, in the conditions that the saccadic gain was larger, the subjects developed an expectation drift (Kowler and Steinman 1979) to the right during their attempt to continue fixation of the FP for one estimated second. Inversely, in the conditions that the saccadic gain was smaller, they showed a leftward drift. This fact means that the larger the eccentricity of the ST on the retina at the beginning the saccade, the smaller the saccade gain became. At least, thus, the saccadic gain change did not occur by the drift causing the change of the eccentricity of the ST.

In the experiment 1, the larger the ST was, the smaller the saccadic gain was. This gain change does not reflect so-called global effect (Findlay 1982).

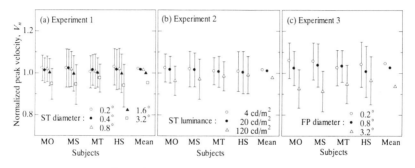

Figure 2. Normalized saccadic peak velocity.

Conditions that produced lower normalized peak velocities also produced lower saccadic gains in all of the experiments conducted in this study. The results of experiment 3 show that a larger fixation point decreases both the amplitude and the peak velocity of the saccades. In the monkey (Sparks and Mays 1983) and cat (Paré et al. 1994), the amplitude of saccades elicited by suprathreshold currents on the superior colliculus was reduced if electrical stimulation occurred during fixation. In the cat, electrical activation of the collicular fixation area was found to mimic well the effects of natural fixation on the elicited gaze shift (Paré et al. 1994). The visual stimulation of the largest fixation point retinotopically may cover the entire collicular fixation area, causing the area to be strongly activated. This activation may reduce the peak velocity as well as the amplitude of the saccades. In addition, the results of experiments 1 and 2 show that larger targets as well as brighter targets decrease the amplitude and peak velocity of the saccades. Peripherally larger or brighter stimulation may strongly elicit a saccade. However, the subject must have actively suppressed saccade occurrence for a short period of time (longer than one second). If fixation causes suppression, this fixation may reduce the amplitude and peak velocity of the elicited saccades.

REFERENCES

Findlay M (1982) Global visual processing for saccadic eye movements. Vision Res 22: 1033–1045

Kowler E, Steinman RM (1979) The effect of expectations on slow oculomotor control - I. Periodic target steps. Vision Res 19: 619–632

Paré M, Crommelinck M, Guitton D (1994) Gaze shifts evoked by stimulation of the superior colliculus in the head-free cat conform to the motor map but also depend on stimulus strength and fixation activity. Exp Brain Res 101: 123–139

Smit AC, Van Gisbergen JAM (1989) A short-latency transition in saccade dynamics during square-wave tracking and its significance for the differentiation of visually-guided and predictive saccade. Exp Brain Res 76: 64–74

Smit AC, Van Gisbergen JAM, Cools AR (1987) A parametric analysis of human saccades in different experimental paradigms. Vision Res 27: 1745–1762

Sparks DL, Mays LE (1983) Spatial localization of saccade targets. I. Compensation for stimulation-induced perturbations in eye position. J Neurophysiol 49: 45–63

11

EFFECTS OF WARNING SIGNALS ON SACCADIC REACTION TIMES AND EVENT-RELATED POTENTIALS

A. Spantekow,[1] P. Krappmann,[1] S. Everling,[2] and H. Flohr[1]

[1]Brain Research Institute
University of Bremen
POB 33 04 40, 28334 Bremen, Germany
[2]Department of Physiology
Queens University
Kingston, Ontario, Canada K7L 3N6

1. INTRODUCTION

Saccadic reaction times (SRTs) are reduced by about 50 ms when the fixation point (FP) is extinguished 200 ms prior to a peripheral target (T) is presented (gap task) as compared to a condition where the FP remains visible continuously (overlap task). Moreover, the gap paradigm favors the occurence of express saccades (SRTs between 80 und 120 ms). Two main explanations have been proposed for the gap effect: the dissappearance of the FP (1) leads to a disengagement of fixation and/or (2) elicits a general warning effect which results in a motor preparation (Klein and Kingstone 1993). Several authors investigated the cortical mechanisms underlying the gap effect by recording event-related potentials in a gap task. It was shown that the disappearance of the FP in a gap task is associated with a negative event-related potential (ERP) during the gap (Everling et al. 1996; Gomez et al. 1996; Csibra et al. 1997; Krappmann et al. 1997). This negative potential was interpreted as being consistent with the motor preparation hypothesis. In this study, we recorded ERPs to examine whether a change of the color of the FP prior to target presentation had the same effects on SRTs, the proportion of express saccades, and ERPs as the disappearance of the FP.

2. METHODS

We recorded ERPs from 6 subjects (4 females and 2 males) performing an overlap task (FP remains visible continuously), a gap task (FP was extinguished 200 ms prior to

Current Oculomotor Research, edited by Becker *et al.*
Plenum Press, New York, 1999.

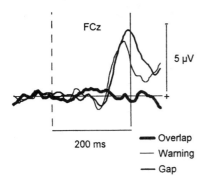

Figure 1. Grand average waveforms recorded at the midline fronto-central electrode (FCz) for the overlap task (thick line), the warning task (thin line), and the gap task (intermediate line) in 6 subjects. Left vertical dashed line indicates the disappearance and the change of the color of the FP, respectively. The right vertical solid line marks the appearance of the peripheral target.

target presentation) and a warning task (the color of the FP was changed 200 ms prior to target presentation). Subjects were instructed to fixate the central FP and to look to the peripheral target as quickly as possible. The electroencephalogram was recorded with a time constant of 10 sec and a low-pass filter of 75 Hz from 19 sites over the scalp. Recordings were digitized with a frequency of 167 Hz.

3. RESULTS

The main results are as follows:

1. The mean SRT for the overlap task, the warning task and the gap task was 199.38 ± 11.2 ms, 150.43 ± 6.9 ms and 130.35 ± 8.7 ms, respectively. SRTs differed significantly depending on the task ($F=21.3$, $p=0.0002$). They were significantly shorter in the gap task than in the warning task ($t=4.9$, $p=0.0046$) and significantly shorter in the warning task than in the overlap task ($t=3.9$, $p=0.0115$).
2. Subjects also elicited significantly different proportions of express saccades in the three tasks ($F=14.5$, $p=0.0011$). Subjects executed significantly more express saccades in the gap task than in the warning task ($t=2.9$, $p=0.0339$) and significantly more express saccades in the warning task than in the overlap task ($t=4.9$, $p=0.0045$).
3. Grand-average wave forms showed a negative potential in the gap and the warning task with a maximum at frontal and central recording sites. This negative potential for both tasks started at the midline fronto-central electrode (FCz) about 50 ms prior to target presentation and reached maximal amplitudes around target presentation. Maximal amplitudes, measured at FCz differed significantly depending on the task ($F=9.1$, $p=0.0057$). However, post-hoc comparison of maximal amplitudes recorded in the gap task and the warning task did not reach significance ($t=0.9$, $p=0.4346$). In the overlap task, the negative potential was absent.

4. DISCUSSION

Our data confirm earlier studies, which have shown that different foveal warning signals can reduce SRTs. ERPs recorded in the gap task and the warning task showed a negative potential over frontal and central cortical areas. This result indicates that the negative potential in the gap task was in fact evoked by the warning signal carried by the advanced offset of the FP. However, our findings of significantly shorter SRTs and a higher proportion of express saccades in the gap task, despite the same negative ERP as in the warning task, suggest that the advanced offset of the FP has an additional effect, which may depend on processes in subcortical structures, probably the superior colliculus (Dorris et al. 1997).

ACKNOWLEDGMENTS

This work was supported by the Deutsche Forschungsgemeinschaft, SFB 517, and EV 32/1-1.

REFERENCES

Csibra G, Johnson MH, Tucker LA (1997) Attention and oculomotor control: a high density ERP study of the gap effect. Neuropsychologia 35: 855–865

Dorris MC, Pare M, Munoz DP (1997) Neuronal activity in monkey superior colliculus related to the initiation of saccadic eye movements. J Neurosci 17: 8566–8579

Everling S, Krappmann P, Spantekow A, Flohr H (1996) Cortical potentials during the gap prior to express saccades and fast regular saccades. Exp Brain Res 111: 139–143

Gomez C, Atienza M, Gomez GJ, Vazquez M (1996) Response latencies and event-related potentials during the gap paradigm using saccadic responses in human subjects. Int J Psychophysiol 23: 91–99

Klein RM, Kingstone A (1993) Why do visual offsets reduce saccadic latencies? Behav Brain Sci 16: 583–584

Krappmann P, Everling S, Spannhuth C, Spantekow A, Flohr H (1997) Electrophysiologic correlates of the gap effect in human subjects: event-related potentials in an oculomotor gap and anti-gap paradigm. Soc Neurosci Abstr 23: 743

12

ADAPTATION TO VISUAL FIELD DEFECTS WITH VIRTUAL REALITY SCOTOMA IN HEALTHY SUBJECTS

W. H. Zangemeister and U. Oechsner

Neurological University Clinic Hamburg, Germany

1. ABSTRACT

Normal Subjects (Ss) show a stairstep/overshoot saccadic strategy similar to hemianopic patients either when confronted with a virtual reality model of an artificial hemianopia using eye position feedback (H3 - VRM), or when achieving eccentric fixation using secondary visual feedback (2ndVFB). Here gaze position is displayed simultaneously with the target and the subject learns either to superpose target and eye position feedback, or to position the gaze feedback target up to 9 deg off the target (eccentric fixation), which helps to keep the "blind side" in sight. Using this technique normal Ss confronted with H3 - VRM as well as hemianopic patients minimize their deficit very fast and efficiently, much faster than without 2ndVFB training.

2. INTRODUCTION

As a new visual technical method secondary visual feedback (2ndVFB) was introduced by Zeevi and Stark in 1979. In 1985 Zangemeister et al. showed that this technique could be used in the treatment of reading disorders, visual discomfort and associated perceptual distortions of patients with hemianopia (Zangemeister et al. 1982). This method permits to instruct and train patients with hemianopia to apply parafoveal, eccentric vision while searching and scanning through pictures, their environment and while reading. Experimentally, normal subjects show a similar behaviour as hemianopics when they learn how to achieve eccentric eye fixation using secondary visual feedback. Here, gaze position is displayed simultaneously with the target and the subject learns to either superpose target and the gaze-feedback target (centric fixation) or to position the gaze-feedback target off the visual stimulus (eccentric fixation, ranging between 1 and 9 deg visual angle). When Ss at first try to achieve eccentric 2ndVFB they apply a stairstep

Current Oculomotor Research, edited by Becker *et al.*
Plenum Press, New York, 1999.

saccadic strategy and/or macrosaccadic square wave oscillations comparable to the hemianopic patients. After some training they adapt and now use slow and fast eye drifts to achieve eccentric fixation and a nystagmic pattern to maintain it. - In the present study a simulation of virtual hemifield blindness in normal human subjects was produced by linking a high accuracy eye position sensor with a computer visual display. This eye controlled system may be classified as a form of virtual reality for safely exploring the effects of visual defects, diseases, and adaptability under experimental control (Bertera 1988).

3. METHOD

A homonymous hemianopic simulated scotoma (VirtH3) was stabilized on the fovea of 10 normal observers while they attempted to maintain a moving target in clear view, or to perform a search and scanning task of 10 sec viewing Five of the subjects were naive and were free to view the target (alternating step or pursuit stimulus, pictures, 10sec viewing, 2min. one set of 9 trials, 15 sets in 40 min.) in any way they chose. Five other subjects had undergone one experimental session a week before, where they had to practice 2ndVFB for 30 Minutes. For the quantification of the term "similarity of eye movements" Markov matrices (Stark and Ellis 1981) and string editing (Stark and Choi 1995; Zangemeister et al. 1995) have been used. Both methods are applied to preprocessed eye movement data. Shortly after the run of the last group of pictures in our simulated "patients" and normal subjects an additional run was appended where our patients had to view the empty VDT and imagine the pictures they just saw for 10 sec in the same sequence and within the same time, each picture 5, 30 and 60 sec after the real picture had appeared on the VDT. This provided us with data on imagined scanpaths in virtual hemianopic "patients" and normal subjects, and thus information as to how at this level of deficiency i.e. visual hemifield defect leads to a distorted visual imagery that otherwise could not be detected.

4. RESULTS AND DISCUSSION

Similarly as in normal 2ndVFB, eccentric eye positioning developed within two minutes of viewing time in all VirtH3-subjects, with a range of eccentricity between 1 and 9 deg off the virtual scotoma location. The durations of correctly positioned fixations became longer during eccentric viewing practice indicating rapid improvements in fixation stability, while fixation durations of incorrect fixation positions became shorter, demonstrating high level adaptation to the virtual scotoma defect.

The types of eye movements that were used by the subjects resembled very closely eye movements used by hemianopic patients to overcome their deficit, and also by normal subjects adapting to 2ndVFB: i.e. the transition from stairstep saccades to overshooting saccades with drifts and glissades for more accurate "fixation". Those normal subjects that had a half hour training session a week before exposure to H3-VRM demonstrated a significantly faster increase of eccentric total viewing time, ecc.fixations and ecc.fixation durations in their "seeing hemifield" (Tab.1). Virtual hemianopics get the pursuit stimulus, about 1 to 2 cycles later than normal subjects.- Using string edit analyses, Brandt and Stark (1997), Zangemeister et al. (1995) and Gbadamosi et al. (1997) were able to demonstrate firm evidence for scanpath sequences of their subjects' eye movements in performing real viewing and visual imagery. As in "real" hemianopic patients our results

Table 1. Eccentric viewing time (VT) in % of
total viewing time; % of eccentric Fixations
(EF), mean duration of single eccentric Fixations
in sec (DSEF) of 10 healthy virtual hemianopic subjects

	No 2nd VFB (n=5)			With 2nd VFB (n=5)		
	VT	EF	DSEF	VT	EF	DSEF
First trial (#1)	5	11	0.280	12	25	0.355
Last trial (#15)	45	52	0.450	73	86	0.525

demonstrate a "convergence of visual imagery": The three sequential visual imageries show a significantly lower similarity to the viewing of the real image than with each other in both groups, virtual hemianopic subjects and normal subjects. The visual imageries of normal subjects as well as of hemianopic patients are quite different from the primary viewing of the real image, and they converge to each other with repetition. The results suggest a "convergence of visualization" in all normal, hemianopic, and virtual hemianopic subjects: eye movement sequences were significantly less similar for viewing and re-visualization (but still significantly above the measure of similarity calculated for random sequences) than those for the imageries among each other. Similarities between consecutive eye movement sequences showed a major difference between real viewing and the first imagery, whereas between the first and the last two imageries there was only a comparatively slight increase in similarity. The matching results for all three goups suggest a strong top-down component in viewing an image: a mental model of the thing viewed is constructed early on, which takes an essential part in controlling eye movements during viewing.

The eccentric fixation stairstep-overshoot optimizing strategy is a general approach that is always applied in coping with random or pseudorandom situations by healthy subjects as well as patients when they face the same problem, i.e. a hemifield scotoma. Therefore it is most likely a "medium level" strategy, that is more subconsciously developed and that can be helped by the above techniques.

Table 2. Comparison of visual imageries (5, 30, 60)
later than real presentation (0) calculated from
median region string similarity indices
(Zangemeister et al. 1995) of 10 normal VirtH3 Ss,
10 real hemianopic patients (from Gbadamisi et al. 1997,
and 10 normal Ss in response to 6 visual stimuli

Similarity index	VirtH3-sS	Real H3 pat.	Nor. Ss
Random	0.20	0.25	0.26
Real image (0) and			
5 sec later (0-1)	0.42	0.45	0.43
30 sec later (0-2)	0.40	0.38	0.42
60 sec later (0-3)	0.41	0.40	0.40
(1 - 2)	0.54	0.52	0.46
(1 - 3)	0.49	0.48	0.47
(2 - 3)	0.51	0.50	0.47

REFERENCES

Bertera JH (1988) Visual search with simulated skotomas in normal subjects. Invest.Ophthalmol. Vis Sci 29: 470 - 478

Brandt S, Stark L (1997) Sponteneous eye movements during visual imagery reflect the content of the visual scene. J Cogn Neurosci 9: 27-38

Gbadamosi J, Oechsner U, ZangemeisterWH (1997) Quantitative analysis of gaze movements during Visual Imagery in hemianopic patients and control subjects. J Neurol Rehabil 3: 165-172

Stark L, Ellis S (1981) Scanpaths revisited: Cognitive   models in active looking. In: Eye Movements, Cognition and Visual Perception, ed.by B. Fisher, C. Monty and M. Sanders, Erlbaum Press, New Jersey, pp193 - 226

Stark L,Choi YS (1996) Experimental metaphysics: the scanpath as an epistemological mechanism. In: Visual attention and aognition, ed. by WH Zangemeister, S Stiehl, C Freksa. Adv Psychol 116: 3-73

Zangemeister WH, Meienberg O, Stark L, Hoyt WF (1982) Eye-head coordination in homonymous hemianopia. J Neurol 225: 243-54 .

Zangemeister WH, Dannheim F, Kunze K (1986) Adaptation of gaze to eccentric fixation in homonymous hemianopia. In: Adaptive processes in visual and oculomotor aystems, ed. by EL Keller, D Zee. Adv in Bio Sci 57: 247-252

Zangemeister WH, Oechsner U, Freksa C (1995) Short-term adaptation of eye movements in patients with visual hemifield defects indicates high level control of human scan path. Optom Vision Science 72: 467-478

Zeevi YY, Peli E, Stark (1979) Study of eccentric fixation with secondary visual feedback. J Opt Soc Am 69: 669-675

SACCADIC SUPPRESSION AND ADAPTATION

Revisiting the Methodology

M. R. MacAskill,[1] S. R. Muir,[2] and T. J. Anderson[1]

[1]Department of Medicine
Christchurch School of Medicine
[2]Department of Medical Physics and Bioengineering
Christchurch Hospital
Christchurch, New Zealand

1. INTRODUCTION

The likelihood of perceiving the displacement of an object which occurs during a saccade is much lower than the likelihood of detecting such a movement during fixation ("saccadic suppression of image displacement", or SSD). The methodology of inducing such unseen intrasaccadic target movements has been used to study adaptive changes in saccadic amplitude (first by McLaughlin (1967), and subsequently by many others including Mack, Fendrich, and Pleune (1978), Erkelens and Hulleman (1993), and Deubel (1995)). SSD was first quantitatively described in an experiment where the entire visual field was displaced (Bridgeman, Hendry, and Stark, 1975). Later studies have often used the displacement of small targets. We suggest that the induction of saccadic suppression with small targets requires more stringent conditions than those established by Bridgeman et al. for movement of the entire visual field.

2. METHOD

In a signal detection study, eye movements of 21 normal subjects (including 3 non-naive (the authors); mean age 24 years; 13 male) were recorded using a Skalar IRIS infra-red limbus tracker. A computer-generated stimulus (a red square target subtending 0.75° on a homogeneous background) was video front-projected on to a large screen. Subjects were instructed to follow the target as it jumped horizontally by 8, 12, 16, 20 or 24°.

During the saccade toward the new target position, the target was displaced centripetally by 1, 2, 3 or 4° in 120 trials (thus displacement ratios ranged from 0.04 to 0.50).

Current Oculomotor Research, edited by Becker *et al.*
Plenum Press, New York, 1999.

An average of 27 ms was required from saccade initiation until the target could be displaced. (This comprised a mean 15 ms to reach and detect the $30°s^{-1}$ velocity threshold indicating saccade initiation, a further 5 ms to move the target, and a mean delay of 7 ms due to screen refresh rates.) As the average saccade duration was 68 ms, this was well within the SSD "critical period". Added to this were set delays of 0, 10, 20, 35, 50, or 65 ms to assess differences in detection between targets displaced intrasaccadically and those displaced after the eyes had come to rest.

On 60 "catch" trials, the target was not displaced during the saccade. Subjects reported awareness of intrasaccadic target displacements by pressing a key.

3. RESULTS AND DISCUSSION

We found that the SSD effect required larger saccade sizes, and smaller intrasaccadic displacements, than is commonly accepted. The conventional rule-of-thumb is that the displacement ratio (the ratio of the intrasaccadic shift to the saccade size) should be no more than one third (Bridgeman et al., 1975). Our results show that for displacements of a small target, a displacement ratio of 0.3 produces minimal suppression (see Figure 1), and we suggest that the ratio used be a value closer to 0.1, in order to ensure that subjects are not consciously aware of the majority of target displacements. Other researchers (e.g. Li and Matin, 1997; McConkie and Currie, 1996; Mack, 1970) have also advocated the use of a displacement ratio of 0.1 when employing such stimuli. Part of the difficulty in agreeing on consistent stimulus parameters is the lack of a definition of what would constitute an appropriate threshold level. The standard psychophysical threshold is arbitrarily set at the 50% detection rate. However, this level is too high for the purposes of studying adaptation to a target manipulation which one wishes the subject to be unaware of (particularly as the false alarm rate in SSD experiments is typically very low). Thus, researchers displacing small targets (with a displacement ratio of $\cong 0.3$) in order to produce adaptation of saccades should be wary. They are possibly examining a conscious strategy rather than an unconscious perceptual learning process. (See Deubel's (1995) comments on Erkelens and Hulleman, 1993.)

Studies of saccadic parametric adaptation should include a signal detection pilot study in order to assess the effectiveness of their intrasaccadic displacement procedures. But even those studies concerned with signal detection *per se* have tended to use a small number of (often non-naive) subjects. In any signal detection task, there exist wide individual differences, perhaps reflecting different response criteria rather than underlying dif-

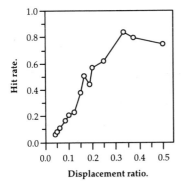

Figure 1. Probability of detecting an intra-saccadic target shift as a function of the ratio of the size of that shift to the size of the saccade made to the target (the "displacement ratio").

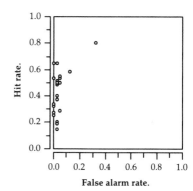

Figure 2. Hit rate vs False alarm rate for detecting intrasaccadic displacements. Each point represents one of 21 subjects, and scores are collapsed across all displacement ratios.

ferences in sensitivity to the stimulus. (That is, some subjects are more liberal or conservative responders than are others.) A lack of knowledge of individual differences in sensitivity and response bias must affect the conclusions one can draw from subjects' reports. This is especially so when only a small number of subjects are employed.

A comparatively large (n=21) number of subjects allowed us to gain an appreciation of individual differences. A subject who is a very liberal responder will have an inflated Hit rate (an indicator of sensitivity), but will consequently also have a higher False Alarm rate (an indicator of response bias). The scattergram (Figure 2) shows that subjects differed primarily in sensitivity rather than in response bias: only two of the 21 subjects had high false alarm rates. Thus it is encouraging that subjects appear to apply much the same response criterion when reporting awareness of intrasaccadic displacements; however there *are* marked individual differences in the sensitivity to those displacements (see also Wallach and Lewis, 1965).

The simultaneous collection of subjective event reports (i.e. keypresses indicating awareness of target displacement) and objective measures (i.e. eye movement recordings) provides a unique opportunity to validate the signal detection methodology (for example, the saccadic system may produce corrective eye movements in response to a target displacement which the subject may or may not be consciously aware of). Subjective reports and manual pointing have already been used to show that different information is available to the motor system and to the conscious level of the perceptual system (Bridgeman et al., 1979). Eye movements are a more direct and precise motor measure than manual pointing, and analysis of data from this perspective continues.

REFERENCES

Bridgeman B, Hendry D, and Stark L (1975) Failure to detect displacement of the visual world during saccadic eye movements. Vision Res 15: 719–722

Bridgeman B, Lewis S, Heit G, and Nagle M (1979) Relation between cognitive and motor-oriented systems of visual position perception. J Exp Psychol Hum Percept Perform 5: 692–700

Deubel H (1995) Separate adaptive mechanisms for the control of reactive and volitional saccadic eye movements. Vision Res 35: 3529–3540

Erkelens CJ and Hulleman J (1993) Selective adaptation of internally triggered saccades made to visual targets. Exp Brain Res 93: 157–164

Li WX and Matin L (1997) Saccadic suppression of displacement - separate influences of saccade size and of target retinal eccentricity. Vision Res 37: 1779–1797

Mack A (1970) An investigation of the relationship between eye and retinal image movement in the perception of movement. Percept Psychophys 8: 291–298

Mack A, Fendrich R, and Pleune J (1978) Adaptation to an altered relation between retinal image displacements and saccadic eye movements. Vision Res 18: 1321–1327

McConkie GW and Currie CB (1996) Visual stability across saccades while viewing complex pictures. J Exp Psychol Hum Percept Perform 22: 563–581

McLaughlin SC (1967) Parametric adjustment in saccadic eye movements. Percept Psychophys 2: 359–362

Wallach H and Lewis C (1965) The effect of abnormal displacement of the retinal image during eye movements. Percept Psychophys 1: 25–29

14

MODELLING PREDICTION IN OCULAR PURSUIT

The Importance of Short-Term Storage

G. R. Barnes and S. G. Wells

MRC Human Movement and Balance Unit
Institute of Neurology
23 Queen Sq., London WC1N 3BG

1. INTRODUCTION

It has been realised since the early work of Dallos and Jones (1963) that predictive behaviour must be present in human ocular pursuit for three main reasons: (1) performance is better in response to predictable periodic target motion than it is to more random stimuli; (2) when pursuing sinusoids, phase errors at frequencies above 0.5Hz are much less than would be expected from the time delay (100ms) in visual feedback (Carl and Gellman 1987); (3) in a linear velocity error feedback system a combination of high gain and a large time delay would lead to an unstable system. But evidence of predictive behaviour is not readily apparent because anticipatory smooth movements cannot normally be generated at will. Over recent years we have carried out experiments designed to facilitate the generation of anticipatory movements and investigate their role in predictive pursuit (Barnes et al. 1987; Barnes and Asselman 1991; Wells and Barnes 1998). The model presented here was developed on the basis of the results from these experiments and attempts to demonstrate how predictive processes reduce phase errors during periodic tracking through the short-term storage of pre-motor drive information and its subsequent release to form anticipatory smooth movements.

2. EXPERIMENTAL EVIDENCE FOR PREDICTION IN OCULAR PURSUIT

2.1. Anticipatory Smooth Eye Movements

Although the presence of predictive mechanisms can be inferred from sinusoidal responses, it is difficult to demonstrate overt predictive behaviour in the control of smooth

Current Oculomotor Research, edited by Becker *et al.*
Plenum Press, New York, 1999.

97

eye movements. Most individuals find it impossible to generate anticipatory smooth movements with a peak velocity of more than about 5°/s in the absence of a moving visual target even if they are aware of the velocity and direction of the movement (Barnes et al. 1987). It is therefore difficult to understand how subjects can initiate a response that would precede the visually driven response and thus overcome the delay in visuomotor processing. However, in recent years we have devised a technique that does allow this predictive behaviour to be reliably observed, even in the absence of a visual target, through the presentation of regularly repeated intermittent motion stimuli of the type illustrated in Fig.1 (Barnes and Asselman 1991; Ohashi and Barnes 1996; Barnes et al. 1997). In this example, the underlying target motion was a triangular wave with a ramp velocity of +/- 36°/s and a frequency of 0.39Hz, but the target was exposed for only 120ms as it passed through the mid-point. Subjects were instructed to pursue the target during this brief exposure period, a task that became progressively easier with repeated presentation. During the first presentation of the target there was a delay (approx. 100ms) before the onset of smooth eye movement. However, after a few presentations, the smooth eye movement was initiated well before (450ms on average) the target came on, at a time when the subject was still in darkness. The timing of peak eye velocity was also brought forward by approximately 50–100ms, just sufficient to overcome most of the time delay in the visual feedback (Ohashi and Barnes 1996). Simultaneously, peak eye velocity increased by a factor of 1.5–2, depending on target velocity and exposure duration. Both the timing and magnitude of eye velocity were found to be dependent on the preceding part of the stimulus (Barnes and Asselman 1991). Consequently, if the target unexpectedly failed to appear, an inappropriate predictive smooth eye velocity trajectory was initiated (PVE, Fig. 1) with a magnitude and timing that were correlated with the response prior to target disappearance. Attempts to generate further PVE's in darkness were ineffective, except when there was a high expectancy of target reappearance, whereupon the anticipatory response could be revived before target onset (Barnes et al. 1997).

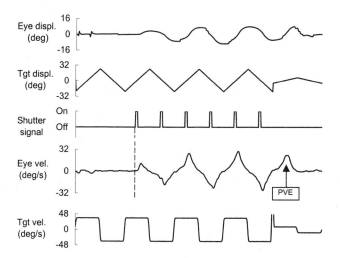

Figure 1. Eye movements evoked by intermittent presentation of a target moving with a triangular waveform (velocity +/-36°/s; frequency 0.39Hz). Target was exposed for 120ms every half-cycle (indicated by shutter signal) as it passed through centre. Eye velocity was obtained after saccade removal. PVE predictive velocity estimate occurring in darkness.

The magnitude of the anticipatory response can be characterised by eye velocity (V100) measured 100ms after target onset (i.e. just before any effect of visual feedback). It has been shown consistently that V100 increases with target velocity; thus, it is not only anticipatory, but also truly predictive in the sense that it is appropriately scaled for expected target velocity. The importance of anticipatory movements in predictive pursuit has frequently been called into question because early studies (Kowler and Steinman 1979; Becker and Fuchs 1985; Boman and Hotson 1988) evoked anticipatory velocities that were only very low (1–2°/s) compared with normal pursuit. But more recent studies have revealed much higher anticipatory velocities (Barnes and Asselman 1991; Kao and Morrow 1994). This modelling study will show that a single mechanism can account for both periodic pursuit and anticipatory movements.

Three particular features of the response have led to the conclusion that the mechanism of prediction involves the temporary storage of pre-motor drive information and its subsequent release under the control of a periodicity estimator so as to act as a predictive estimate of ensuing target velocity. First, build-up of velocity with repetition implies the charging of an internal store. It cannot arise from direct summation, since each individual transient response may decay between presentations and change direction. Secondly, release of this internally stored information would account for the ability to generate anticipatory responses, which normally cannot be produced in darkness. We have recently shown that anticipatory movements even occur in the presence of a structured background (Barnes et al. 1997), which would be totally impossible without prior stimulation. Thirdly, the occurrence of the PVE (Fig. 1) when the stimulus unexpectedly fails to appear can be explained as output from the internal store, the timing of which is determined by the periodicity estimator.

2.2. The Longevity and Independence of the Store

We now have evidence that this store may have a limited life span, its contents decaying exponentially over a period of 5–10s (Wells and Barnes 1998). Results in Figure 2

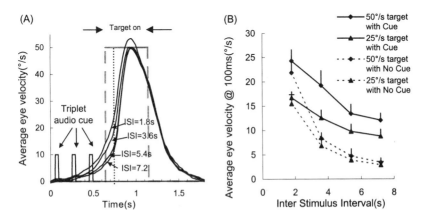

Figure 2. (A). Mean smooth eye velocity trajectories of 8 subjects to repeated presentation of target (velocity 50°/s) for 500ms, preceded by triplet audio timing cue. Inter-stimulus interval (ISI) ranged from 1.8–7.2s. Dotted line - 100ms marker. (B). Eye velocity 100ms after target onset versus ISI for target velocities of 25 and 50 deg/s with or without audio cues.

are from an experiment in which varying lengths of time from 1.8–7.2s were left between target presentations. For the longest inter-stimulus intervals time estimation is known to deteriorate and it was thus not unexpected that the anticipatory eye velocity might also decline. However, V100 still declined, though less markedly, even when a triplet audio cue gave accurate timing information prior to target onset (Fig.2). Moreover, the effect occurred for both unidirectional and bi-directional stimuli so, from this and other evidence (Kowler 1989), it seems probable that the store is not specific to a particular direction, but may be directed under voluntary control. We also have strong evidence that cues for timing the release of the store do not have to be associated with the periodicity of the visual motion stimulus. If the time between motion stimuli is randomised, but time-to-onset cues are provided by an independent audio source, subjects are still able to generate high velocity anticipatory smooth movements (Barnes and Donelan 1997) time-locked to the audio cues.

2.3. Volitional versus Reflex Behaviour and the Role of Positional Feedback

Anticipatory eye movements can also be observed during passive stimulation of the oculomotor system, that is, when the subject simply stares at the moving display (Barnes and Asselman 1991; Ohashi and Barnes 1996). In fact, experiments have shown that most of the non-linear features of active pursuit can also be observed during passive stimulation, but the gain of such responses is always less than for active pursuit (Barnes and Hill 1984; Pola and Wyatt 1985). So, it appears that active pursuit largely involves augmentation of the basic reflex gain associated with passive stimulation, a feature that is probably necessary when pursuing a selected target against a structured background (Worfolk and Barnes 1992).

In recent experiments (Barnes et al. 1995) we have investigated the role of these volitional mechanisms and their use of stored information, by examining the ability of subjects to produce smooth eye movements with a stabilised image. Using the intermittent presentation paradigm, subjects initially pursued the target during the exposure period in the normal closed-loop mode. Then, during a dark period between presentations, the target image was stabilised on the fovea using the calibrated eye movement signal to drive the target directly so that any subsequent target movement was driven by the eye alone. Subjects continued to make smooth eye movements alternately to left and right, with a velocity proportional to that in the preceding closed-loop phase. These results demonstrate that subjects can volitionally generate repeated predictive smooth movements, based on stored information. Our hypothesis is that this is only possible in the stabilised mode because there is no conflict between the predictive estimate and the visual feedback, since retinal error remains at zero.

Other experiments with stabilised images have shown that although stored information can be used, it is not always necessary to control the velocity of the smooth eye movement (Kommerell and Taümer 1972). If the stabilised image contains a number of targets at different eccentricities smooth movements can be generated in alternate directions by directing attention to targets on either side of the foveal target in time with an audio cue (Barnes et al. 1995). At frequencies above 0.4Hz this induces a pseudo-sinusoidal smooth eye movement that is remarkably like normal smooth pursuit, even though no external target drive is present. Peak velocity tends to increase with eccentricity of the centre of attention so that this appears to represent a form of positional feedback dependent on the locus of attention.

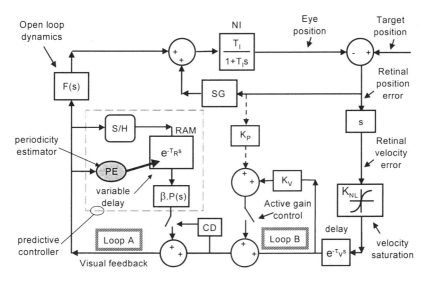

Figure 3. Ocular pursuit model. S/H - sample/hold module -sampling interval=0.16s; RAM - re-afferent memory simulated by variable delay network (T_R=0; β=0.95 for initial transient - t<T/2; T_R=T/2-$τ_v$; β= -0.95 for steady-state periodic - t>T/2, where t = time; T = stimulus period; $τ_v$ = visual feedback delay = 0.1s); CD-conflict detector; PE-periodicity estimator. SG-Saccade generator. Non-linear feedback gain - K_{NL}= $(1+ε/2)^{-0.5}$, ε = retinal velocity error. F(s) = 0.5/(1+0.15s). P(s) = 1/(1+0.15s). NI - neural integrator - T_I = 20s. K_V=4. K_P= 1.

3. DEVELOPMENT AND MODE OF OPERATION OF THE MATHEMATICAL MODEL

3.1. Raising the Gain for Active Pursuit while Maintaining Stability

A model (Fig. 3) has been developed on the basis of the information described above; it is slightly modified from a previous version (Barnes 1994). Its operation will now be described.

If the subject views a target that is initially stationary but then moves unexpectedly, the retinal velocity error feedback system will generate an eye movement that follows the target motion, thereby reducing retinal velocity error. But during passive stimulation this direct pathway has a low feedback gain, particularly for a small stimulus and results in a low-gain (0.6–0.7) closed-loop response. If the subject decides actively to pursue the moving target, closed-loop gain for the smooth component increases to 0.9–1, implying an effective increase in the feedback gain. This function is accomplished in the model by the feedforward loop B, activation of which raises velocity feedback and possibly also introduces positional error feedback. However, it has long been realised that increasing feedback gain to a level of 10–20 that would be required to achieve this closed-loop gain would result in instability (Dallos and Jones 1963). A simple way to raise the gain and maintain stability is to introduce a low-pass filter into the feedback pathway that effectively attenuates the high frequency (>0.4Hz) components of the stimulus waveform. There are a number of ways of achieving this effect. One that has gained increasing popularity is the internal positive feedback system first proposed by Yasui and Young (1975) and subsequently elaborated by others (Lisberger and Fuchs 1978; Robinson et al. 1986).).

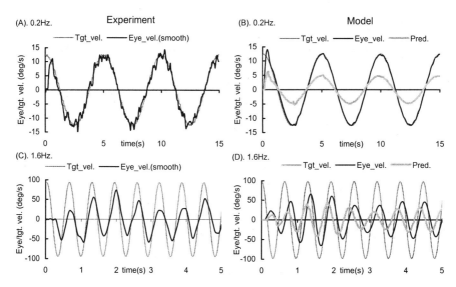

Figure 4. Experimental and simulated smooth pursuit velocity responses to sinusoidal target motion at frequencies of 0.2Hz and 1.6Hz. Peak target displacement +/-10°. Pred.=output of internal reafferent feedback (Loop A).

Although this has been conceptualised as an internal representation of target velocity, which feeds back an efference copy of eye velocity, its essential action is that of a low-pass filter. If the positive feedback loop contains a finite time delay (or a filter P(s) as in the model of Fig. 3) and a gain element that is less than unity it provides the features of a rather special low-pass filter for which the time constant increases as the gain of the internal loop more closely approaches unity. In the proposed model this is one of the functions carried out by Loop A. We have referred to this as 'reafference feedback' since it is evident from recent experiments (Barnes et al. 1997) that it is feedback of a post-sensory but pre-motor drive signal, not feedback of a copy of the eye movement itself.

Another way in which gain can be raised whilst maintaining stability is to introduce positional error feedback and, as indicated earlier, there is some evidence for this. If present, it offers the advantage of allowing zero velocity error to be achieved (i.e. unity velocity gain), although only at low frequencies. The relative merits of position feedback will be discussed later. Unfortunately, the penalty of introducing stability by either of the means described is that they create large phase errors in the closed-loop response at frequencies above 0.4Hz as we shall see later (Figure 5).

3.2. The Steady-State Predictive Response

So how can phase errors be reduced whilst maintaining stability? On the basis of the experimental evidence presented it is suggested that the internal reafference feedback pathway (Loop A) effectively operates in two ways. Initially, during either active or passive stimulation, the velocity estimate is sampled and stored in RAM, but is played out directly, with negligible delay. This provides a direct increase to the gain of the feedback, but has the stabilising effect discussed above. However, when there is a regular periodicity

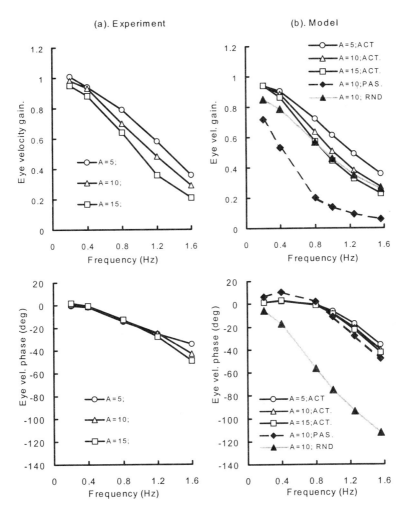

Figure 5. (a). Mean gain and phase of smooth eye velocity from 20 normal humans during active pursuit of sinusoid with peak displacement (A) of +/-5,10 or 15deg. (b). Model simulations. ACT:-gain and phase of active pursuit: A=+/-5,10 or 15deg; RND:-gain and phase evoked by direct reafferent feedback alone ($T_R=0$). PAS:- passive stimulation ($K_V=0$).

to the stimulus, this velocity information can be stored for a longer period and subsequently released as a predictive velocity estimate. It is envisaged that sampled velocity estimates for each half-cycle of the drive to the oculomotor system are stored in the short-term memory (RAM) and released from the store in the next half-cycle under the control of the periodicity estimator (PE), as suggested by the experimental findings outlined above. The specific manner in which this store (RAM) operates is not known at present. A simple way to simulate it is as a variable delay element, with a delay equivalent to one half-cycle of the stimulus and a gain that remains close to unity but changes polarity depending on the expected direction of target motion. So, once stimulus periodicity is reliably established, the delay (T_R) changes from zero for a non-periodic stimulus to a finite value for periodic stimuli. It is possible to show that the system response will remain stable unless the timing estimate is grossly in error and that it effectively operates as a band-pass filter tuned to the frequency of the periodic stimulus.

There is strong supportive evidence for this type of switching behaviour from the response of the saccadic system. When following a regular square wave target displacement at frequencies around 0.5Hz, subjects initially respond with a latency of some 250ms, but after a few cycles start to make predictive saccades based not on current visual feedback, but on information previously stored and released under the control of a periodicity estimator.

4. MODEL SIMULATIONS

4.1. Responses to Sinusoidal Target Motion Stimuli

4.1.1. Waveform Simulation. Typical smooth eye velocity responses to sinusoidal stimuli at two frequencies are shown in Fig. 4 after removal of saccadic components. At the lower frequency (0.2Hz) eye velocity begins to match target velocity within the first quarter cycle with little phase error thereafter. In this subject's response there is a considerable oscillation of eye velocity at a frequency of approximately 2–3Hz, as noted previously (Robinson et al. 1986). For a 1.6Hz stimulus there is a considerable delay (nearly one half-cycle) before any response is made and initially there is a large phase lag, which is evident from the difference in time between the first trough of the response and the corresponding trough of the stimulus. However, after two cycles of stimulation phase lag has significantly decreased, a feature that could not be explained by a linear feedback system and must result from prediction.

In the model simulations, responses were obtained by closing the switch for active gain control (i.e. K_v=4), but without invoking positional feedback (i.e. K_p=0). This effectively raises open-loop gain to 2.5. In the initial part of each response (1/2 cycle), before PE has had time to assess the periodicity of the stimulus, the predictive controller enhances the velocity drive with direct positive feedback (i.e. ß= 0.95). Beyond this time, PE estimates the duration of one half period of the stimulus, which is then used to set the value of T_R. The direction of the internal drive provided by the predictive controller is reversed by setting ß= -0.95. So, after the first half-cycle, the drive is provided by playing back the drive for the previous half cycle, but with reversed polarity. In these examples the sampling interval was set at 160ms throughout the frequency range, but an almost identical response can be obtained if a much coarser sampling is carried out at lower frequencies. At frequencies above 0.8Hz a realistic simulation can be achieved with only one sample per half-cycle (see Fig.6). The most important feature of the simulations is that they indicate how the model is able to overcome the time delays in the visual feedback. Because the release of the internal predictive drive is timed to occur just before the expected arrival of visual feedback, phase error of eye velocity is rapidly reduced after the PE obtains its first estimate of periodicity. This is achieved within the first cycle at 0.2Hz, but may take 2–3 cycles at higher frequencies. In the steady-state, the internal drive effectively takes over the major part of the control and only uses visual feedback to check that it is correct or to make small adjustments to the current drive and thereby update the internal estimate.

4.1.2. Frequency Characteristics of the Model. Gain and phase characteristics for model and experimental responses are compared in Fig. 5 for sinusoidal stimuli with a peak displacement (A) of +/-5,10 or 15 degrees. Peak velocity thus increased with fre-

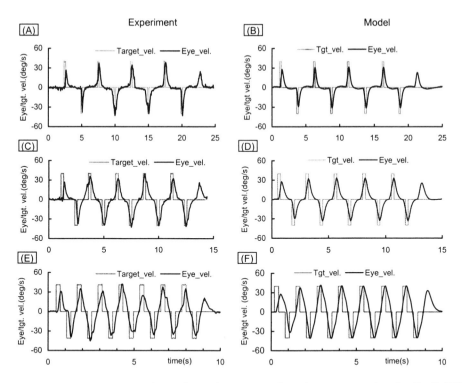

Figure 6. Experimental and simulated smooth pursuit responses to intermittent target motion stimuli with ISI's of 2.5s (A,B), 1.25s (C,D) & 0.625s (E,F). Target velocity=40°/s.

quency and at higher frequencies was well into the range at which saturation effects in the visual feedback (represented by K_{NL}) became effective. As a result, smooth eye velocity gain exhibited a decrease with increasing displacement at the higher stimulus frequencies, in accord with the experimental results. The gain and phase generated by the model at different frequencies are of the same order as those found experimentally, although the model produced slightly less phase error around 1Hz.

The effect that the predictive mechanism has on the phase error at higher frequencies can be demonstrated by comparing the results obtained when the predictive response is controlled by the periodicity estimator (ACT, Figure 5) with those obtained through the activity of the direct positive reafferent feedback (i.e. $T_R=0$: RND, Figure 5). It is evident that adding prediction has little effect on the gain of the response, but a dramatic effect on phase. Without prediction, the phase lag would have been approximately 115° for a 1.6Hz stimulus, whereas prediction reduced this to 45°. Implementation of the model of Robinson et al. (1986) results in phase errors similar to those for the non-predictive system, because this model makes no attempt to simulate predictive control.

The most important objective of the predictive system thus appears to be to reduce phase errors at high frequency. Because the gain of the reafferent memory pathway remains high, this phase minimisation can be achieved even when open-loop gain is reduced, whereas in a linear system phase error would increase with decreasing gain. The model simulates this effectively; when K_V is zero, closed-loop gain decreases at all frequencies (Figure 5), but the phase error remains similar to that when K_V is at its normal value. This represents the response obtainable during passive stimulation and gain and phase values are comparable with those obtained experimentally (Barnes and Hill 1984; Pola and Wyatt 1985). Dissociation between gain and phase has been observed in some patients with cerebral lesions (Lekwuwa and Barnes 1996) who have low gain without increased phase error. The part played by positional feedback in pursuit has not been illustrated but would not appear to be significant. Although it raises gain slightly at low frequency, phase error increases unrealistically at 1.6Hz, even for small values of positional gain (e.g. K_p=1). Moreover, unless the positional threshold for saccade initiation is elevated during pursuit, the saccadic system dominates positional error correction, thus almost nullifying the effect of positional feedback.

4.2. Responses to Intermittent Target Presentation

The response of the model to intermittent presentation of a target moving at constant velocity in each direction is compared with experimental responses in Fig.6 for an exposure duration of 240ms at three pulse intervals (2.5,1.25 and 0.625s). This shows the manner in which the anticipatory eye velocity builds up with repetition in a similar way to the experimental response. The initial response is delayed by 100ms, but in the steady-state, eye velocity begins well before target onset. Between presentations, absence of visual feedback opens the feedback loop so that eye velocity is determined by the open-loop dynamic characteristics F(s) and thus decays with a time constant of 0.15s. The examples in Fig. 6 show the important effect of changing the duration between presentations. At intervals of 2.5s the anticipatory velocity and the transient decay of the response are quite separate for each presentation, although, at present, there is no provision to simulate the decay with long intervals noted earlier (see Fig.2). But, as frequency increases, each response merges with the next, so that at 0.8Hz, the response appears as a continuous pseudo-sinusoidal waveform. Note that the model also correctly simulates the appropriately-timed appearance of the predictive velocity estimate when the target disappears. Other effects, such as changes in peak eye velocity with target velocity and pulse duration are also effectively simulated by the model.

5. DISCUSSION

What has been described is a simplified representation of the mechanism for controlling predictive behaviour in pursuit. It is based on the hypothesis that prediction is achieved by storing a copy of the pre-motor drive, derived from prior stimulation, and replaying it through an internal reafferent feedback system to boost the basic visual feedback under the control of a separate timing device. This arrangement allows high gain to be achieved rapidly with stability and minimal phase error. Positional feedback may play a small part in raising gain at low frequencies. Despite its simplicity, the model can effectively simulate a wide variety of transient and steady-state response characteristics, including some not shown here. It would probably be more realistic to represent RAM as a discrete short-term storage element that holds the stored information until it is released by the periodicity estimator (PE). The time delay element used here simulates the effect of such a buffer for periodic stimuli, but cannot simulate more complex waveforms. It is not known at present how precisely waveform trajectories are stored in practice, but model simulations indicate that a relatively coarse representation (e.g. 4 samples/half-cycle) may be all that is required at low frequencies. An important feature of the model is that it is wholly self-contained; predictive behaviour is generated from within the model itself by replaying what the system did previously. It is not dependent, for example, on the existence of an internal sine wave generator, and could replicate any periodic waveform. Nor is it dependent on obtaining an internal representation of target velocity as suggested by Yasui and Young (1975).

REFERENCES

Barnes GR. (1994) A model of predictive processes in oculomotor control based on experimental results in humans. In: Information processing underlying gaze control. Ed:

Delgado-Garcia JM. Pergamon Press: Oxford. pp. 279–290.

Barnes GR, Asselman PT (1991) The mechanism of prediction in human smooth pursuit eye movements.. J Physiol (Lond) 439: 439–461

Barnes GR, Donelan AS (1997) Evidence for segregation of timing and velocity storage in ocular pursuit. J.Physiol (Lond) 505P:79–80P

Barnes GR, Donnelly SF, Eason RD (1987) Predictive velocity estimation in the pursuit reflex response to pseudorandom and step displacement in man. J Physiol (Lond) 389:111–136

Barnes GR, Goodbody SJ, Collins S (1995) Volitional control of anticipatory ocular pursuit responses under stabilised image conditions in humans. Exp Brain Res 106: 301–317

Barnes GR, Grealy MA, Collins CJS (1997) Volitional control of anticipatory ocular smooth pursuit after viewing, but not pursuing, a moving target: evidence for a re-afferent velocity store. Exp. Brain Res. 116:445–455

Barnes GR, Hill T (1984) The influence of display characteristics on active pursuit and passively induced eye movements. Exp Brain Res 56: 438–447

Barnes GR, Rathbone K, Sira M. (1997). Effects of a structured background on anticipatory ocular pursuit. J.Physiol. (Lond) 505P:113P

Becker W, Fuchs AF (1985) Prediction in the oculomotor system: smooth pursuit during transient disappearance of a visual target. Exp Brain Res 57: 562–575

Boman DK, Hotson JR (1988) Stimulus conditions that enhance anticipatory slow eye movements. Vision Res 28: 1157–1165

Carl JR, Gellman RS (1987) Human smooth pursuit: stimulus-dependent responses. J Neurophysiol 57: 1446–1463

Dallos P, Jones R (1963) Learning behaviour of the eye fixation control system. IEEE Trans Autom. Contr. AC-8: 218–227

Kao GW, Morrow MJ (1994) The relationship of anticipatory smooth eye movements to smooth pursuit initiation. Vision Res. 34(22):3027–3036

Kommerell G, Taümer R (1972) Investigations of the eye tracking system through stabilised retinal images. In: Bizzi E (ed) Bibl.ophthal. Karger. Basel, pp 288–297

Kowler E (1989) Cognitive expectations, not habits, control anticipatory smooth oculomotor pursuit. Vision Res 29: 1049–1057

Kowler E, Steinman RM (1979) The effect of expectations on slow oculomotor control-II. Single target displacements. Vision Res 19: 633–646

Lekwuwa GU, Barnes GR (1996) Cerebral control of eye movements. II. Timing of anticipatory eye movements, predictive pursuit and phase errors in focal cerebral lesions. Brain 119:491–505

Lisberger SG, Fuchs AF (1978) Role of primate flocculus during rapid behavioural modification of vestibulo-ocular reflex. I. Purkinje cell activity during visually guided horizontal smooth-pursuit eye movements and passive head rotation. J Neurophysiol 41:733–763

Ohashi N, Barnes GR (1996) A comparison of predictive and non-predictive ocular pursuit under active and passive stimulation conditions in humans. J.Vestib. Res.6: 261–276

Pola J, and Wyatt HJ (1985) Active and passive smooth eye movements: Effects of stimulus size and location. Vision Res 25: 1063–1076

Robinson DA, Gordon JL, Gordon SE. (1986) A model of the smooth pursuit eye movement system. Biol. Cybern. 55: 43–57

Wells SG, Barnes GR (1998) Fast, anticipatory smooth-pursuit eye movements appear to depend on a short-term store. Exp Brain Res. (In press).

Worfolk R, Barnes GR (1992) Interaction of active and passive slow eye movement systems. Exp Brain Res 90:589–598

Yasui S, Young LR (1975) Perceived visual motion as effective stimulus to pursuit eye movement system. Science 190: 906–908

15

PARIETO-TEMPORAL CORTEX CONTRIBUTES TO VELOCITY STORAGE INTEGRATION OF VESTIBULAR INFORMATION

J. Ventre-Dominey, N. Nighoghossian, and A. Vighetto

INSERM U94
Neurology Hospital
Lyon, France

1. ABSTRACT

We previously demonstrated that the parieto-temporal cortex modulates vestibulo-ocular function in monkey (Ventre and Faugier-Grimaud 1986). To date, this question has not been addressed in man. In this study, the vestibulo-ocular reflexe (VOR) was investigated in a group of 6 patients with unilateral lesion of the parieto-temporal cortex (4 patients with right-sided lesion, 2 with and 2 without hemineglect, and 2 patients with left-sided lesion) and compared to a group of 8 control age-matched subjects. VOR was induced by sinusoidal rotation at different frequencies (0.02, 0.05 and 0.1 Hz) and by constant velocity rotation (50 deg/sec) around the vertical axis. VOR responses were analyzed in terms of left vs right hemispheric lesion, with vs without hemineglect. VOR was quantified by analyzing slow phases of the nystagmus induced in the different conditions of rotation. Our preliminary data demonstrate a VOR asymmetry in the lesion group, quantified by measuring the directional preponderance, DP (Positive DP = Directional preponderance away from the lesion; Negative DP = Directional preponderance towards the lesion).

DP was significantly decreased for the VOR time constant and the nystagmus frequency, in the group of patients with a right lesion (ANOVA main group effect: $p < 0.05$). While no VOR velocity bias (mean shift= 0.63 deg/sec; sd=1) was found in the normal group, a velocity bias was revealed with sine rotation in the patient groups. This VOR bias was significant towards the lesioned side, especially in the right group and more pronounced in the presence of neglect (ANOVA, main group effect: $p < 0.05$). VOR gain in the patient groups was not different from the control group. These results showed a VOR directional preponderance toward the lesion, mainly in the patient group with right cortical lesion associated to hemineglect.

We suggest that in man, the effects of a parieto-temporal cortex lesion on VOR are closely related to the hemispheric lateralization and the presence of a neglect syndrome.

Current Oculomotor Research, edited by Becker *et al.*
Plenum Press, New York, 1999.

These data are discussed in terms of a cortical influence on the brainstem network involved in velocity storage integration and spatial reconstruction.

2. INTRODUCTION

Evidence from several experimental contexts has been provided about the role of cortex in vestibulo- ocular function. First, Foerster (1936) and Penfield and Jasper (1954) described vestibular sensation during electrical stimulation of the parietal cortex in patients. Electrophysiological evidence later implicated several cortical areas in vestibulo-ocular integration (Kornhuber et al. 1964; Fredrickson et al. 1966; Becker et al. 1979; Kawano et al. 1984; Grusser et al. 1990). Our behavioural animal studies were the first to demonstrate the existence of an efferent mechanism involving the posterior parietal region in a vestibulo-ocular control (Ventre et al. 1984; Ventre 1985a; Ventre 1985b; Ventre and Faugier-Grimaud 1986). Indeed, we showed that unilateral lesions of the parietal cortex (namely area 7a) induced an asymmetry of the optokinetic and vestibulo-ocular reflexes. Finally, the existence of direct projections from the parieto-temporal cortex onto the vestibular and prepositus hypoglossi complex in monkey firmly established the existence of an efferent cortical mechanism linked to visuo-vestibular ocular functions in animal (Ventre and Faugier-Grimaud 1988; Faugier-Grimaud and Ventre 1989; Akbarian et al. 1994). Human studies related to the role of cortex in vestibular function in man are still very sparse. Imaging studies, during caloric labyrinthine stimulation in normal subjects, have shown an increase in focal blood flow in different cortical regions, particularly the parieto-temporal cortex (Friberg et al. 1985; Bottini et al. 1994). Brandt et al (1995) reported the case of one patient with a lesion of the posterior insula, who experienced rotational vertigo, nausea and unsteady gait and presented a contraversive tilt of the perceived vertical. Moreover, in patients with focal parietal and frontal lesions, Israel et al. (1995) demonstrated that specific regions of the cortex are implicated in the generation of vestibularly-derived goal-directed saccades. Based on these observations in humans, it emerges that vestibular inputs are integrated over a cortical network involving frontal and parieto-temporal sub-regions whose respective roles in vestibular function are not fully understood. Indeed, the question of an efferent cortical control onto vestibulo-ocular function in man remains unknown.To address this question, we investigated vestibulo-ocular dysfunction in patients with unilateral temporo-parietal cortex lesions.

3. MATERIALS AND METHODS

3.1. Clinical Examination

Before vestibulo-ocular testing, each subject underwent a complete neurological examination, an ophthalmological (visual accuracy, visual field completion) and ORL examination (caloric test). Visuo-spatial hemineglect was assessed by using 3 different tasks: 1) the line bisection test requiring to mark the midline of a line drawn on a paper, 2) the line crossing requiring to cross all the lines equally distributed on the 2 halves of a paper and 3) the reproduction of different sketched objects (clock, daisy.) or simple pictures with symmetrical features. All these neuropsychological tests were performed by presenting in front of the subject the midline of the paper aligned with the body axis. These tests were performed by the controls and the patients and a visuo-spatial hemineglect was assessed when the subject made errors, usually in the left hemispace, in 2 of the tests presented, in addition to the neurological clinical observations.

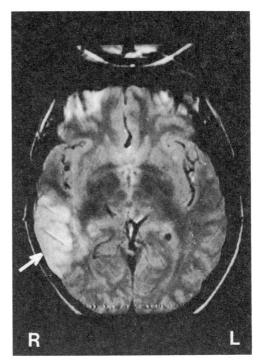

Figure 1. Transaxial MRI showing an example of the hemispheric lesion location (arrow) in the parieto-temporal cortex patient MJL of the right group with hemineglect). R: Right hemisphere. L: Left hemisphere.

3.2. Material

We investigated the vestibulo-ocular functions in a group of 6 right-handed patients with unilateral lesion of the parieto-temporal cortex due to vascular, ischaemic or haemorrhagic stroke (3 males and 3 females; mean age: 54 years, range: 38- 66 years). The group of patients was divided into 3 sub-sets: one group of 2 patients with a right-sided lesion with hemi-neglect, one group of 2 patients with right-sided lesion without hemi-neglect and another group of 2 patients with a left-sided lesion. The patients were recruited in the neurological clinic of the Lyon Neurology Hospital.

Computerized tomography (CT scan) and magnetic resonance imaging (MRI) assessed the location of the cortical lesion which always involved the superior part of the posterior temporal lobe and the inferior part of the posterior parietal lobe related to the superficial posterior sylvian artery territory (Fig. 1). All patients were screened for no history of psychiatric, ORL and ophthalmological disorders (except hemianopia) and of neurological disorders other than their current cerebral stroke (Table 1).

The patients group was compared to a group of 8 healthy age-matched subjects (mean= 46 years; range= 28–69 years; 4 males and 4 females) with no history of psychiatric, neurological, ORL and ophtalmological disorders.

Before vestibulo-ocular testing, all the subjects gave their informed consent to participate in the study.

3.3. Methods

In the patient groups, the vestibulo-ocular reflexe (VOR) was recorded about 1 month after the onset of the neurological symptoms (mean: 36 days, range: 10- 120 days).

Table 1. Characteristics of patients with unilateral cortical lesions

Subjects	Sex	Age	Lesion	Side	Hemianopia	Hemineglect
MJL	M	52	Parietal stroke	R	—	—
BJ	M	58	Parieto-Temporal stroke	R	—	—
BY	F	60	Occipito-Parieto-Temporal stroke	R	Yes	Yes
HP	F	66	Parieto-Temporal stroke	R	—	Yes
LL	F	52	Occipito-Parieto-Temporal stroke	L	Yes	—
CM	M	39	Parietal angioma	L	—	—

The subject was seated in a rotatory chair in the dark, in front of a panel supporting LEDs. Head movements were restricted by maintaining the head against a head rest by a frontal strap.

Eye movements were recorded by direct current electro-oculography (DC-EOG). Cutaneous electrodes were placed on the outer canthi of the orbits for horizontal eye movements recording and on the upper and the lower orbital ridge for vertical eye movements recording. The EOG signals were amplified and filtered (40 Hz) and then collected on a PC computer for further analysis.

The horizontal EOG signal was calibrated on saccades to visual targets (10, 20 and 30 deg in the right and left visual hemifields). In case of hemianopia (2 patients), the visual targets were displayed in the normal hemifield and the EOG calibration curve was extrapolated into the hemianopic hemifield. EOG calibration was performed at the beginning and at the end of the session and twice during the session. Before vestibular stimulation, spontaneous eye movements were recorded in the dark.

Vestibulo-ocular reflex (VOR) was induced by rotation of the subject around the vertical axis:

a. By sinusoidal rotation: The chair was sinusoidally rotated with a peak angular velocity of 50 deg/sec and at different frequencies (0.02, 0.05 and 0.1 Hz). At each frequency, VOR was continuously recorded over 5 cycles of rotation.

b. By velocity step: The chair was suddenly rotated at constant velocity (acceleration 100 deg/sec^2; constant velocity: 50 deg/s) and after 90 sec of rotation, the chair was stopped (deceleration: 100 deg/sec^2). The 2 directions of rotation (Clockwise: CW and Counterclockwise: CCW) were tested in 2 successive trials. For each trial, VOR was recorded in response to the chair acceleration as the per-rotatory nystagmus and in response to the decceleration (chair stop) as a post-rotatory nystagmus.

3.4. Data Analysis

Eye movements velocity was digitally calculated by an interactive software using the two-point central difference algorithm (50 msec step size). Quick phases were then removed by an algorithm using velocity and acceleration thresholds (Denise et al. 1996). Different parameters were quantified as following:

a. For sine responses: -1) A sinusoidal adjustment was performed on the slow phase velocity curve and a linear regression between eye and head velocities provides the gain values for each direction of rotation. -2) VOR bias was calculated as the intercept of the regression line.

b. For per- and post-rotatory responses: -1) VOR gain was calculated as the ratio between maximal slow phase velocity and constant chair velocity -2) VOR time constant was measured as the time when the area under the slow phase velocity curve reaches 63 % of the total area (Denise et al. 1996) and -3) finally, the nystagmus frequency was analysed. For each parameter, the mean value between the 2 per- and post-rotatory phases was calculated to be used for further statistical analysis.

As the cortical lesions were lateralized in different hemispheres, we expressed the data in terms of ipsilateral and contralateral to the hemispheric lesion. To quantify VOR asymmetry, we calculated the directional preponderance (DP) for each parameter, as:

$$DP = \frac{(Contralateral\ Performance\ -\ Ipsilateral\ Performance\ )*100}{(Contralateral\ Performance\ +\ Ipsilateral\ Performance)}$$

Positive DP = Directional preponderance away from the lesion

Negative DP = Directional preponderance towards the lesion

For each parameter, statistical analysis was computed by using multifactorial ANOVA analysis and LSD post-hoc comparison. The factors were: the group (control, patient) and the hemisphere (control, right and left). Inside the patient group, we analysed the neglect factor effect on each parameter. All statistical analysis were performed by the STATISTICA software package.

4. RESULTS

No spontaneous nystagmus was found in the dark, in the patients and in the controls. VOR performance was asymmetrical in the patient groups as compared to the control group.

During sinusoidal rotation, VOR was significantly biased towards the lesioned side in the patient groups as compared to the control group (main group effect: $F(1,11)= 5.3$, $p < .05$). This effect likely corresponds to an offset in the vestibulo-ocular velocity due to the lesion. As shown in Fig. 2, the VOR bias was more significant in the right hemispheric lesion and specifically with visuo-spatial neglect (neglect effect in patient groups: $F(1,4)= 7.8$, $p < .05$).

During constant velocity rotation, VOR time constant was asymmetrical, strongly reduced with rotation away from the lesion in the patient group (contra: 15.9 sec; sd= 4.5 versus ipsi: 10.6 sec; sd= 3.3). As shown in Fig. 3, the directional preponderance (DP) of the time constant was significantly decreased in the patient group as compared to the control group (main group effect: $F(1, 11)= 7.4$, $p= .02$). This asymmetry in time constant was greater with right-sided lesion (DP= -23% ; sd= 14) than with left-sided lesion (DP= -11%; sd= 9) (main hemisphere effect: $F(1,2)= 5.4$, $p= .025$). The time constant symmetry was more affected in the patient group with neglect (DP= -33%; sd= 12) (neglect effect in patient group: $F(1, 4)= 7.8$, $p< .05$). VOR asymmetry was also observed in the reduction of the DP of nystagmus frequency in the patient groups (main group effect: $F(1,11)=$,

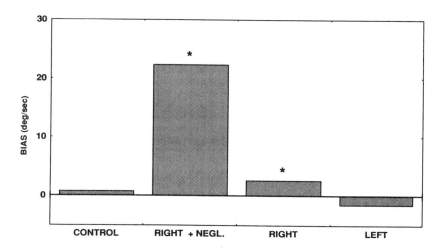

Figure 2. Bar graph of VOR velocity bias in the different groups: the control group and the patient groups with a right lesion and hemineglect (RIGHT+NEGL.), with a right lesion (RIGHT) and with a left lesion (LEFT). * P < 0.05.

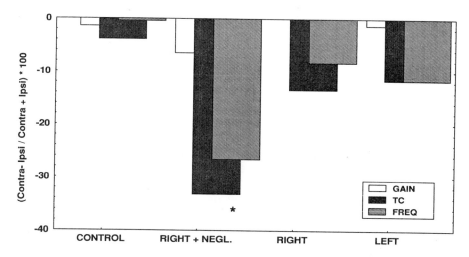

Figure 3. Bar graph of the directional preponderance of the VOR gain, the time constant (TC), the nystagmus frequency (FREQ) in the different groups: the control group and the patient groups with a right lesion and hemineglect (RIGHT+NEGL.), with a right lesion (RIGHT) and with a left lesion (LEFT). * P < 0.05.

F(1,11)=7.6, p= .02). LSD post-hoc comparison showed a significant effect of the right lesion with neglect on the nystagmus frequency (p< .05) (Fig. 3).

After removal of the VOR velocity bias, no significant asymmetry was found in VOR gain in the patient group (DP= -2.6%; sd= 5) and in the control group (DP= -1.5%; sd= 6) (Fig. 3).

5. DISCUSSION

In this preliminary study, we demonstrate a VOR asymmetry after unilateral lesion of the parieto-temporal cortex in human. The VOR imbalance was expressed as a slow phase velocity bias and a directional preponderance, mainly of the VOR time constant and the nystagmus frequency, towards the side of the lesion. VOR gain was normal.

In accordance with our previous animal studies (Ventre et al. 1984; Ventre 1985a; Ventre 1985b; Ventre and Faugier-Grimaud 1986), these data indicate that the parieto-temporal region of the cerebral cortex in man is directly implicated in the maintenance of vestibulo-ocular balance. In our patients, the cortical lesion specifically perturbed the low frequency aspects of the VOR, expressed as a velocity bias component and a time constant asymmetry. Such a role of the cortex in dynamic low frequency VOR components observed in human is comparable to the predominant deficits we observed at low frequency rotation after cortical lesion in cat and monkey (Ventre 1985b; Ventre and Faugier-Grimaud 1986).

While our previous animal studies revealed VOR gain disorders, the current human study exhibits only a vestibulo-ocular offset and a deficit in VOR time constant. This difference might have several explanations related to 1) an adaptive recovery of VOR gain after lesion: in our patients, a post-lesional compensatory mechanisms might have easily occured during the time (1 month on average) elapsed between the cerebral stroke and the VOR registration, 2) differences in the location of the lesion as the cortical lesion in our patients extended to the temporal lobe (equivalent of the retro-insular cortex: Faugier-Grimaud and Ventre 1989; Akbarian et al. 1994), and 3) species differences in the specificity and the complexity of human cortex versus primate and non primate cortex. Human cortex is characterized by a hierarchical and lateralized organization not found in primate. Indeed, the right hemisphere in man is specialized in processing of spatial information and right posterior cortical lesions often disturb visuo-spatial orientation in man, not reported in the primate with the same type of lesion. In fact, our preliminary results in patients with right-sided lesion of parieto-temporal cortex showed a strong correlation between vestibular imbalance and visuo-spatial disorders as the VOR deficits were more pronounced in the hemineglect patients. In this view, we can suggest that in human, the deficits in VOR following right parieto-temporal cortex damage might be closely linked to the deficits observed in visuospatial behaviour. In this context of cortical visuospatial processing, the vestibular inputs informing the cortex of head displacements, might be crucial for continuous updating of the visuospatial maps during body motion.

Supporting this interpretation, the main issue of this study is that the parieto-temporal cortex subserves low frequency dynamic properties of vestibulo-ocular function. We know that low frequency dynamic VOR properties are closely related to the integrity of a central vestibular storage mechanism (Raphan et al. 1979). Several behavioural and electrophysiological studies (Raphan and Cohen 1988; Wearne et al. 1997) argue for the existence of a multidimensional velocity storage mechanism organized in a network distributed bilaterally between the two vestibular nuclei complexes. By visuo-vestibular cross-coupling experiments, Raphan and Cohen (1988) suggested that this velocity storage integrator might not only store temporal information coming from visual, vestibular and postural velocity estimators but that it also stores spatial information along the vertical axis.

We conclude that the parieto-temporal cortex, implicated in the internal spatial representation, belongs to a network that achieves the multimodal storage integrator continously sollicitated during head and body displacements. However, such an hypothesis merits further experiments upon vestibulo-ocular function in a larger population of patients with localized lesions in the cerebral cortex.

REFERENCES

Akbarian S, Grusser OJ, Guldin WO (1994) Corticofugal projections to the vestibular nuclei in Squirrel monkeys: Further evidence of multiple cortical vestibular fields. J Comp Neurol 332: 89–104.

Becker W, Deecke L, Mergner T (1979) Neuronal responses to natural vestibular and neck stimulation in the anterior suprasylvian gyrus of the cat. Brain Res 165: 139–143.

Bottini G, Sterzi R, Paulesu E, Vallar G, Cappa SF, Erminio F, Passingham RE, Frith CD, Frackowiak G (1994) Identification of the central vetsibular projections in man: a positron emission tomography activation study. Exp Brain Res 99: 164–169.

Brandt T, Bötzel T, Yousry T, Dieterich M, Schulze S (1995) Rotational vertigo in embolic stroke of the vestibular and auditory cortices. Neurology 45: 42–44.

Denise P, Darlot C, Ignatiew-Charles P, Toupet M (1996) Unilateral peripheral semicircular canal lesion and off-vertical axis rotation. Acta Oto-laryng (Stockh.) 116: 361–367.

Faugier-Grimaud S, Ventre J (1989) Anatomic Connections of inferior parietal cortex (area 7) with subcortical structures related to vestibulo-ocular function in monkey. J Comp Neurol 280: 1–14.

Friberg L, Olsen TS, Roland PE, Paulson OB, Lassen NA (1985) Focal increase of blood flow in the cerebral cortex of man during vestibular stimulation. Brain 108: 609–623.

Foerster, O (1936) Sensible corticale Felder. In: Handbuch der Neurologie, Bumke O, Foerster O (eds) Vol. VI. Springer, Berlin pp 358–449.

Fredrickson JM, Figge U, Scheid P, Kornhuber HH (1966) Vestibular nerve projection to the cerebral cortex of the Rhesus monkey. Exp Brain Res 2: 318–327.

Grusser OJ, Pause M, Schreiter U (1990a) Localisation and responses of neurons in the parieto-insular vestibular cortex of awake monkeys (Macaca Fascicularis). J Physiol 430: 537–557.

Kawano K, Sasaki M, Yamashita M (1984) Response properties of neurons in posterior parietal cortex of monkey during visual-vestibular stimulation: visual tracking neurons. J Neurophysiol 51: 340–351.

Israel I, Rivaud S, Gaymard B, Berthoz A, Pierrot-deseilligny C (1995) Cortical control of vestibular-guided saccades in man. Brain 118: 1169–1183.

Kornhuber HH, Da Fonseca JS (1964) Optovestibular integration in the cat's cortex: a study of sensory convergence on cortical neurons. In: The Oculomotor System. Bender MB (ed) Hoeber, New-York, pp 239–279

Penfield W, Jasper H(1954) Epilepsy and functional anatomy of the brain. Boston Little, Brown, pp 408–409.

Raphan T, Matsuo V, Cohen B (1979) Velocity storage in the vestibulo-ocular reflex arc (VOR). Exp Brain Res 35: 229–248.

Raphan T, Cohen B (1988) Organizational principles of velocity storage in three dimensions: the effect of gravity on cross-coupling of optokinetic after-nystagmus. Ann N Y Acad Sci 545: 74–92.

Ventre J, Flandrin M, Jeannerod M (1984) In search for the egocentric reference. A neurophysiological hypothesis. Neuropsychologia 22: 797–806.

Ventre J (1985a) Cortical control of oculomotor functions. I Optokinetic nystagmus. Behav Brain Res 15: 211–226.

Ventre J (1985b) Cortical control of oculomotor functions. II Vestibulo-ocular reflex and visual-vestibular interaction optokinetic nystagmus. Behav Brain Res 17: 221–234.

Ventre J, Faugier-Grimaud S (1986) Effects of posterior parietal lesions (area 7) on VOR in monkeys. Exp Brain Res 62: 654–658.

Ventre J, Faugier-Grimaud S (1988) Projections of the temporo-parietal cortex on vestibular complex in the macaque monkey. Exp Brain Res 72: 653–658.

Wearne S, Raphan T, Cohen B (1997) Contribution of vestibular commissural pathways to spatial orientation of the angular vestibulo-ocular reflex. J Neurophysiol 78: 1193–1197.

16

THREE-DIMENSIONAL PRIMATE EYE MOVEMENTS DURING LATERAL TRANSLATION

M. Quinn McHenry,[1] Bernhard J. M. Hess,[3] and Dora E. Angelaki[1,2]

[1]Department of Anatomy
[2]Department of Surgery (Otolaryngology)
University of Mississippi Medical Center
2500 N. State St., Jackson Mississippi 39212
[3]Department of Neurology
University Hospital Zürich
CH-8091 Zürich, Switzerland

1. INTRODUCTION

Natural head movements provide a rich vestibular stimulus containing both rotational and translational components. Reflexive eye movements elicited by head motion provide a unique opportunity to study sensorimotor function. The oculomotor response to linear motion (translational vestibulo-ocular reflex, TVOR) is kinematically more challenging than that to rotation. In general, compensatory eye movements during translational motion are different for each eye and exhibit a dependence on the position of the target of interest. The distance of a desired fixation point also imposes kinematic requirements on the TVOR (Virre et al. 1986; Paige 1989, Schwarz et al. 1989, Paige and Tomko 1991a,b; Schwarz and Miles, 1991, Snyder and King 1992, Telford et al. 1997).

To further complicate the TVOR, ambiguity exists in the signals arising from the otolith organs, the vestibular organs sensitive to linear acceleration. Translational accelerations are physically indistinguishable from the acceleration of gravity. Otolith afferents in the squirrel monkey respond identically to static tilts with respect to gravity and centrifugal acceleration (Fernandez and Goldberg 1976). While the otolith response during translation and tilt may be identical, the ideal compensatory eye movements in each case are different. A sinusoidal lateral translation requires a horizontal eye movement for compensation. However, a sinusoidal roll rotation that provides an equivalent otolith stimulus requires a torsional movements. Quantification of the horizontal and torsional eye modulation during lateral translation may provide insight into the neural mechanisms contributing to the TVOR.

Current Oculomotor Research, edited by Becker *et al.*
Plenum Press, New York, 1999.

Prior to investigating the underlying neural mechanisms responsible for generating eye-position dependent translation-evoked eye movements, the normal behavior of the TVOR must be understood. While rotational vestibulo-ocular reflexes have been extensively investigated, TVOR responses are less frequently studied and usually restricted to a narrow frequency range. The results here represent preliminary observations of the primate TVOR in response to steady-state sinusoidal translational motion in a frequency range from 0.16 to 30 Hz in the dark and following fixation of targets at different viewing distances.

2. METHODS

Five juvenile rhesus monkeys provided data presented here. Each animal underwent aseptic surgical procedures under isoflurane anesthesia to implant a dual scleral eye coil in each eye and a delrin head ring to fix the head during experiments. Before implantation, each eye coil was precalibrated (Hess et al. 1992). The head implant was secured to the skull using stainless steel screws and dental acrylic with the animal's head stereotaxically aligned. All animal procedures were in accordance with NIH guidelines.

Following adequate recovery time, animals were trained to fixate LED targets for juice rewards. Following successful fixation of the target for a random period of 500–1000 ms, the target light was extinguished while an auditory cue remained. The reward was contingent upon sustained fixation for a variable period up to 2 s after the light was turned off. Adequate fixation was determined with position windows of ~1° which required the animal to maintain vergence.

2.1. Experimental Protocols

Animals participated in experiments only after sufficient training. Animals were seated in a chair with their heads pitched 18° down to align the horizontal semicircular canals with the horizontal plane. The chair was mounted inside the motion delivery system (Acutronics, Inc.) and the animal's head was rigidly fixed to the support structure. The coordinate system was defined such that a positive lateral motion was to the animal's right. A three-axis accelerometer was rigidly mounted to the fiberglass support structure which secured the animal's head ring to the sled. Eye coil, sled position and velocity feedback, and accelerometer signals were low pass filtered (200 Hz, 6 pole Bessel) and digitized at 833.3 Hz using a CED1404 data acquisition system (Cambridge Electronic Design). Before each experiment, the animals fixated a series of vertical targets to calibrate the eye coils (Hess et al. 1992).

2.1.1. Dark Protocols. Lateral sinusoidal acceleration stimuli in darkness were initiated manually through a computer interface. A light was occasionally turned on between trials to maintain alertness which was monitored by viewing eye position traces on an oscilloscope. Stimuli consisted of 0.16, 0.2 Hz (0.1g peak amplitude), 0.3 Hz (0.2 g), 0.37 Hz (0.3 g), 0.5, 0.7, 1, 1.5, 2, 3, 4, 5, 6, 8, 10, 12, 13, 18, 20, 25 and 30 Hz (0.4 g). Between 3 and 50 steady-state cycles of data were recorded depending on the frequency, and each stimulus was repeated at least 3 times in each animal. Data were gathered during lateral translation with the animal in two orientations, upright and supine. Animals were reoriented using a servo-controlled rotation axis. In one animal, responses were also recorded in the upright orientation while the room lights were illuminated and with most visual targets at a distance of ~3 m.

2.1.2. Target Protocol. The same LED target array used for training was used during experiments. Target distance was varied between 10 and 40 cm. Under computer control, the target aligned between the eyes was illuminated. Fixation of the target was determined with binocular position windows of ~1°. After fixation for a random period of 500–800 ms, the sled began moving and the position window size was automatically increased. An acceleration constraint was in effect during the stimulus to exclude trials containing a fast eye movement. Trials in which eye position was maintained in the position window and all eye movements were below the acceleration threshold resulted in behavioral reinforcement with juice. Between trials, a light was turned on inside the animal's environment to maintain alertness. Stimulus frequency was randomly varied among 4, 5, 6, 8, 10, 12, 13, 18, 20, 25, and 30 Hz at a fixed peak amplitude of 0.4 g. At least three repetitions of each frequency and viewing distance were gathered.

2.2. Data Analysis

Eye position data were converted offline into rotation vectors using each day's calibration. The three components of eye velocity were computed and filtered. Fast phases of responses gathered in the dark or with the room lights illuminated were removed using a semi-automated procedure. Trials with a target containing a fast phase were discarded. The steady-state portion of the response was manually selected for each trial and these cycles were averaged together. Stimulus and response amplitude and phase were computed by fitting a sinusoid to both stimulus and response using a nonlinear least squares algorithm.

3. RESULTS

Steady-state sinusoidal translation along the interaural axis generated robust horizontal eye movements at all frequencies and amplitudes examined (Figure 1). Torsional modulation was smaller than horizontal modulation at all frequencies. Vertical modulations were small and inconsistent.

3.1. TVOR in Complete Darkness

Horizontal sensitivity, expressed as slow phase velocity/stimulus velocity (°/s/cm/s), and phase (re: stimulus velocity) for all animals in complete darkness have been plotted as a function of stimulus frequency in Figure 2. Each point represented a single trial. Horizontal sensitivity consistently increased with increasing frequency in all animals. Phase remained close to 0° (compensatory) but developed phase lags at high frequencies. Low frequency phase characteristics were more variable but tended to lag although phase leads were present in some responses.

3.2. Effects of Head Orientation

Mean horizontal and torsional response sensitivity in both upright and supine orientations were plotted in Figure 3. When expressed as slow phase velocity/stimulus acceleration (°/s/g), horizontal sensitivities were constant across frequency with a slight decrease at higher frequencies. Torsional phase was close to 0° for frequencies above 1 Hz and developed phase leads for lower frequencies. Given the coordinate system definition, a torsional phase of 0° refers to a positive torsional velocity (superior pole of the eye toward the right) during a positive translational velocity (toward the animal's right). The

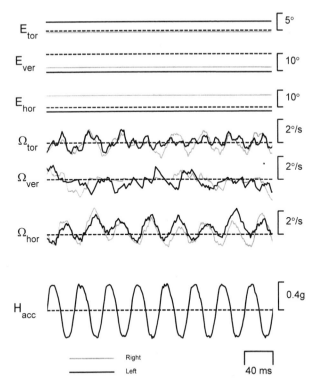

Figure 1. Example of primate TVOR in response to lateral, steady-state sinusoidal translation at 25 Hz with a peak acceleration of ~0.4 g. The top 3 traces show binocular torsional (E_{tor}), vertical (E_{ver}) and horizontal (E_{hor}) eye position. Torsional (Ω_{tor}), vertical (Ω_{ver}) and horizontal (Ω_{hor}) velocities are plotted below. The bottom trace shows stimulus acceleration (H_{acc}) along the motion axis measured with an accelerometer mounted on the animal's head. Dashed lines indicate zero position and velocity.

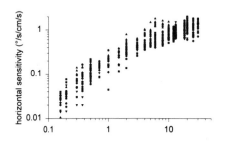

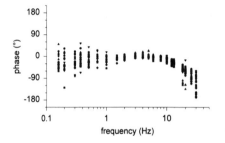

Figure 2. Right eye horizontal sensitivity and phase as a function of stimulus frequency during lateral translation. Each point represents the fit of several cycles from a single trial. Responses from each animal are represented by a different symbol. Response sensitivity and phase have been expressed relative to stimulus velocity.

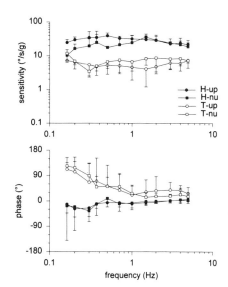

Figure 3. Right eye horizontal (solid symbols) and torsional (open symbols) sensitivities and phases in upright (circles) and supine (squares) orientations. Sensitivities have been expressed as slow phase velocity relative to stimulus acceleration. Phases have been expressed relative to stimulus velocity.

compensatory torsional response to the perceived tilt due to the otolith ambiguity between translational and gravitational acceleration would have exhibited a phase of 180°. No statistically significant differences in sensitivity or phase existed between upright and supine conditions over the frequency range tested.

3.3. TVOR in an Illuminated Room

Horizontal slow phase velocity sensitivity and phase for one animal in complete darkness (dotted line) and with the room lights on (mean +/- standard deviation) have been plotted in Figure 4. While sensitivity in the dark increased with increasing frequency as described above, sensitivity in the light remained constant at ~0.2 °/s/cm/s and was independent of frequency. Horizontal slow phase velocity was in phase with stimulus velocity (0°) in the light across most frequencies, but developed a slight phase lag at the highest frequencies tested.

3.4. Effects of Viewing Distance

Mean horizontal response gain (expressed as slow phase velocity/ideal response velocity) for each animal as a function of stimulus frequency has been plotted in Figure 5 for target distances of 10, 20 and 40 cm. Gain increased with increasing frequency and approached (10 cm) or exceeded (40 cm) unity gain (dotted line) at frequencies over 20 Hz. Otherwise, response magnitudes were consistently below the requirements for ideal compensation. While gain increased as target distance increased, sensitivity (°/sec/cm/sec) decreased with increasing viewing distance (not shown).

4. DISCUSSION

Robust eye movements were evoked during lateral translation even in complete darkness at all frequencies tested, from 0.16 to 30 Hz. Responses were most robust at high

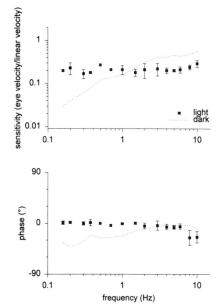

Figure 4. Right eye horizontal sensitivity and phase during lateral translation in complete darkness (dashed line) and with room lights illuminated (solid squares). Sensitivity and phase have been expressed relative to stimulus velocity. Data have been plotted as mean +/- standard deviation.

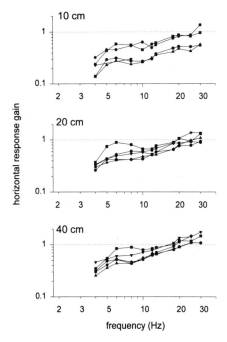

Figure 5. Right eye horizontal response gain as a function of stimulus frequency for viewing distances of 10, 20, and 40 cm. Gains were computed as slow phase velocity relative to the ideal velocity required to maintain fixation. Dotted lines represent ideal compensation (gain=1).

frequencies at which visual mechanisms for gaze stabilization would be less effective. Response magnitude has been represented in three ways, as acceleration sensitivity (°/s/g), velocity sensitivity (eye velocity/stimulus velocity) and gain (measured eye velocity/ideal eye velocity). Acceleration sensitivity relates the reflex output (eye velocity) to the otolith sensory input (linear acceleration). Velocity sensitivity and gain relate reflex output to the actual motion, both related to the objective of the reflex. Since the ideal response magnitude depends on viewing distance and eccentricity, gains could not be calculated for trials without the behavioral control of target fixation.

4.1. TVOR in the Dark and Light

With sensitivity expressed in °/s/g, the dynamics of the reflex can be described as follows (Figure 3). In the mid frequency range (~0.5 – 2 Hz), horizontal response sensitivity remained relatively independent of frequency with values ~30 °/s/g. At lower frequencies (< 0.5 Hz), sensitivity decreased. At higher frequencies (> 2 Hz), sensitivity also slightly decreased with increasing frequency. The most conspicuous aspect of the reflex dynamics was a functional relationship between sensitivity and phase: between ~0.5 – 10 Hz, horizontal eye velocity was in phase with stimulus velocity but sensitivity was relatively independent of frequency only when expressed relative to stimulus acceleration.

The effective viewing distance can be estimated from the velocity sensitivity (°/s/cm/s equivalent to °/cm). Given a lateral translation x and the resulting eye position change á, the viewing distance is $D=x$/tan á which may be approximated as x/á for small angles. In the light (Figure 4), the sensitivity remained ~0.2°/s/cm/s across the frequencies tested. This corresponded to a viewing distance of ~3 m which was the approximate distance of most visual targets in the lab. At frequencies above 3 Hz in the dark, sensitivity was ~0.4°/s/cm/s which corresponded to a viewing distance of ~1.5 m. In addition to the vestibular component at low frequencies, visual mechanisms probably augmented the responses with the room lights illuminated such that response sensitivity and phase were constant across the frequencies examined.

4.2. Effects of Orientation

One explanation of the torsional modulation during lateral translation is a misinterpretation of the translational acceleration along the interaural axis as a roll rotation with respect to gravity. If true, the same motion delivered while supine should not elicit a torsional modulation. However, torsional sensitivity is unchanged during upright (open circles) and supine (open squares) orientations (Figure 3) suggesting that the torsional modulation is a response to lateral translation, not to a reorientation of the gravitoinertial acceleration vector.

4.3. Effects of Viewing Distance

The horizontal eye modulation during lateral translation while viewing close targets was generally inadequate to compensate completely (gain < 1, dotted line Figure 5). Only at the highest frequencies and longest distances did the gain reach or exceed unity. Expressed as gain, the responses increased as viewing distance increased. When expressed as sensitivity, responses increased with inverse viewing distance (not shown). While the TVOR is scaled by inverse viewing distance, the increased demands of fixating closer targets were not totally met.

Viewing distance, linked closely with vergence, exerts a strong influence on the TVOR as seen with the behavioral control of target fixation. This effect is also demonstrated in the responses with the room lights on. Under these conditions, the animal had a rich visual environment at a distance of ~3 m and probably fixated at this distance prior to the stimulus. It has been proposed that the TVOR in the dark defaults to a viewing distance of ~1 m at high frequencies (Angelaki in press).

5. CONCLUSIONS

The TVOR is a robust sensorimotor reflex that participates in symphony with visual mechanisms to stabilize gaze during linear head movements. The complex kinematic dependencies on viewing parameters such as target distance make the TVOR an intriguing system for further investigation.

This work was supported by grants from NIH (EY10851), NASA (NAGW-4377), the Air Force Office of Scientific Research (F-49620).

REFERENCES

Angelaki DE (in press) Three-dimensional organization of otolith-ocular reflexes in rhesus monkeys. III. Responses to linear motion. J Neurophysiol.

Fernandez C and Goldberg JM (1976) Physiology of peripheral neurons innervating otolith organs of the squirrel monkey. I. Response to static tilt and to long-duration centrifugal force. J Neurophysiol 39:970–984.

Hess BJM, Van Opstal AJ, Straumann D, Hepp K (1992) Calibration of three-dimensional eye position using search coil signals in the rhesus monkey. Vision Res 32:1647–1654.

Paige GD (1989) The influence of target distance on eye movement responses during vertical translation. Exp Brain Res, 77:585–593.

Paige GD and Tomko DL (1991a) Eye movement responses to linear head motion in the squirrel monkey I. Basic characteristics. J Neurophysiol 65:1170–1182.

Paige GD and Tomko DL (1991b) Eye movement responses to linear head motion in the squirrel monkey II. Visual-vestibular interactions and kinematic considerations. J Neurophysiol 65:1183–1196.

Schwarz U, Busettini C and Miles FA (1989) Ocular responses to linear motion are inversely proportional to viewing distance. Science 245:1394–1396.

Schwarz U and Miles FA (1991) Ocular response to translation and their dependence on viewing distance: I. Motion of the observer. J Neurophysiol 66:851–864.

Snyder LK and King WM (1992) Effect of viewing distance and location of the axis of head rotation on the monkey's vestibuloocular reflex I. Eye movement responses. J Neurophysiol 67:861–874.

Telford L, Seidman DH, Paige GD (1997) Dynamics of squirrel monkey linear vestibuloocular reflex and interactions with fixation distance. J Neurophysiol 78:1775–1790.

Virre E, Tweed D, Milner K and Vilis T (1986) A re-examination of the gain of the vestibuloocular reflex. J Neurophysiol 56:439–450.

17

SMOOTH PURSUIT TO A MOVEMENT FLOW AND ASSOCIATED PERCEPTUAL JUDGMENTS

Yue Chen,[1] Robert M. McPeek,[2] James Intriligator,[3] Philip S. Holzman,[1] and Ken Nakayama[1]

[1]Department of Psychology
Harvard University
Cambridge, Massachusetts
[2]Smith-Kettelwell Eye Research Institute
San Francisco, California
[3]Department of Neurology
Beth Israel Deaconess Medical Center
Boston, Massachusetts

1. INTRODUCTION

Smooth pursuit is typically regarded as foveal tracking of simple targets and is therefore usually examined with stimuli such as a small moving dot. In real world situations, however, it is rare to encounter such perceptually minimal stimuli. Can smooth pursuit follow a complex object, such as a movement flow that contains ambiguous local but unambiguous global pattern of motion? Does this type of eye tracking always correspond to the motion perception of the same complex moving target? Our results show that one can smoothly pursue a movement flow even when the detection of this driving signal requires significant integration of information across space and time. Additionally, the generation of smooth pursuit appears to require sensory signals slightly stronger than that for perceiving coherent motion.

2. SMOOTH PURSUIT TO THE RANDOM DOTS OF SHORT DOT LIFETIME

Smooth pursuit usually occurs when the position and /or motion of target is obvious and explicit. While tracking a moving dot, for example, observers move continuously their focus along a series of spots (or trajectory) where the target travels. It is unclear whether the smooth pursuit system can also be engaged when only implicit information is available to eye tracking. In the present context, the term "implicit" is being used to signify absence of individual and constant low-level stimulus features such as position or velocity. This

Current Oculomotor Research, edited by Becker *et al.*
Plenum Press, New York, 1999.

experiment shows that a dynamic random-dot pattern can generate smooth pursuit eye movements even when the motion information is defined globally.

Three observers followed the movement flow presented on a computer monitor. A trial starts with fixation of a central circle. The observer pressed a key to trigger two events - stimulus presentation and the eye movement recording. After a random delay, the stimulus for eye tracking appeared on screen, moving either left or right at a constant speed (selected from 3–14 deg/s). The stimulus field extended 24 deg horizontally and 6 deg vertically. The monitor frame rate was 67 Hz and the moving pattern on each trial lasted 150 frames (i.e. 2250 ms). A similar random-dot pattern was recently used to elicit smooth pursuit (Watamaniuk & Heinen, 1994; Bullmore et al. 1995). However, it is conceivable that the tracking task could be accomplished by selecting and following one dot from the whole flow. We therefore controlled the dot lifetime (60 ms and 600 ms) to prevent the possible tracking of any individual dots, instead of the global flow. The nominal value of motion coherence is 100% if all the dots moved uniformly and had an infinite dot lifetime. Because 20% of the dots in the present experiment were replaced for every dot lifetime period, the actual coherence ranged between 80% and 100%. The horizontal movement of one eye was measured using an infrared Eye Trace System (Ober2). Eye position signals were digitized at a sampling rate of 250 Hz and stored for off-line analysis. A bite bar, made of dental impression material for each observer, was used to minimize head movement.

All three observers initiated smooth pursuit to the random dot patterns of both long and short dot lifetimes (Fig. 1). Smooth pursuit was more robust when the target moved at a speed above 5 deg/s; the initial eye acceleration (defined as second derivative of eye position signals averaged across a time window starting 150 ms after onset of the target and lasting for 150 ms) increased with target velocity. Initial catch-up saccades, as typically seen with single dot tracking, were absent, suggesting that foveation of individual dots did

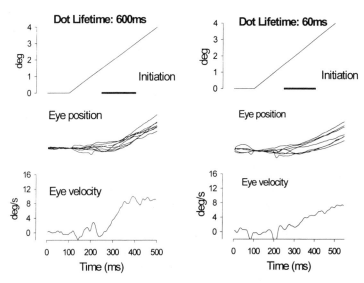

Figure 1. Representative smooth pursuit responses to a dynamic random dot pattern of short (60 ms) and long (600 ms) dot lifetimes.

not occur. It should be pointed out that the transience of dot life (e.g. 60 ms) virtually excluded the feasibility of using a particular dot continuously. Therefore, the accurate tracking must be based on global information integrated across space and time.

3. A COMPARISON BETWEEN SMOOTH PURSUIT AND MOTION PERCEPTION

Does eye tracking reflect the perceived motion ? We assessed the relation between oculomotor and perceptual responses by measuring simultaneously smooth pursuit and direction judgment of perceived motion to the same random-dot stimulus. This experiment shows that there was no exact correspondence between the directions of initial eye tracking and of perceived motion when the motion signals were relatively weak but, nevertheless, above the detection threshold.

The procedure in Experiment 2 was similar to that used in Experiment 1, with the following variations. On each trial, the motion coherence was randomly set to be 10, 20, 40, or 80% and the speed was fixed at 10 deg/s. In this experiment, the observers performed two tasks - to follow the movement flow with their eyes, as in the previous experiment, and also to make a judgment whether direction of motion was to the left or to the right.

Observers occasionally failed to generate smooth pursuit in the direction of the coherent motion (opposite), as expected if the signals of the stimulus were below perceptual threshold. Observers also initiated smooth pursuit in the opposite direction around 150 ms and then reversed its direction (i.e. in the direction of coherent motion) about 500 ms after target onset (reverse) (Figure 2). This initial tracking in wrong direction was observed, unexpectedly, with stimuli for which observers could make accurate perceptual judgments (e.g., 20–40% coherence). A trial-by-trial comparison verifies that the tracking in the wrong direction does not completely correlate with the incorrect perceptual judgment. At 20% coherence, for example, the observers made incorrect perceptual judgments only in about 40% of the trials on which initial smooth pursuit was made in the wrong directions (opposite and reverse); indicating that the initiation of smooth pursuit in correct direction needs slightly stronger coherent motion signals than does the perceptual judgment. A qualitative observation suggests that those trials with correct perceptual judgment but incorrect initial smooth pursuit were frequently accompanied in the preceding trials with strong coherent motion in opposite direction.

4. GENERAL DISCUSSION

Previous research has shown that smooth pursuit may be elicited with an unconventional moving target, such as a perceived "contour" that has no primary physical stimulation at or near to the fovea (e.g. Steinbach, 1976), and may be affected by cognitive factors like expectation (e.g. Kowler, 1988). The evidence from this study suggests that grouping of individual elements of a global object (like the movement flow) may also play a decisive role in generating eye tracking. Additionally, imperfect correspondence between initiation of smooth pursuit and perception of coherent motion argues that non-sensory signals like previous events may modify the generation of smooth pursuit.

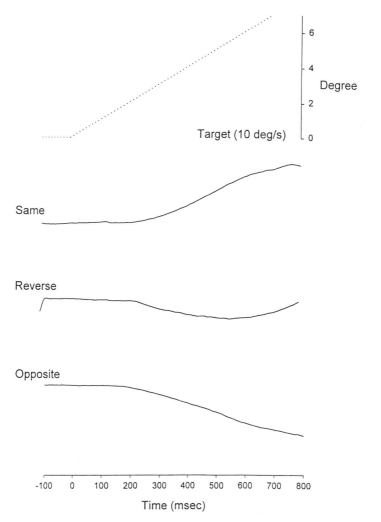

Figure 2. Three types of initial smooth pursuit responses to a movement flow of 20% coherence.

REFERENCES

1. Watamaniuk S & Heinen S (1994) Smooth pursuit eye movements to dynamic random-dot stimuli *Society for Neuroscience Abstract* 24th: 317
2. Bullmore M, Fendrich R, Wessiger CW & Johnson CA (1995) Pursuit eye movements for random dot motion stimuli. *Investigative Ophthalmology and Vision Science* 36:S206
3. Steinbach M. (1976) Pursuing the perceptual rather than the retinal stimulus. *Vision Research* 16, 1371–1376.
4. Kowler E (1989) Cognitive expectations, not habits, control anticipatory smooth oculomotor pursuit. *Vision Research* 29, 1049–1057.

REACTION TIMES OF SMOOTH PURSUIT INITIATION IN NORMAL SUBJECTS AND IN "EXPRESS-SACCADE MAKERS"

H. Kimmig,[1] J. Mutter,[2] M. Biscaldi,[2] B. Fischer,[2] and T. Mergner[1]

[1]Neurologische Universitätsklinik
Freiburg, Germany
[2]AG Hirnforschung Institut für Biophysik der Universität
Freiburg, Germany

1. INTRODUCTION

Introducing a temporal gap between extinction of fixation point (FP) and occurrence of a visual target (T) is known to reduce the reaction time (RT) of saccades performed from FP to T. In this 'gap paradigm', as it is called, the frequency distribution of saccadic RTs is typically bimodal with an early peak of very short latency saccades (express saccades, ES) and a second peak of regular saccades (Fischer and Boch 1983). There are considerable inter-individual differences. A large proportion of ES has been taken to indicate a weak fixation system which normally inhibits the generation of reflexive saccades, a finding in a subpopulation of dyslexic children (Biscaldi et al. 1996). Moreover, repeated practice of this paradigm may increase the percentage of ES in some normal subjects. Also, target eccentricity plays a role (ES are missing with eccentricities <1°; Weber et al. 1992). Finally, the phenomenon depends on gap duration; for instance, if FP extinction coincides with T appearance ('simultaneous paradigm') ES become rare and the RT distribution becomes unimodal.

Considerably less is known about RTs of smooth pursuit eye movements. Merrison and Carpenter (1995) reported a bimodal RT distribution for smooth pursuit movements, and this, surprisingly, in a 'simultaneous paradigm' with moving T. On the other hand, Krauzlis and Miles (1996a,b) found a shortening of pursuit RTs when introducing a gap, but the RT distribution in their experiments was unimodal. This discrepancy is still unsolved.

We assessed pursuit RTs for a number of different paradigms and report here on findings for a 'simultaneous paradigm'. We compared three subject groups for which we assumed differences in their saccadic RT distributions:

Current Oculomotor Research, edited by Becker *et al.*
Plenum Press, New York, 1999.

i. 'Naive subjects' who never before performed eye movement tests (they typically show a low percentage of ES)

ii. 'trained subjects' from whom we knew that they make a relatively high percentage of ES

iii. so-called express-saccade makers ('ES-makers'; see above). The latter subjects previously were found to make almost exclusively ES in the gap paradigm and to produce more than 30% ES in an overlap paradigm (FP not extinguished at time of T appearance; Biscaldi et al. 1996; Cavegn and Biscaldi 1996). We asked whether the distribution of pursuit RTs systematically varies across these three groups.

2. METHODS

We measured pursuit RT of 11 naive subjects producing a normal number of ES in a gap paradigm ('naive'), 7 trained subjects ('trained'), known to produce a high percentage of ES, and 8 'ES-makers'. For the pursuit task we used a 'simultaneous ramp' paradigm (fixation time, 1400 ms; ramp velocity 6, 12 or 20 deg/s; eccentricity at end of movement always 12°, either right or left). Eye movements were recorded with an infrared light reflection technique and stored in a computer for off-line analysis.

3. RESULTS

In all three subject groups the first pursuit RTs occurred at 80–90 ms and the RT distribution showed a first peak at 100–110 ms. In the naive and trained subject groups a second, broader peak occurred at approximately 150 ms. 'ES-maker' did not show a clearly separated second peak in the distribution of pursuit RTs; the second peak seemed to be merged with the first one, such that their distribution appeared skewed towards longer latencies. Mean reaction times amounted to 138±17 ms in the naive group, 139±31 ms in the trained group and 132±18 ms in the 'ES-maker' group. Statistically, there was no difference between groups (p=0.2). When considering only the very fast pursuit RTs (upper limit, 120 ms), the percentage of these amounted to 35±18% in the naive group, 41±25% in the trained group and 45±22% in the 'ES-maker' group. Again, there was no statistically significant difference between groups (p=0.6).

4. DISCUSSION

Whereas it is possible to separate the three subject groups by the amount of ES in a saccadic gap paradigm, these groups do not differ with respect to smooth pursuit RTs in a 'simultaneous ramp' paradigm. The results might be interpreted as follows:

i. Although the trained subjects had much experience in saccade paradigms, they were naive with respect to pursuit; obviously, the training of saccadic RT tasks does not shorten pursuit RTs.

ii. It is known that 'ES-maker' produce less or no ES if the target eccentricity becomes very small (Weber et al. 1992, Biscaldi et al., 1996). Note, however, that in our 'simultaneous ramp' paradigm there is essentially no initial target eccen-

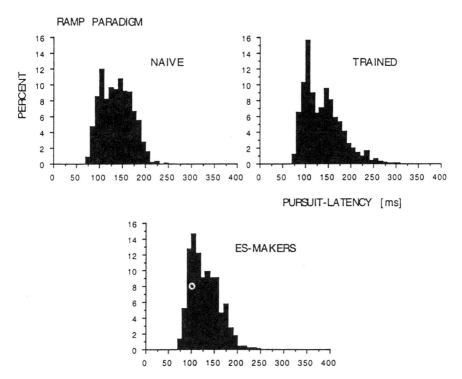

Figure 1. Frequency distributions of smooth pursuit reaction times in a 'simultaneous ramp' paradigm for the three subjects groups.

tricity. Thus, we have to consider the possibility that the rules that are established for ES do not apply to pursuit.

iii. Yet, all three groups showed a considerable proportion of very fast pursuit RTs which are in the range of ES. Two of the three groups even showed a bimodal distribution of RTs, which resembled those of saccadic RTs. We therefore speculate that certain parts of the mechanisms responsible for the bimodal saccadic RT distribution are, in some way, also acting on the pursuit system, i.e. on the release of fixation/attention (Mayfrank et al. 1986). In the study of Merrison and Carpenter (1994) pursuit RT was also measured in a 'simultaneous ramp' paradigm. These authors assumed a distinct 'express smooth pursuit response' and suggest a similarity with the saccadic system. We, in contrast, consider the express RTs for pursuit as the normal case and the longer RTs an exception; in the other pursuit paradigms we used (not reported here) the distribution was essentially unimodal, like in the study of Krauzlis and Miles (1996b). We would hold that pursuit onset is more reflexive in nature than that of saccades: Try to make an anti-pursuit movement!

REFERENCES

Biscaldi M, Fischer B, Stuhr V (1996) Human express saccade makers are impaired at suppressing visually evoked saccades. J Neurophysiol 76: 199–214

Cavegn D, Biscaldi M (1996) Fixation and saccade control in an express-saccade maker. Exp Brain Res 109(1):101–116.

Fischer B, Boch R (1983) Saccadic eye movements after extremely short reaction times in the monkey. Brain Res 260:21–26.

Krauzlis RJ, Miles FA (1996a) Decreases in the latency of smooth pursuit and saccadic eye movements produced by the "gap paradigm" in the monkey. Vision Res 36(13):1973–85.

Krauzlis RJ, Miles FA (1996b) Release of fixation for pursuit and saccades in humans: evidence for shared inputs acting on different neural substrates. J Neurophysiol 76(5):2822–33.

Mayfrank L, Mobashery M, Kimmig H, Fischer B (1986) The role of fixation and visual attention in the occurrence of express saccades in man. Eur Arch Psychiatr Neurol Sci 235: 269–275.

Merrison AF, Carpenter RH (1995) "Express" smooth pursuit. Vision Res 35(10):1459–62.

Weber H, Aiple F, Fischer B, Latanov A (1992) Dead zone for express saccades. Exp Brain Res 89:214–222.

19

ACTIVE REPRODUCTION OF PASSIVE ROTATIONS AND CONTINGENT EYE MOVEMENTS

I. Israel and I. Siegler

Laboratoire de Physiologie de la Perception et de l'Action
CNRS-Collège de France, Paris

1. INTRODUCTION

It has been shown (Metcalfe and Gresty, 1992) that subjects can return to their initial orientation after a passive rotation in complete darkness. The presentation of a visual target straight ahead before the imposed rotation further improves the accuracy (Israël et al. 1996). In order to perform the return task with no memorized reference, the subjects must have reproduced, in the opposite direction, the imposed motion. Therefore, subjects should also be able to reproduce an imposed motion in the same direction, as it has been demonstrated for linear displacements (Berthoz et al. 1995; Israël et al. 1997).

Furthermore, whereas it has been suggested that suppressing the vestibulo-ocular reflex (VOR) does not influence self-rotation estimate (Israël et al. 1996), the eye movements during such a task have never specifically been examined. We then decided to investigate the VOR during both imposed (passive) and reproduced (active) rotations.

2. METHODS

The subject was seated on a mobile robot (Robuter™, Robosoft, France) delivering rotations about the vertical axis. Robot motion was controlled by a remote computer or by the subject with a joystick. Robot position was continuously measured by optical odometry.

Eye movements were measured with an infra-red system (IRIS, Skalar). The subject was surrounded by an opaque curtain ensuring complete darkness, wore headphones delivering a wide band noise, and had his/her head firmly maintained between two soft cushions.

A passive whole-body rotation was imposed, and after a free delay the subject had to reproduce the same angle in the same direction, driving the robot with the joystick. The velocity profile of the stimulus was triangular, and angles were 80°, 167° and 340°. 24 young healthy subjects participated to the experiment.

Current Oculomotor Research, edited by Becker *et al.*
Plenum Press, New York, 1999.

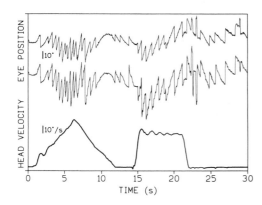

Figure 1. Example of a 340° trial (60°/s stimulus peak velocity). Bottom thick trace = robot velocity. Top thin traces = position of each eye.

3. RESULTS

3.1. Performance

For all subjects, the correlation between imposed and reproduced angles was significant (p < 0.01). Slopes of the corresponding regression lines ranged from 0.5 to 1.3, with a mean of 0.8 ± 0.2. Overall amplitude ratio (reproduction/stimulus angle) was 1.0 ± 0.2, decreasing from 1.1 ± 0.3 to 0.9 ± 0.2 with increasing stimulus angle.

Subjects mostly used trapezoidal velocity profiles with short acceleration and deceleration phases (Fig.1). Plateau velocity significantly increased with the angle. The ratio of response plateau to stimulus peak velocity remained below unity, decreasing from 0.8 ± 0.2 at 80° to 0.6 ± 0.1 at 340°.

Since the imposed rotations had a triangular velocity profile, stimulus duration and angle were interdependent, and we wondered whether the subjects used duration as an information to execute the reproduction. Indeed, the mean slope of the stimulus-response duration regressions was 0.9 ± 0.4, and mean duration ratio remained approximately constant (close to unity) across angles.

In a control experiment, subjects were first submitted to the same stimuli of variable duration (VD) as in the main experiment, and then to another set of stimuli with triangular velocity profiles but with a constant duration (CD) of 9 s. In VD the mean slope was 0.8 ± 0.2, and in CD it was 0.7 ± 0.2, which indicates that the reproduction of stimulus angles was less accurate in CD than in VD. Furthermore, the mean amplitude ratio was significantly (p = 0.01) higher in VD (1.0 ± 0.3) than in CD (0.9 ± 0.3).

3.2. Eye Movements

Many subjects did not exhibit post-rotatory nystagmus (PRN) after the smallest angle (80°), and neither after the greatest stimulus angle (340°) for some of them. Some did not even exhibit per-rotatory nystagmus at 340°. Moreover some subjects did not wait the end of PRN (when present) to start reproduction (Fig.1), whereas among the subjects who did not exhibit PRN, most of them waited more than 4 s before to start reproducing.

VOR gain was very variable: individual mean values ranged from 0.2 to 0.85. VOR gain decreased when the angle increased (p = 0.04), during the reproduction but not during the stimulus. Furthermore, VOR gain was significantly lower during reproduction than during stimulus (p = 0.01). So the larger the angle, the smaller the mean VOR gain during reproduction and the larger the difference between stimulus and reproduction. This could be due to the difference in velocity profiles during reproduction (trapezoidal) and stimulus (triangular).

In an additional control experiment, trials with two successive passive rotations each were applied. The two rotations had the same angle but different velocity profiles. The first rotation had a triangular velocity profile as in the main experiment. The velocity profile of the second rotation was chosen so as to mimic subjects response to the corresponding stimulus in the main experiment. We found the same mean values of VOR gain during "stimulus" and "reproduction" profile as in the main experiment.

4. DISCUSSION

In previous experiments with linear motion (Berthoz et al. 1995) it was found that the velocity profile of the stimulus was played back during the reproduction, which is not the case in the present experiment. It could be that the output of the semi-circular canals (angular velocity) is directly time-integrated to yield angular position perception, so that velocity is not recorded.

The slope of the regression line between stimulus and response is lower in the present experiment (0.8) than in a return task (0.66), with the same condition of complete darkness (Israël et al. 1996). The change of direction required in return may have disturbed the subjects. Another possibility is that the subjects did try to use the memory of their initial self-orientation, which seems to move closer during self-driven rotation in the absence of external reference (Israël et al. 1995); indeed, when this reference had been presented, for return, the slope was 0.81 (Israël et al. 1996).

VOR gain decreases when the angle increases in reproduction only, and is higher during stimulus than reproduction. This can be explained by the velocity profile, triangular for the stimulus and trapezoidal during the reproduction. The constant velocity part of a trapezoidal profile induces a decrease of VOR gain, which is not the case in a triangular profile. However, these rotations also differ insofar as unlike the stimulus, the reproduction is an 'active' task. This characteristic could either influence the subject's alertness inducing an increase of VOR gain (Kasper et al. 1992), or elicit a decrease of gain due to the interference of the concurrent task with the perception being measured (Guedry, 1974). In the control experiment, VOR gain is the same during the reproduction profile, whether it is passively or actively travelled. Therefore, both 'active task' effects could well take place, compensating each other, and overwhelmed by the velocity profile effect.

A striking observation is the dissociation between the post-rotatory nystagmus and the delay awaited by the subjects before to start the reproduction. Whereas we thought that this "free delay" would provide an incidental measure of post-rotatory sensations duration, this shows that ocular nystagmus is not a valid index of these sensations.

Finally, the main result is that there is no correlation whatsoever between the performance in the reproduction task and the gain of the VOR. While VOR has been compared to a concurrent magnitude estimator for motion perception (Israël et al. 1993), the present results demonstrate that in complete darkness, the VOR does not contribute to angular self-motion perception, which actually validates its role of perception estimator.

ACKNOWLEDGMENTS

This work was supported by the GIS "Sciences de la Cognition" (France) and HFSP (RG-71/96B).

REFERENCES

Berthoz A, Israël I, Georges-François P, Grasso R, Tsuzuku T (1995) Spatial memory of body linear displacement: What is being stored ? Science 269: 95–98

Guedry FE (1974) Psychophysics of vestibular sensation. In: Kornhuber HH (ed) Handbook of Sensory Physiology; Vol. VI/2. Springer Verlag, Berlin, Heidelberg, New York, pp 3–154

Israël I, Fetter M, Koenig E (1993) Vestibular perception of passive whole-body rotation about horizontal and vertical axes in humans: goal-directed vestibulo-ocular reflex and vestibular memory-contingent saccades. Exp Brain Res 96: 335–346

Israël I, Sievering D, Koenig E (1995) Self-rotation estimate about the vertical axis. Acta Otolaryngol (Stockh) 115: 3–8

Israël I, Bronstein AM, Kanayama R, Faldon M, Gresty MA (1996) Visual and vestibular factors influencing vestibular "navigation". Exp Brain Res 112: 411–419

Israël I, Grasso R, Georges-Francois P, Tsuzuku T, Berthoz A (1997) Spatial memory and path integration studied by self-driven passive linear displacement .1. Basic properties. J Neurophysiol 77: 3180–3192

Kasper J, Diefenhardt A, Mackert A, Thoden U (1992) The vestibulo-ocular response during transient arousal shifts in man. Acta Otolaryngol (Stockh) 112: 1–6

Metcalfe T, Gresty MA (1992) Self-controlled reorienting movements in response to rotational displacements in normal subjects and patients with labyrinthine disease. Ann NY Acad Sci 656: 695–698

20

STATIC VESTIBULO-OCULAR BRAINSTEM SYNDROMES

Three-Dimensional Modeling and Stimulation

S. Glasauer, A. Weiß, M. Dieterich, and Th. Brandt

Neurologische Universitätsklinik und Zentrum für Sensomotorik
Klinikum Großhadern
LMU München

1. INTRODUCTION

Vestibular brainstem syndromes can be classified clinically according to the three main planes of action (Brandt and Dieterich 1994) of the vestibulo-ocular reflex (VOR): horizontal (yaw), frontal (roll), and sagittal (pitch). Ocular signs of a tone imbalance of the VOR in the roll plane include skew deviation, skew torsion, and torsional nystagmus; in the pitch plane, they are conjugate vertical deviation and downbeat or upbeat nystagmus. Since the neuronal circuit of the VOR operates in both co-ordinate systems of the sensors (otoliths and semicircular canals) and of the actors (ocular muscles), the same upward neuronal pathways have to be used for ocular movements in the roll and pitch planes (Brandt and Dieterich 1995). It is only the different activation patterns of these pathways which determine the plane of action (roll or pitch).

As a result of animal experiments (anatomic and electrophysiological) revealing the ipsilateral and contralateral, excitatory and inhibitory connections (Büttner and Büttner-Ennever 1988) between the individual semicircular canals and otoliths, on the one hand, and the ocular muscles, on the other (3-neuron reflex arcs), it is possible to model the VOR in three planes. While building on earlier models of the VOR which addressed the phasic aspects of the VOR, i.e., nystagmus and eye velocity (Robinson 1982; Vilis and Tweed 1988), our model focuses on different aspects: (1) it explains the effect that the "graviceptive" inputs have on the static eye position; (2) its aim is to yield a detailed bilateral modeling of the brainstem structures involved (vestibular and oculomotor nuclei) as well as their well-known anatomic interconnections.

Current Oculomotor Research, edited by Becker *et al.*
Plenum Press, New York, 1999.

2. MODELING

2.1. The Influence of Gravity on Static Eye Position and Listing's Plane

According to the data on the relationship between the orientation of Listing's plane and head position in monkeys (Haslwanter et al. 1992), the effect of head position on static eye position is solely determined by utricular afferents. Markham (1989) and Bucher et al. (1992) draw the same conclusion from ocular counterroll studies in humans (a shift of Listing's plane is equivalent to static ocular counterroll). Findings of Citek and Ebenholz (1996) on the "straight-ahead" eye position for different body positions in humans support this, although vertical version may require additional saccular input. In summary, for static ocular counterroll, the change of primary position is approximately proportional to lateral head acceleration with a gain of about 5 deg/g. A corresponding relationship holds for the tilt of Listing's plane in response to head pitch.

In the following, we assume that utricular input determines the static position of Listing's plane and thus ocular counterroll and vertical version. The eye muscle innervation m can be related to eye position by $r=T*(m-m_{ref})$, where r is the eye position rotation vector, T the transformation matrix of the anatomical mapping (Robinson 1982), and m_{ref} the muscle innervation vector in reference position (Haustein 1989). m is regarded as the difference between agonist and antagonist muscle activity and can be interpreted as motoneuron activity due to the proportional relationship of muscle innervation and pooled motoneuron activity (Hepp and Henn 1985).

While eye position depends on the muscle innervation m, a change of Listing's plane by utricular input requires that both T and m_{ref} are modified (non-corresponding superposition, Haustein 1989). Accordingly, the torque produced by the eye muscle pairs depends linearly on the innervation m and quadratically on a superimposed static neuronal input c_{ag} and c_{ant} to both agonist and antagonist muscle pairs from the utricular afferents. Primary eye position thus can be written as $r_{ref}=T*m_{ref}=G*U*a$ where G is a gain matrix and U a matrix describing the mapping of head acceleration a onto the utricle. In terms of superimposed static innervation, the primary position is $r_{ref}=T*(c_{ag}^2-c_{ant}^2)$. Hence, the required static neuronal input to the eye muscles is $c_{ag}^2-c_{ant}^2=T^{-1}*G*U*a$. These simple relationships already permit simulation of the static changes of Listing's plane in response to head tilts.

2.2. The Effect of Peripheral and Central Lesions

To simulate unilateral lesions, we must rewrite the present model for left and right sides and introduce anatomical connections and brainstem centers between otoliths and muscles. We assumed that the well known canal-ocular pathways (3-neuron reflex arcs) are shared by the, yet unknown, static otolith-ocular projections. The relative weight of parallel pathways, such as the ascending tract of Deiters (ATD), the brachium conjunctivum (BC), or the medial longitudinal fasciculus (MLF) is not known; therefore, we must make further assumptions that can be tested with data from patients after acute lesions of the peripheral nerve or in different regions of the brainstem. Acute unilateral vestibular lesions lead to ocular torsion of both eyes toward the affected side and skew deviation. Therefore, it can be assumed that both left and right utricles project to both eyes. This assumption was corroborated by electrical stimulation of the utricular nerve in the cat (Suzuki et al. 1969): stimulation of the left utricular nerve resulted in eye muscle contractions of the ipsilateral medial rectus (MR), superior rectus (SR), and superior oblique (SO) and the contralateral lateral rectus (LR), inferior rectus (IR), and inferior oblique (IO). This fits well the model outlined above; the projection of one utricle apparently excites the ipsilateral agonists and the contralateral antagonists.

A peripheral lesion on the ipsilateral side can be modeled to be equivalent to full inhibition of one utricle, corresponding to a utricular acceleration input of more than 2 g (Fernandez and Goldberg 1976). Assuming this, a simulated peripheral ipsilateral lesion will produce conjugate ocular torsion of about 5 deg in both eyes and vertical skew deviation of about 5 to 6 deg with a different sign for both eyes. Larger values, as sometimes found in patients, can be easily achieved by assuming a higher acceleration value for complete inhibition of the utricle.

Simulation of brainstem lesions, such as those involved in Wallenberg's syndrome, require further model refinement. Assuming that the mapping of utricular afferents to the eye muscle coordinate system is done in the vestibular nuclei, we can define the pathways within the brainstem. The known excitatory connections from the vestibular nuclei fit perfectly to the necessary excitatory connections from both sides in our model. For purposes of the simulation, the parallel pathways mentioned above (BC, MLF) have been given the same relative strength. Now we can simulate a lesion of the ipsilateral MLF above the crossing of the midline : this will weaken the projections to the ipsilateral IR and contralateral SR and disconnect the ipsilateral IO and the contralateral SO. The simulation yields 5.5 deg of intorsion and 2.5 deg of upward skew of the contralateral eye and 4.9 deg of extorsion and 4.5 deg of downward skew of the ipsilateral eye. These values are similar to those found in patients.

3. DISCUSSION

With the present model, we were able to simulate the effect of vestibular and brainstem lesions on static eye positions. Surprisingly, otolith activity alone is, according to our model, sufficient to explain skew deviation and ocular torsion not only qualitatively, but even quantitatively. Thus, our relatively simple model confirms earlier hypotheses about the otolithic origin of these clinical signs (e.g., Zee and Hain 1993; Dieterich and Brandt 1992).

The assumptions of the model are rather simple: static head roll causes a shift of Listing's plane (ocular counterroll) and static forward/backward head pitch causes a tilt of Listing's plane. The utricular afferent information is projected via the vestibular nuclei and the oculomotor nuclei to the eye muscles, presumably to the tonic muscle fibers, in an asymmetric fashion (non-corresponding superposition) as suggested by Haustein (1989). Hence, utricular information causing static eye position deviations is supposed to interact with voluntary gaze commands only at the level of eye mechanics, thereby changing Listing's plane without affecting voluntary gaze commands. Peripheral lesions are then simulated by inhibition of the affected utricle, brainstem lesions by inhibiting the corresponding motoneurons.

Further refinement of our model is, however, necessary. Inhibitory pathways, commissural pathways between the vestibular nuclei, resting discharge of the various nuclei, and co-contraction of the eye muscles have to be included to predict more realistically the clinical signs of various lesions of the vestibular nerve and the otolith-ocular pathways.

REFERENCES

Brandt Th, Dieterich M (1994) Vestibular syndromes in the roll plane: topographic diagnosis from brainstem to cortex. Ann Neurol 36: 337–347

Brandt Th, Dieterich M (1995) Central vestibular syndromes in roll, pitch and yaw planes. Neuro-Ophthalmology 15: 291–303

Bucher UJ, Mast F, Bischof N (1992) An analysis of ocular counterrolling in response to body positions in three-dimensional space. J Vest Res 2: 213–220

Büttner U, Büttner-Ennever JA (1988) Present concepts of oculomotor organization. In: Büttner-Ennever JA (ed) Neuroanatomy of the oculomotor system. Elsevier, Amsterdam, pp 3–32

Citek K, Ebenholz SM (1996) Vertical and horizontal eye displacement during static pitch and roll postures. J Vest Res 6: 213–228

Dieterich M, Brandt Th (1992) Wallenberg's syndrome: lateropulsion, cyclorotation, and subjective visual vertical in thirty-six patients. Ann Neurol 31: 399–408

Fernandez C, Goldberg JM (1976) Physiology of peripheral neurons innervating otolith organs of the squirrel monkey. II. Directional selectivity and force-response relations. J Neurophysiol 39: 985–995

Haslwanter Th, Straumann D, Hess BJM, Henn V (1992) Static roll and pitch in the monkey: shift and rotation of Listing's plane. Vision Res 32: 1341–1348

Haustein W (1989) Considerations on Listing's law and the primary position by means of a matrix description of eye position control. Biol Cybern 60: 411–420

Hepp K, Henn V (1985) Iso-frequency curves of oculomotor neurons in the rhesus monkey. Vision Res 25: 493–499

Markham Ch (1989) Anatomy and physiology of otolith-controlled ocular counterrolling. Acta Otolaryngol Suppl 468: 263–266

Robinson DA (1982) The use of matrices in analyzing the three-dimensional behavior of the vestibulo-ocular reflex. Biol Cyb 46: 53–66

Suzuki JI, Tokamasu K, Goto K (1969) Eye movements from single utricular nerve stimulation in the cat. Acta Otolaryngol 68: 350–362

Vilis T, Tweed D (1988) A matrix analysis for a conjugate vestibulo-ocular reflex. Biol Cyb 59: 237–245

Zee DS, Hain TC (1993) Otolith-ocular reflexes. In: Sharpe JA, Barber HO (eds) The vestibulo-ocular reflex and vertigo. Raven Press, New York, pp 69–78

21

PROPRIOCEPTIVE EVOKED EYE MOVEMENTS

G. Schweigart, F. Botti, A. Lehmann, and T. Mergner

Department of Neurology
University of Freiburg, Germany

Stimulation of neck afferents by torsion of the head relative to the trunk elicits the cervico-ocular reflex (COR; Barany 1906, 1918/19; Jürgens and Mergner 1989) and rotations of the lower trunk or the legs relative to the stationary upper body also elicit reflexive eye movements (Grahe 1926, Warabi 1978; Botti et al. 1995). We reevaluated these proprioceptive eye responses since their functional relevance was unknown so far.

Seven adult healthy subjects participated. Stimuli consisted of horizontal rotations:

  i. Whole body rotation (vestibular stimulus, VEST)
 ii. En bloc rotation of shoulders, pelvis and feet relative to the stationary head (neck proprioceptive stimulus, NECK)
iii. Rotation of pelvis and feet relative to the stationary shoulders and head (trunk proprioceptive stimulus, TRUNK; torsion about the spinal column mainly at lower thoracic levels)
 iv. Rotation of the feet relative to the pelvis (leg proprioceptive stimulus, LEG).

Usually, sinusoidal stimuli were used and either peak angular displacement or stimulus frequency was kept constant (±8°, Fig. A,B or 0.05/0.2 Hz, Fig. C, resp.). In addition, a transient smoothed position ramp stimulus profile was used with NECK ('cosine bell velocity', Fig. D). Horizontal and vertical eye movements were recorded using an infra-red device (IRIS, Skalar; sampling rate, 100 Hz). After eliminating saccades >0.2° and eye blinks and after drift correction we evaluated the horizontal slow components. Eye responses evoked by sinusoidal stimulation were analyzed in terms of gain and phase using the fundamental waves of a fast Fourier transformation.

Sinusoidal NECK or TRUNK evoked an eye response with the slow component in the direction of the relative movement of the head (Fig. A), while the response to LEG was oriented in the opposite direction (i.e. in that of the feet, Fig. B). In contrast, the gain behavior of all three responses was similar, with very low median gain at mid- to high frequencies but increasing gain at low frequencies (tested down to 0.0125 Hz; for comparison, responses to VEST are shown in B). This gain behavior, however, is mainly due to a gain non-linearity for low angular velocities rather than depending on frequency (cf. Fig.

Current Oculomotor Research, edited by Becker *et al.*
Plenum Press, New York, 1999.

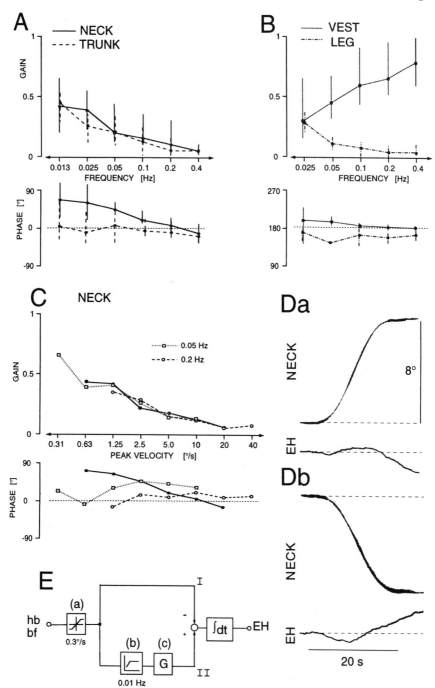

Figure 1. A-C, Gain and phase values of eye responses are shown with respect to (relative) head movement. Values obtained with sinusoidal horizontal rotations are plotted as a function of stimulus frequency (A,B; peak amplitude, 8°; interconnected median values and their 95% confidence intervals) or of peak stimulus velocity (C, mean values obtained with NECK). D, Cumulative desaccaded slow eye-in-head position (EH; grand averages) to a smoothed ramp-like NECK stimulus (superpositions of individual stimuli) towards the right (a) and the left (b). E, Model of proprioceptive input to the gaze stabilizing network (hb, bf: head-on-body and body-on-feet velocity, resp.). Further details in text.

C for NECK; similar results were obtained for LEG, not shown). During transient NECK (Fig. D) the neck response, noticeably, consisted of two components - an initial head-directed eye shift (phasic component, anti-compensatory) followed by a shift in the opposite direction (compensatory tonic component).

We suggest that proprioceptive stimulation evokes two responses: (i) A tonic component shifts the eye in the direction of the trunk or feet thereby stabilizing the eye, by compensating for slow head movements in the dark. (ii) A phasic component of opposite direction, which can neutralize the tonic one and which may be useful during reorienting gaze shifts in humans. The phasic component was only found in the neck response and not in the leg response. One simple model (Fig. E) successfully simulated the results of both leg and neck responses during sinusoidal and transient stimulation. Since the eye responses were weak, the proprioceptive input in the model is restricted to low velocities by a velocity saturation (a). Then, the signal is fed into the gaze network via two pathways (I, II) which differ in their dynamics (high pass filter b in II) and directional sign. The model simulates either leg or neck responses by selecting an appropriate weight for the gain (c) of pathway II.

ACKNOWLEDGMENT

Supported by DFG Me 715.

REFERENCES

Barany R (1906) Augenbewegungen durch Thoraxbewegungen ausgelöst. Zbl Physiol 20: 298–302

Barany R (1918/1919) Über einige Augen- und Halsmuskelreflexe bei Neugeborenen. Acta Otolaryngol (Stockh) 1: 97–102

Botti FM, Schweigart G, Mergner T (1995) Eye movements evoked by leg-proprioceptive and vestibular stimulation. In: Findlay JM et al. (eds) Eye Movement Research, Elsevier Science BV, pp 109–118

Grahe, K. (1926) Beckenreflexe auf die Augen beim Menschen und ihre Bedeutung für die Drehschwachreizprüfung des Vestibularapparates. Z Hals-Nasen-Ohrenheilk 13: 613–616

Jürgens R, Mergner T (1989) Interaction between cervico-ocular and vestibulo-ocular reflexes in normal adults. Exp Brain Res 77: 381–390

Warabi T (1978) Trunk ocular reflex. Neurosci Lett 9: 267–270

22

PURSUIT-DEPENDENT DISTRIBUTION OF VERGENCE AMONG THE TWO EYES

Casper J. Erkelens

Helmholtz Institute
Utrecht University, P.O. Box 80.000
3508 TA Utrecht, The Netherlands

1. ABSTRACT

Recordings of eye movements show that fixations of monocular and binocular details of a moving stereogram induce different smooth eye movements. Simulations show that such eye movements cannot be explained by existing models of smooth pursuit and vergence. Examination of their dynamics shows that the smooth eye movements are composed of voluntary smooth pursuit and involuntary vergence. The distribution of smooth pursuit among the two eyes is fixed, however, the distribution of vergence is adjustable. Distribution of vergence depends on the eye that fixates the pursued target. The consequence of the adjustable distribution of vergence is that the oculomotor system uses eye-of-origin information of the pursued target for the control of vergence.

2. INTRODUCTION

Recently, Erkelens & van Ee (1997a,b) investigated the laws of binocular visual direction under dynamic viewing conditions. In their study, the subjects viewed large random-dot stereograms of which the half-images oscillated in counterphase. Recordings of eye movements showed that fixation of monocular and binocular details of the moving stereogram induced different smooth eye movements. The top part of Fig. 1 shows a stereogram similar to the one used by Erkelens & van Ee (1997b). If subjects are asked to fixate the monocular line that is visible to the left eye, their eye movements (Fig. 1, bottom) appear to be asymmetrical. The left eye pursues its stimulus much better than does the right eye, although the left and right half-images including the line oscillate with the same frequency and amplitude. The line oscillates in phase with the random-dot pattern of the left half-image so that there is no relative retinal motion.

Current Oculomotor Research, edited by Becker *et al.*
Plenum Press, New York, 1999.

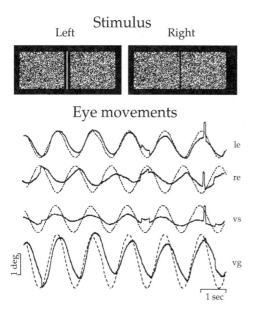

Figure 1. Eye movements induced by an oscillating stereogram (stimulus) consisting of two random-dot half-images and a vertical line visible to the left eye (le), right eye (re), version (vs) and vergence (vg) are measured by the scleral coil technique during fixation of the monocular line.

Tracking by the left eye is superior in amplitude and phase to tracking by the right eye. Tracking by the right eye is superior if the monocular line is presented in the right half-image. In order to understand this tracking behaviour, smooth eye movements are simulated by a simple model which incorporates a smooth pursuit and a vergence subsystem. The smooth pursuit subsystem generates eye movements in response to the left-right oscillations of the monocular line. In accordance to Hering's law of equal innervation, the smooth pursuit subsystem causes movements of the two eyes that are equal in amplitude and direction. In the model, smooth pursuit has a gain of 0.95 and a phase lag of 5 degrees in response to the target frequency of 0.75 Hz. These values are similar to those measured in pure pursuit tasks (Yasui & Young, 1984). The vergence subsystem responds to the disparity induced by the left-right oscillations of the random-dot stereogram. In accordance to Hering's law of equal innervation, the vergence subsystem causes movements of the two eyes that are equal in amplitude and opposite in direction. In the model, vergence has a gain of 0.65 and a phase lag of 40 degrees in response to the target frequency of 0.75 Hz. These values are similar to those of vergence induced by full-field oscillating stereograms (Erkelens & Collewijn, 1985).

The measured (Fig. 1) and simulated (Fig. 2) eye movements show striking differences. Tracking by both eyes is much better than predicted by the model. Tracking of the version target (vs) is much worse than predicted. Tracking of the vergence target (vg) is well predicted by the model. The simulations show that the eye movements in response to the oscillating stereogram cannot result from the addition of conjugate smooth pursuit and disjunctive vergence. Violating Hering's law of equal innervation by manipulating the output signals of the model shows that two different asymmetrical distributions of smooth pursuit and vergence can describe the observed eye movements equally well. In one version of the model, called model A, the smooth pursuit signal is sent exclusively to the eye viewing the monocular line and half of the vergence signal is sent to the other eye. In the other version, called model B, the pursuit signal is sent to both eyes (i.e. pursuit follows Hering's law of equal innervation) and the vergence signal is sent exclusively to the eye which does not view the monocular line. In an experiment, the validity of these two alter-

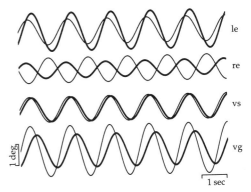

Figure 2. Stimulation of eye movements produced by a symmetrical (conjugate) pursuit subsystem in conjunction with a symmetrical (disjunctive) vergence subsystem. Target (thin lines) and eye movements of the left eye (le), right eye (re), version (vs) and vergence (vg) are simulated during pursuit of the monocular line.

native models is investigated by changing the stimulus conditions. The stereogram of Fig. 1 is used as the stimulus, however, the random-dot half-images and the monocular line are oscillated with different frequencies.

3. METHODS

3.1. Subjects

Two subjects participated in the experiments. None of them showed any visual or oculomotor pathologies other than refraction anomalies. The subjects had normal or corrected-to-normal vision. They were checked for normal stereo vision by means of partially decorrelated random-dot test images (Julesz, 1971). The subjects were experienced in stereoscopic experiments.

3.2. Eye Movement Recording

The positions of the two eyes were measured with scleral sensor coils (Skalar Delft, The Netherlands) connected to an electromagnetic system for recording eye movements (Skalar S3020) based on amplitude detection. The dynamic range of the recording system was from d.c. to better than 100 Hz (3 dB down), noise level less than + 3' and deviation from linearity less than 1% over a range of + 25 deg. The head position of the subjects was restricted by a chin rest and a head support. Horizontal and vertical positions of the eyes were digitised on-line at a frequency of 512 Hz and stored in digital format with a resolution of 3'. In the off-line analysis, eye position signals recorded in calibration trials were used to calibrate the eye position signals of all trials. Vergence was calculated by subtracting the right target and eye positions from the left ones. Version was calculated by averaging the right and left target and eye positions.

3.3. Stimuli

The half-images were generated at a frequency of 70 Hz by an HP 750 graphics computer and back-projected on a fronto-parallel translucent screen by a projection TV (Barco Data 800). The subject was seated about 1.5 m in front of the screen. One image was projected on the screen after passing through a green filter and was observed by the right eye through a green filter. Red filters were used to make the other image visible exclusively to the left eye. Between stimuli the screen was blanked for two seconds. The subjects were not restricted in their head and eye movements. The stereogram was viewed in a completely dark room. Figure 1 shows the stereogram that was used in the various experiments. The anaglyphic stereogram contained two equal squares (20 x 20 deg) filled with black (50%) and white random dots (dot size: 16 x 16'). In the half-images the two squares were placed next to each other with gaps of 16' and 32' respectively. The half-images oscillated as a whole in counterphase with each other with a fixed frequency of 0.75 Hz and an amplitude of 40', resulting in peak-to-peak vergence changes of 160'. Despite the oscillations, the subjects perceived a completely stationary stereogram during binocular viewing. The two random-dot patterns were perceived to be at fixed positions side by side, one pattern appearing a little closer than the other. A vertical line (16' x 30 deg) was placed either in the left or in the right half-image. The line oscillated with a frequency of 0.75 Hz in phase with the half-image viewed by the same eye (Fig. 1) or with a frequency of 0.125 Hz (Fig. 3).

4. RESULTS

4.1. Pursuit and Vergence of Different Frequencies

Pursuit of the monocular line by the left eye (le) is affected by the different frequency of the random-dot patterns (Fig. 3). Although the line oscillates at a slow frequency of only 0.125 Hz, pursuit is less accurate than if line and random-dot pattern oscillate at the same high frequency of 0.75 Hz (compare the signals le in Figs 1 and 3).

The movement of the left eye shows a small oscillation of 0.75 Hz superimposed on the slow oscillation of 0.125 Hz. The movement of the right eye shows the reverse pattern, a small drift-like oscillation of 0.125 Hz is superimposed on the fast oscillation of 0.75 Hz. Both frequency components are also present in the version signal. The vergence movements differ from the left eye, right eye and version movements in that vergence shows only one frequency component, namely, the frequency of 0.75 Hz of the random-dot pattern motion.

4.2. Simulations of Pursuit and Vergence

The eye movements shown in Fig. 3 are simulated by the models A and B in which the smooth pursuit subsystem controls the tracking of the eyes in response to the motion of the monocular line and the vergence subsystem responds to the oscillations of the ran-

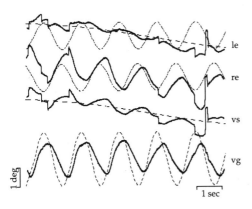

Figure 3. Eye movements induced by the oscillating stereogram shown in Fig. 1. Target (dashed lines) and eye movements of the left eye (le), right eye (re), version (vs) and vergence (vg) were recorded during fixation of the slowly oscillating line.

dom-dot patterns. The dynamics of these subsystems are given in the introduction section. In model A, the pursuit signals are sent only to the eye viewing the monocular line. Half of the vergence signal is sent only to the other eye.

Figure 4 shows the simulated eye movements produced by model A. As a consequence of the strict separation of smooth pursuit and vergence, the left and right eyes oscillate at different frequencies. Version and vergence show both frequencies, the low smooth-pursuit frequency and the high vergence frequency. This behaviour is essentially different from the eye movements shown in Fig. 3 in which the left eye, right eye and version show oscillations containing two frequency components and vergence oscillates at a single frequency. The differences between simulated and recorded eye movements show that a complete separation of smooth pursuit and vergence does not explain the asymmetrical eye movements.

In model B, the pursuit signals are sent to both eyes simulating a purely conjugate system and the vergence signal is sent only to the eye that does not view the monocular line.

Figure 5 shows the simulated eye movements produced by model B. As a consequence of the asymmetrical vergence distribution, the left eye oscillates only at the low pursuit frequency. The right eye movement shows both frequencies because this eye receives the smooth pursuit and the vergence signals. Version shows both frequency components too. Vergence only show the high frequency component because the smooth-pursuit signals are sent to both eyes which after subtraction do not appear in the vergence movements. This behaviour is rather similar to the eye movements shown in Fig. 3 in which the right eye and version show oscillations containing two frequency components and vergence oscillates at a single frequency. The left-eye movements of the model are not fully realistic. The recorded eye movements show slight oscillation at the high vergence frequency which are absent in the simulations. A much better result requires only a minor adjustment of the model. In model B, the vergence signal is exclusively sent to the right eye. However, if a slightly different distribution is used, namely 10% of the vergence signal to the left eye and 90% to the right eye, the simulated signals are very similar to the recorded ones in all respects. The signals of the left eye, right eye and version show both frequency components and vergence oscillates at a single frequency.

5. DISCUSSION

5.1. Smooth Pursuit and/or Vergence?

The eye movement recordings of Fig. 1 show that fixation of monocular details of a symmetrically oscillating stereogram induces asymmetrical smooth eye movements. An

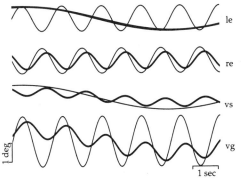

Figure 4. Simulations of eye movements produced by an asymmetrical pursuit subsystem in conjunction with an asymmetrical vergence subsystem. Target (thin lines) and eye movments of the left eye (le), right eye (re), version (vs) and vergence (vg) are simulated during pursuit of the monocular line.

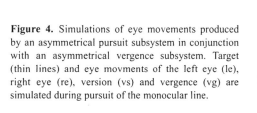

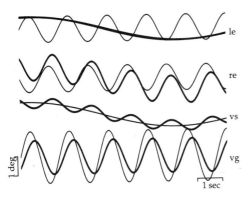

Figure 5. Simulations of eye movements produced by a symmetrical (conjugate) pursuit subsystem in conjunction with an asymmetrical vergence subsystem. Target (thin lines) and eye movments of the left eye (le), right eye (re), version (vs) and vergence (vg) are simulated during pursuit of the monocular line.

obvious question is: are these eye movements a combination of smooth pursuit and vergence or is the smooth pursuit subsystem not involved in the task and are we just looking at asymmetrical vergence movements? This question is relevant in particular because the subjects do not perceive any motion of the line or random-dot patterns if the left half-image, including the line, and the right half-image oscillate in counterphase (Erkelens & van Ee, 1997a,b). Thus, the subjects see a stationary line, which does not have to be voluntarily pursued, against a stationary background. If the line and the random-dot patterns oscillate with different frequencies, the subjects see a line oscillating in a combination of two frequencies against a stationary random-dot pattern. The conviction that Fig. 1 shows combinations of smooth pursuit and vergence is based on the dynamics of the movements. The left eye oscillates without hardly any phase lag relative to its target, whereas the right-eye oscillation shows a phase lag of about 40 deg. The zero phase lag of the left eye is characteristic of smooth pursuit (Carpenter, 1988) and the phase lag of the right eye is characteristic of vergence induced by large stereograms (Erkelens & Collewijn, 1985). If we would assume that the eye movements were generated by a single vergence subsystem producing asymmetrical movements, we would expect equal phase lags of the movements of both eyes.

5.2. Adjustable Distribution of Vergence

Interaction between smooth pursuit and vergence has been studied previously to investigate the validity of Hering's law of equal enervation (Miller, Ono & Steinbach, 1980; King & Zhou, 1995; Enright, 1996). In these studies the targets were smooth pursuit and vergence stimuli at the same time. In the present study the stimuli of smooth pursuit and vergence are separated; the oscillating monocular line is only a stimulus for smooth pursuit; the symmetrically oscillating random-dot patterns are only stimuli for vergence. The eye movements and the simulations clearly show that smooth pursuit is a conjugate system. The distribution of vergence among the two eyes appears to be adjustable. If the smooth pursuit subsystem tracks a monocular target, the vergence responses are predominantly induced in the eye to which the smooth pursuit target is not visible. Adjustable distribution of vergence is a clever mechanism in the control of smooth eye movements. The mechanism allows accurate tracking of the monocular target without interference by vergence induced by the surround. The adjustable distribution of vergence does not affect stereopsis negatively because the limit of binocular fusion depends on the difference between the eye movements which remains unaffected. Thus, during pursuit of a monocular

Figure 6. A flow diagram of the control of smooth eye movements. It contains essential elements and signals involved in the interaction between smooth pursuit and vergence. Thick lines mark the signals involved in the adjustable distribution of vergence.

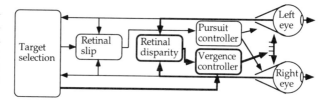

target the adjustable distribution of vergence permits optimal reduction of retinal slip and retinal error of the pursued target in combination with optimal reduction of disparity of the surround.

5.3. Consequences for the Control of Vergence

The fact that the distribution of vergence among the two eyes is adjustable has implications for the organisation of the oculomotor system. The monocular line is not a stimulus of the vergence subsystem. This means that adjustment of the distribution cannot be a mechanism of the vergence subsystem itself but must be imposed on this subsystem.

Figure 6 shows a simple scheme of the control signals involved in the generation of smooth eye movements. An attentional mechanism selects the target, i.e. the monocular line, from the visual field. The target can induce retinal slip and retinal error which are used for the control of smooth pursuit. In general, target selection plays a role in the control of vergence too (Erkelens & Collewijn, 1991). However, the monocular target does not induce retinal disparity which implies that the target is irrelevant for the control of vergence. Vergence movements are induced by disparity of the random-dot surround. The distribution of vergence among the eyes can be controlled by mechanisms involved in the selection of the target. Another option is that the distribution of vergence is adjusted by the smooth pursuit subsystem. The major difference between the two types of control is that adjustment is limited to smooth eye movements if it is controlled by the smooth pursuit subsystem. Adjustment of the distribution can be generalised to saccadic eye movements if it is controlled by mechanisms involved in target selection. A consequence of the adjustable distribution of vergence is that the control mechanism needs to have access to eye-of-origin information of the target. Howard and Rogers (1995) are convinced that eye-of-origin information must be available to the vergence system. The conviction is based on the observation that the eyes make appropriate vergence responses to crossed and uncrossed disparities, even in open-loop situations (Howard, 1970). However, the same argument can be given for appropriate depth perception. Appropriate vergence and depth perception only show that eye-of-origin information must be implicitly present in binocular neurones. The present results show a new phenomenon, namely that eye-of-origin information of a target which is irrelevant for vergence is used to control the distribution of vergence among the two eyes.

REFERENCES

Carpenter R.H.S. (1988). Movements of the eyes. London: Pion Limited.
Enright J.T. (1996) Slow-velocity asymmetrical convergence: a decisive failure of "Hering's law". Vision Research 36, 3667–3684.

Erkelens C.J. & Collewijn H. (1985). Eye movements and stereopsis during dichoptic viewing of moving random-dot stereograms. Vision Research 25, 1689–1700.

Erkelens C.J. & Collewijn H. (1991). Control of vergence gating among disparity inputs by voluntary target selection. Experimental Brain Research 87, 671–678.

Erkelens C.J. & van Ee R. (1997a). Capture of visual direction: an unexpected phenomenon in binocular vision. Vision Research 37, 1193–1196.

Erkelens C.J. & van Ee R. (1997b). Capture of visual direction of monocular objects by adjacent binocular objects. Vision Research, 37, 1735–1745.

Erkelens C.J., van der Steen J., Steinman R.M. & Collewijn H. (1989). Ocular vergence under natural conditions. I. Continuous changes of target distance along the median plane. Proceedings of the Royal Society of London B236, 417–440.

Julesz B. (1971). Foundations of cyclopean perception. Chicago, Ill.: University of Chicago press.

Howard I.P. (1970). Vergence, eye signature, and stereopsis. Psychonomic Monograph Supplements 3, 201–204.

Howard I.P. & Rogers B.J. (1995). Binocular vision and stereopsis. pp. 600–602. New York, NY.: Oxford University Press.

King W.M. & Zhou W. (1995)Initiation of disjunctive smooth pursuit in monkeys: evidence that Hering's law of equal innervation is not obeyed by the smooth pursuit system. Vision Research 35, 3389–3400.

Miller J.M., Ono H. & Steinbach M.J. (1980) Additivity of fusional vergence and pursuit eye movements. Vision Research 20, 143–147.

Yasui S. & Young L.R. (1984) On the predictive control of foveal eye tracking and slow phases of optokinetic and vestibular nystagmus. Journal of Physiology (London) 347, 17–33.

23

COUPLED PERTURBATION EFFECTS DURING 3D TARGET-TRACKING INDICATING A SHARED CONTROL STAGE FOR SACCADES AND VERGENCE

J. A. M. Van Gisbergen and V. Chaturvedi

Department of Medical Physics and Biophysics
University of Nijmegen
The Netherlands

1. INTRODUCTION

The oculomotor field has a tradition of specialised studies that concentrate either on one of the various types of version eye movements, such as saccades, or on vergence movements. In the case of the saccadic and the vergence systems, it is often assumed that these can be regarded as distinct oculomotor subsystems that generate conjugate and disconjugate binocular command signals, respectively, and that their neural control systems at the premotor level are largely separate. When studied in isolation, there are indeed striking differences between the temporal characteristics of these systems. These distinctions are clearly reflected in the general layout of saccade and vergence models. Models of the saccadic system stress that saccades are too fast to allow direct visual feedback, that the system is not continuous but has to be switched on and off, and contain specific proposals about the neuronal circuitry implementing this gating mechanism. By contrast, vergence models have often assumed that these slow eye movements are directly guided by visual feedback and that they are generated by a continuous system. A number of recent studies have compared the dynamic behaviour in combined saccade-vergence movements with the temporal characteristics of pure saccades and pure vergence movements. This work showed that the combined version-vergence movement is not simply a linear summation of the required components executed in isolation. A general finding is that the dynamical characteristics of the combined movements cannot be predicted from either component alone: the saccadic component appears to be slower (Collewijn et al. 1995) and the vergence component is faster than when either movement is executed in isolation (Enright 1984, 1986; Erkelens et al. 1989; Maxwell and King 1992). The latter phenomenon, which has been widely studied, is known as saccadic-vergence facilitation. These developments have led to combined mod-

Current Oculomotor Research, edited by Becker *et al.*
Plenum Press, New York, 1999.

els in an attempt to account for these interactions. One explanation for saccade-vergence en-hancement dismisses the notion that saccades are always conjugate and proposes that this system can contribute a fast depth component by generating unequal saccades in the two eyes (Erkelens et al. 1989; Zhou and King 1997). Another suggestion is that pause cells, long thought to be exclusively engaged in saccade initiation, can modulate the activity of the vergence system (Zee et al. 1992; Mays and Gamlin 1995). All these studies, which im-ply that the systems responsible for movements in direction and depth operate in a dynami-cally coherent fashion, have left open the equally interesting question of how the brain can ensure that both will opt for the same target. While it is obvious that binocular eye move-ments require precise coordination for achieving successful bifoveal fixation of interesting stimuli, remarkably little is known on how this is achieved. It appears that the typical ex-perimental design with a single target is unsuitable for studying this problem. Instead, one has to confront the oculomotor system with a situation requiring target selection in 3D, a task which has never been the object of study so far. By contrast, there is a considerable body of knowledge on the behaviour of the saccadic system in a target selection task. This work has shown that the initial saccadic response to a target-nontarget pair is not necessarily directed to either one or the other stimulus but may show a compromise saccade directed in between when the spatial separation is not too large (Findlay 1982; Ottes et al. 1985). The system shows a clear speed-accuracy trade off allowing it to avoid errors by prolonging its latency. The ability for target selection has previously also been shown in the vergence sys-tem (Erkelens and Collewijn 1991).

We have investigated the behaviour of the system when confronted with a target-nontarget pair in 3D visual space, arranged in a spatial arrangement which forced each subsystem to make a response that could be rated as correct to incorrect, or as anything in between. In this way it was possible to assess to what extent target selection in the two subsystems was coupled. A complete report will appear elsewhere (Chaturvedi and Van Gisbergen, 1998). We have also undertaken neurophysiological experiments in the supe-rior colliculus (SC) to learn more about the neural substrate of combined saccade-ver-gence movements. While the monkey was engaged in a tracking task, electrical stimulation was used as a perturbation to test whether the colliculus might be involved in both saccade and vergence control.

2. METHODS

Eye movements were recorded binocularly from seven subjects using methods de-scribed in Chaturvedi and Van Gisbergen (1997). All trials began by requiring fixation of a green stimulus at straight ahead with a target vergence of 7.5 deg. After the fixation light was extinguished, subjects were either presented with a single green target (80%) or a green stimulus-red nontarget stimulus pair (20%). The target stimulus in both types of trial appeared randomly at one of the eight corners of a 3D LED array which had the fixation point at its centre. In direction, these stimuli always required a horizontal displacement of 20 deg, either to the left or to the right, and a vertical refixation of 10 deg, either up or down. Since the green target was simultaneously presented in depth at a nearer or a farther plane, the task additionally required a 2.5 deg movement in either a converging or diverg-ing direction. The single-target trials served to collect a large number of control responses in order to characterise unperturbed target-selection responses. In the double-stimulus tri-als, the red nontarget always appeared on the same horizontal side as the green target but with diametrically opposite vertical and depth coordinates. For example, in a trial where the green stimulus appeared in the right-far-up location, the red nontarget stimulus would be presented at the right-near-down position. Thus, the task for the oculomotor system required an up-down choice by the saccadic system and a far-near selection from the vergence system. Note that, in theory, this task could lead to discordant responses where the one system made a correct decision while the other erred, causing a binocular response which would bring the eyes to a location where there was no stimulus at all. In the example given above, the combination of a correct saccade and an incorrect vergence movement would bring the eye to right-near-up, both away from the green and the red stimulus. Since little would be learned if subjects would simply make no errors, they were encouraged to make short-latency responses.

In the analysis of the data we concentrated on the characteristics of the first movement which was defined as the change in binocular refixation occurring between the onset of the first and the onset of the second saccade. In trials where a second saccade did not appear, offset was taken at 200 msec after onset. With this definition, the refixation included both the intra- and post-saccadic vergence response. In order to be able to pool data from the eight different target-nontarget configurations, it was necessary to find a way of normalising the data. Exploiting the fact that the target-nontarget configurations always appeared on the same horizontal side of the 3D LED array, but on opposite corners (see above), we defined a gain measure which expressed the ratio between the actual displacements in the refixation and the required displacements. To illustrate, a gain value of +1.0 indicates that the response in the first movement was precisely on target whereas a gain of -1.0 denotes a fully incorrect response to the red nontarget. Since, not surprisingly, the horizontal saccade components were nearly always correct, only the gain of the vertical saccade component (which reflects the choice made by the saccadic system) and that of the vergence component will be discussed further.

For the neurophysiological experiments, two monkeys were trained to refixate a visual target when it jumped from a central location in a far plane to a peripheral location in a nearer depth plane. In 20% of these tracking trials, the oculomotor system was perturbed by applying electrical stimulation (50 msec pulse train at 500 Hz) at a caudal site in the deeper layers of the SC. Invariably, electrical stimulation, by itself, produced only a saccade vector with no vergence. The location of the visual target was chosen to ensure that the required saccade had an amplitude comparable to the electrically-induced saccade but with a direction offset of some 45 deg. Electrical stimulation, just above threshold for consistently evoking a saccade, was applied at various points in time after presentation of the visual target.

3. RESULTS

3.1 Target-Selection Experiments in Humans

Before the double-stimulus trial responses can be properly evaluated, it is essential to obtain a good picture of the characteristics of control responses. As expected, the saccadic response to the single target locations had straightforward temporal profiles with mean gain values close to +1 (range among subjects: 0.88 - 1.00). By contrast, the vergence response had a more complex time course, due to the effect of transient divergence, and showed both intra- and post-saccadic contributions. Despite this complexity, the total vergence contribution at the end of the first movement of the control responses had mean gains varying from 0.92 to 1.01 in our subjects, indicating that they were almost normometric, similar to the saccades. We found, nevertheless, many diverse combinations of intra and postsaccadic vergence contributions, which ranged from responses where the in-

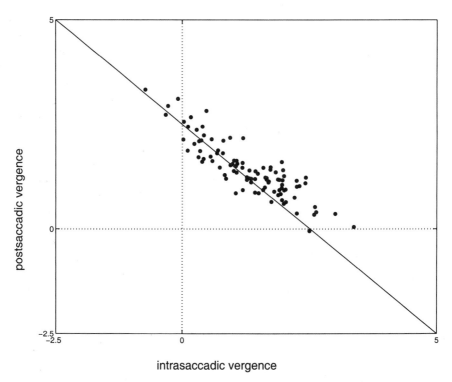

Figure 1. Relative contributions of the intrasaccadic portion and the postsaccadic episode to converging control responses in the first movement. Intrasaccadic vergence reflects the vergence occurring during the primary saccade. Postsaccadic vergence refers to the movement between the offset of the first saccade and the end of the first movement (onset second saccade). Note that there is a wide distribution in the sizes of the intrasaccadic and the postsaccadic phase. The bold line (slope -1) indicates all possibilities of how the sum of the two components can yield an accurate total movement, corresponding to the required vergence change of 2.5 deg. The data points (subject JVG) can be seen to straddle this line. A similar phenomenon was seen in other subjects.

trasaccadic part was almost negligible and the postsaccadic contribution was substantial, to others where the intrasaccadic portion predominated. Figure 1 provides a picture of this variability by showing the relative contributions of intrasaccadic and postsaccadic vergence of the converging responses to nearby control targets. It is clear that if we had taken primary saccade offset as the end criterion, the intrasaccadic portion of the response would, in a number of cases, hardly have shown any net convergence at all. Since a similar scenario was observed for diverging responses we found that, at the time of primary saccadic offset, it was often difficult to discriminate between near and far target refixations. Accordingly, it appears that by limiting the initial response to the duration of the (fast) saccade one would not be able to obtain a correct impression of the vergence component of the binocular refixation. Instead, the first movement concept, as we defined it, does not have this problem as the large post-saccadic vergence contribution makes up for the shortcomings of the intra-saccadic episode, thereby separating the characteristics of near and far responses. In the ensuing analysis our attention will, therefore, be focused on the first movement as reflecting the initial refixation response.

Before discussing the gain values obtained in double-stimulus trials, it is instructive to look at some selected examples of the raw data that illustrate the range of response vari-

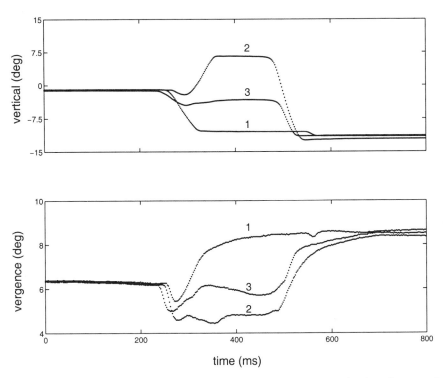

Figure 2. Illustrative examples of responses from subject JVG to a target-nontarget stimulus pair presented on the left side of the fixation point. In all cases shown here, the green target was located downward in the near plane while the red nontarget was presented upward in the far plane.

ability encountered. Trace 1 in Figure 2 shows an example of a correct binocular response that brought the eyes close to the target. Trace 2, by contrast, shows an incorrect saccadic response followed by a large corrective movement later in the trial. The vergence response, which has a more complex temporal profile due to transient divergence, shows the same pattern. The most remarkable response is shown in trace 3 which is typical of a compromise response (averaging) in both the saccadic and in the vergence component. Note also that, in both trials 2 and 3, the vergence response does not correct its error right away but pauses before it executes a corrective movement to the target, timed to be in conjunction with the corrective saccade. This pattern is typical for all subjects and seems to further justify the first movement concept as the basic element of action in a system with a step-by-step mode of operation. The saccade and the vergence response in these examples show concordant behaviour in the sense that the degree of error in performance seems to be correlated. To further explore the validity of this impression, we analysed to what extent the gain values of saccadic and vergence responses were correlated.

By plotting gain values of vertical saccade gain and vergence gain against each other, it is possible to characterise the entire set of first movement responses, in double-stimulus trials, in a concise fashion (see Figure 3). To facilitate interpretation of this figure, we have labelled the responses shown earlier in Figure 2. As expected, the nearly correct response (1) is seen to have gain values close to +1 for both the saccade and vergence, the almost wholly incorrect response (2) has strongly negative gains while the averaging response has intermediate gain values closer to 0. The conclusion to be drawn

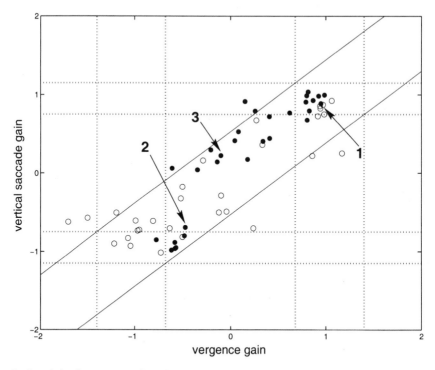

Figure 3. Correlation between saccade and vergence responses to double stimulus in subject JVG. Dotted lines are based on the 95% confidence limits of control responses in the same subject. Converging and diverging responses, denoted by filled and open symbols, respectively, show the same pattern.

from the total data set is that the saccade and vergence components show the entire gamut of behaviour from correct to incorrect and, equally interesting, that this variability in the two systems is highly coupled. Indeed, the correlation coefficient characterising this linkage between saccadic and vergence target selection had a consistently high value, not only in these data ($r = 0.86$), but also in all other subjects investigated in this study (range 0.78 - 0.94). The fact that intermediate gain values were common in both the saccadic and the vergence component clearly shows that the saccadic system retains its averaging tendency in short-latency responses when the response is accompanied with a vergence eye movement. Remarkably, this property is equally prevalent in the vergence response where it has not been shown so directly before. However, in some of our subjects, averaging was absent or rare in both the saccadic and the vergence response. These subjects tended to make responses with an all-or-nothing characteristic in that their binocular movements were either directed to the target or all the way to the nontarget, a bistable response pattern found earlier in the saccadic system for large stimulus separations. It should also be added that averaging, as well as incorrect responses, became rare when subjects were emphatically instructed to avoid errors, but such improved performance inevitably occurred at the cost of increased latencies, much in line with the speed-accuracy trade-off earlier demonstrated in the saccadic system. We found the trade-off to be much the same for both saccades and vergence, indicating that these shared characteristics reflect a common stage, operating at a level where 3D information is available.

It is also of interest to emphasise what was not found in the experiments. Close in-spection of Figure 3 reveals that discordant responses, where one system made the correct response to the green target (gain near +1) while the other chose the red nontarget (gain near -1), simply did not occur. Similar findings were obtained in all other subjects except one where discordant behaviour was seen on very rare occasions. That the behaviour of sac-cades and vergence in the target selection task was not independent could be shown more formally with a chi-square test in which the actual number of observed responses in the various cells shown in Figure 3 was compared to the expected number if both systems would have behaved independently. The chi square value was found to be significant at the p = 0.01 level, showing that the null hypothesis, supposing independence, should be re-jected.

3.2 Neurophysiological Perturbation Experiments in Monkeys

Signals reflecting stimulus location in 3D space have been found in various regions of the visual cortex (for review see Trotter 1995) and in area LIP of the parietal cortex (Gnadt and Mays 1995). Since it is known that LIP carries depth information to the SC (Gnadt and Beyer 1998), the question arises whether the colliculus may be involved in the control of vergence movements, along with its well-established role in saccade control. Our approach in the neurophysiological experiments was to perturb the oculomotor sys-tem by SC electrical stimulation at a time when the monkey was preparing, or had just in-itiated, a 3D refixation to a newly presented target. Our goal was to see whether any effects on vergence, besides the expected change in saccade responses, could be demon-strated. As explained above (Methods), the experiment was designed to ensure that the control responses to separate electrical (E) and visual (V) stimulation yielded responses with clearly distinct saccade and vergence directions. We consistently found that E-control trials yielded the saccade expected on the basis of the stimulated site in the SC motor map, but did not show any vergence response. Accordingly, one might suppose that electrical stimulation, applied in conjunction with a visual target in 3D (EV trials), would only inter-fere with the required saccadic response, leaving vergence unaffected. Two key observa-tions in the perturbation experiments suggest a different story.

First, presenting the E-stimulus in the stage of response preparation, before the ani-mal would normally initiate a response to the V-stimulus, caused an electrically-triggered movement (EV-response) which had a vergence component directed toward the visual tar-get along with the expected saccade (see Figures 4 and 5). Stimulation very early in the preparation phase (just after target onset) elicited no vergence and just a saccadic compo-nent that was almost identical to the control E-response. When the electrical stimulus was shifted to a late stage in the preparation phase, just before the monkey would have initi-ated the movement, we observed a consistent trend that both the saccade and the vergence component of the movement reflected a growing influence of the visual target and became less dominated by the E-stimulus which again triggered the response. This suggests that the EV-response, in both subsystems, represents a weighted average between the presum-ably relatively constant effect of the E-stimulus and the gradually emerging effect of the V-stimulus.

Second, when the E-stimulus was delayed long enough so that the monkey had al-ready initiated the movement (VE-response), the accompanying vergence response was modified in midflight, causing it to remain markedly smaller than in the absence of E-stimulation. In these cases, the 3D movement initially followed the V-control trajectory

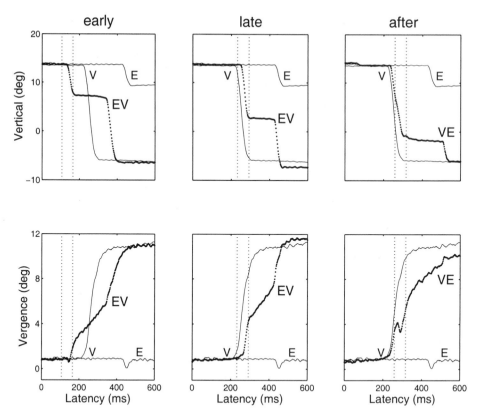

Figure 4. Responses in three trials where the electrical stimulus train (dotted lines) was timed to occur at an early stage of response preparation, shortly after the presentation of the visual stimulus (left-hand panel), at a late stage of preparation (middle panel) and after the monkey initiated the movement (right-hand panel). Control responses (E and V) are denoted by continuous thin lines while the EV and VE responses are shown in bold dotted lines. Note that in the trial where the E-perturbation occurred early, the EV response is still E-dominated but shows a clear effect of the visual stimulus, both in the saccade and in vergence. This effect of the V-stimulus is still more pronounced in the middle panel where the response is again E-triggered. In the trial where the movement was initiated by the monkey (right-hand panel), an initial vergence response with the same time course as the V-control can be observed. The applied E-stimulus subsequently causes a major vergence perturbation which accompanies a concomitant modification in the metrics of the saccade.

(see Figures 4 and 5). Subsequently, both the saccade and the vergence response deviated transiently in the direction of the E-control trajectory.

4. DISCUSSION

If the execution of refixations in 3D involves distinct oculomotor systems (see Introduction) the question arises how the brain can ensure that these subsystems select the same target in a richly-filled natural environment. The results of our behavioural experiments, demonstrating strong coupling in target selection by the two oculomotor subsystems, are most parsimoniously explained by assuming a common selection system operating at a level where 3D information is available. Although the task imposed a simple two-alternative choice, the actual response, in both subsystems, showed a wide range

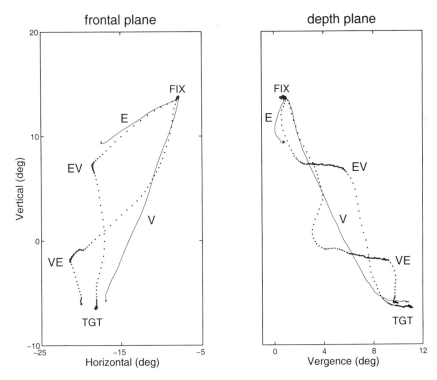

Figure 5. Trajectories of combined saccade-vergence movements projected on the frontal plane and the depth plane to show the perturbation effects elicited by electrical stimulation in the superior colliculus. Response EV corresponds to the left-hand panel in Figure 4. Response VE was visually initiated but perturbed in midflight (right-hand panel in Figure 4). Control trajectories E and V are shown as thin continuous lines. Note that the EV response first shows an E-dominated compromise. The VE response initially proceeds along the V-trajectory, as expected, and then veers off as a result of the electrical perturbation which affects both the amplitude of the vertical saccade component and of the vergence response. FIX and TGT denote the location of the fixation point and the visual target, respectively.

of compromising behaviour. Thus, it appears that this characteristic is not an exclusive property of the saccadic system where it has been studied extensively (see Introduction). The fact that the degree of averaging may vary stochastically from trial to trial, but in a highly coupled fashion in the two subsystems, supports the notion of a shared central control stage for both. So far, little can be said with certainty about where in the brain this shared selection process may be embodied. Since area LIP contains neurons with 3D tuning curves (Gnadt and Mays 1995), which have a capacity for representing target and non-target stimuli differently (Platt and Glimcher 1997), this region seems a very interesting candidate for further exploration.

The neurophysiological perturbation experiments have revealed two distinct effects of electrical SC stimulation on vergence, involving the initiation (WHEN) and the metric-specification (WHERE) systems, respectively, which were not expressed when E-stimulation was applied in isolation. That the saccade component showed similar behaviour is not surprising in view of earlier combined EV stimulation studies in the SC (Glimcher and Sparks 1993) and fits the classical picture which depicts the SC as a saccade-related area. Likewise, our finding that E-stimulation, by itself, evoked a saccade but did not cause any change in vergence is in line with the classical concept that the SC specifies a desired saccadic displacement but is not involved in vergence control.

Whether the newly-discovered vergence effects are a direct reflection of signal processing inside the SC or whether they arise indirectly cannot be determined at this moment. Assuming the former, we will now discuss a hypothetical collicular coding scheme that seems to allow a simple interpretation of our findings. As to the WHEN effect on the vergence system, the simplest explanation would be that the saccadic and the vergence system share a common gating system. This possibility has been proposed before (Zee et al. 1992; Mays and Gamlin 1995) and is supported by our finding (unpublished observations) that electrical stimulation of the rostral pole of the SC can prevent a 3D refixation. Any explanation of the vergence WHERE effects in the perturbation experiments should allow for the fact that such effects were absent when SC electrical stimulation was applied in isolation. Further challenges are to understand how averaging in the vergence response may come about and how tonic vergence affects the outcome of E-stimulation (Billitz and Mays 1997).

It has been shown that the monkey SC has access to depth information from the parietal cortex (Gnadt and Beyer 1998) and a recent study in the cat has shown that many cells in the superficial layers have binocular visual receptive fields with various types of disparity-sensitivity profiles (Bacon et al. 1998). Unfortunately, there are no published reports on the characteristics of movement fields for refixations with a depth component. Let us assume that deeper layer movement cells make use of the depth information available to the SC and that their movement fields are 3D. To be specific, assume further that each movement field is tuned so as to be matched with the depth tuning of the binocular receptive field of the same cell. This means that the rule that visual receptive field and movement field are matched, which is well-established for 2D, is now extended to 3D. If, at a given location in the SC map, movement cells sharing the same direction preference in the HV plane but differing in their depth preference are randomly intermingled, it is easy to see that their indiscriminate activation by electrical stimulation would yield a net depth command signal equalling zero. Based upon population coding, the final outcome in EV trials would be a weighted average of the signal carried by the population of E-activated neurons and the population of V-activated cells. As we saw, the E-population would vote for the locally represented saccade and a zero desired vergence displacement. The V-population would vote for a different saccade vector and a vergence component leading the eyes to the target. From this point of view, the absence of a vergence movement in E-control responses should not be falsely interpreted as an indication that the SC is only concerned with saccades and is therefore simply silent about what vergence should do. On the contrary, we propose that the population of E-activated cells emphatically demands a 3D movement with zero vergence and that it is this insistence on a zero vergence movement which could be the cause of a major disturbance in the vergence component of EV responses. It is not immediately clear how this hypothesis might explain the divergence effects as a result of E-stimulation during near target fixation (Billitz and Mays 1997). The experiments reported here were done during far-plane fixation. Clearly, in the absence of single unit studies showing that SC movement cells are actually tuned in depth, the present interpretation of our findings can only be preliminary.

ACKNOWLEDGMENT

This study was supported by the Foundation for Life Sciences (SLW) and the Netherlands Organization for Scientific Research (NWO).

REFERENCES

Bacon BA, Villemagne J, Bergeron A, Lepore F, Guillemot JP (1998) Spatial disparity coding in the superior colliculus of the cat. Exp Brain Res 119: 333–344.

Billitz MS, Mays LE (1997) Effects of microstimulation of the superior colliculus on vergence and accommodation. Invest Opthalmol Vis Sci 38: S984.

Chaturvedi V, Van Gisbergen JAM (1997) Specificity of saccadic adaptation in three-dimensional space. Vision Res 37: 1367–1382.

Chaturvedi V, Van Gisbergen JAM (1998) Shared target selection for combined version-vergence eye movements. J Neurophysiol , accepted for publication.

Collewijn H, Erkelens CJ, Steinman RM (1995) Voluntary binocular gaze-shifts in the plane of regard: dynamics of version and vergence. Vision Res 35: 3335–3358.

Enright JT (1984) Changes in vergence mediated by saccades. J Physiol Lond 350: 9–31.

Enright JT (1986) Facilitation of vergence changes by saccades: influences of misfocused images and of disparity stimuli in man. J Physiol Lond 371: 69–87.

Erkelens CJ, Collewijn H (1991) Control of vergence: gating among disparity inputs by voluntary target selection. Exp Brain Res 87: 671–678.

Erkelens CJ, Steinman RM, Collewijn H (1989) Ocular vergence under natural conditions. II. Gaze shifts between real targets differing in distance and direction. Proc R Soc Lond B236: 441–465.

Findlay JM (1982) Global processing for saccadic eye movements. Vision Res 22: 1033–1045.

Glimcher PW, Sparks DL (1993) Effects of low-frequency stimulation of the superior colliculus on spontaneous and visually guided saccades. J Neurophysiol 69: 953–964.

Gnadt JW, Mays LE (1995) Neurons in monkey parietal area LIP are tuned for eye-movement parameters in three-dimensional space. J Neurophysiol 73: 280–297.

Gnadt JW, Beyer J (1998) Eye movements in depth: what does the monkey's parietal cortex tell the superior colliculus? Neuroreport 9: 233–238.

Maxwell JS, King WM (1992) Dynamics and efficacy of saccade-facilitated vergence eye movements in monkeys. J Neurophysiol 68: 1248–1260.

Mays LE, Gamlin PDR (1995) Neuronal circuitry controlling the near response. Curr Opin Neurobiol 5: 763–768.

Ottes FP, Van Gisbergen JAM, Eggermont JJ (1985) Latency dependence of colour-based target vs nontarget discrimination by the saccadic system. Vision Res 25, 849–862.

Platt ML, Glimcher PW (1997) Responses of intraparietal neurons to saccadic targets and visual distractors. J Neurophysiol 78: 1574–1589.

Trotter Y (1995) Cortical representation of visual three-dimensional space. Perception 24: 287–298.

Zee DS, Fitzgibbon EJ, Optican LM (1992) Saccade-vergence interactions in humans. J Neurophysiol 68: 1624–1641.

Zhou W, King WM (1997) Monocular rather than conjugate saccade burst generators in paramedian pontine reticular formation (PPRF). Soc Neurosci Abstr 23: Part I, 7.

24

LISTING'S PLANE ORIENTATION WITH VERGENCE

Effect of Disparity and Accommodation

Z. Kapoula,[1] M. Bernotas,[2] and T. Haslwanter[3]

[1]Laboratoire de Physiologie de la Perception et de l'Action
CNRS-College de France UMR 9950
11 place Marcelin Berthelot, 75005 Paris, France
[2]University of Siauliai
Faculty of Technology
Vilniaus St. 141, 5400 Siauliai, Lithuania
[3]Department of Neurology
University Hospital Tübingen
Hoppe Seyler Str. 3, D-72076 Tübingen, Germany

1. INTRODUCTION

According to Listing's law, all eye positions can be reached from the reference position by rotations about axes which lie in a plane, provided the head is stationary (Helmholtz 1867; Ruete 1853). It is known that when the eyes converge upon proximal targets Listing's law still holds but Listing's plane rotates temporally. This causes elevation-dependent torsion: the eyes intort for up proximal gaze and extort for down proximal gaze (Mikhael et al. 1995; Minken and Van Gisbergen 1994; Mok et al. 1992; Van Rijn and Van den Berg 1993). In the following, we will call the tilt of Listing's plane as a function of vergence *Listing's Plane Vergence Tilt (LPVT)*. The functional significance of the LPVT is not clear. In his comprehensive study, Tweed (1997) gives several possible interpretations. A first hypothesis would be that LPVT is a strategy for motor efficiency, allowing to keep the eyes in an eccentric position with minimal effort. A second hypothesis associates that tilt with a functional role for binocular vision, e.g. to obtain binocular single vision of lines orthogonal to Listing's plane or, more likely, to reduce the cyclodisparities of the visual planes themselves. A third hypothesis states that it might be both a strategy for motor efficiency as well as a strategy subserving binocular visual function.

To gain insight on the functional significance for vision we examined whether the LPVT depends on the visual conditions, namely on the stimuli driving convergence of the

Current Oculomotor Research, edited by Becker *et al.*
Plenum Press, New York, 1999.

165

eyes. The main stimuli driving vergence are binocular disparity and blur (disfocused images). Blur induces accommodation, convergence, and pupil constriction (the well known near triad, for a review see Semmlow and Hung, 1983). The amount of accommodative convergence is described by the ratio Accommodative Convergence/Accommodation (AC/A), which is about 3 to 4 in normals, see Von Noorden (1990). Mutually, convergence can influence accommodation; this coupling is known as Convergence Accommodation/Convergence ratio (CA/C). These reciprocal interactions and couplings are well integrated in current thinking and modelling of the vergence system (for reviews see Schor and Kotulak, 1986; Mays and Gamlin 1995). In the present study disparity was manipulated alone or together with accommodation and the orientation of Listing's plane was measured. If LPVT is the result of a motor strategy the gain of the rotation (tilt of Listing's plane/convergence) should be the same regardless of the stimulus driving convergence. We report here that this is not the case. Disparity-vergence alone changed the orientation of Listing's plane for all subjects almost immediately. Addition of accommodation did not induce significant change in the vergence angle of the two eyes. Yet, Listing's plane orientation changed immediately; the change was idiosyncratic for different subjects.

2. MATERIALS AND METHODS

2.1. Subjects

Three subjects (two male and one female), were studied. Their ages were 20, 30 and 38 yr. Each subject underwent complete neuro-ophthalmologic examination. Subject PB had a small hyperopia of +0.5 D in the left eye that stayed uncorrected during the experiment. Binocular vision of subjects was normal (stereoacuity was 60 sec arc or better in the TNO random dot test). Subjects participated in the experiment after giving informed consent.

2.2. Testing Conditions

In a dichoptic viewing setup, three subjects sat 1 m in front of a flat, translucent screen. The head was stabilised by a bite bar with individually fitted dental impression of the subject's upper teeth. Two projectors were used to project a grid subtending (33° x 33°). To separate the images for each eye, the polarisation of the two beams differed by 90°, and the subjects had an appropriate polariser in front of each eye. The room was completely dark, and the subject could see only the projected grids. Two X-Y mirror-galvanometers (General Scanning CCX660) were used to position the grids on the screen (for more details see Kapoula et al. 1996). Subjects were asked to look at the different nodes of the grid. They made vertical saccades (16° up, 16° down) along the midline and among tertiary positions. Three conditions were run:

1. *Far viewing:* The two grids were centered on a screen, placed at 1 m from the subject. Subjects fused them and saw a single grid. The expected horizontal vergence angle was 3.4°.
2. *Partial simulation of close viewing:* The grids were cross-offset on the screen by 13.5° for two subjects (FK and PD) and 8.6° for subject PB (the left eye grid shifted to the right the right eye grid shifted to the left). This caused convergence of the eyes. Accommodation and convergence were in conflict in this situ-

ation. Accommodation, at least at the beginning of this condition, was at 1 m, i.e. at the distance of the physical screen.

3. *Quasi-complete simulation of close viewing:* The grids remained cross-offset, as in the prior condition, and a -3 diopters spherical lens was inserted in front of each eye to adjust accommodation to convergence.

In both conditions, the simulated viewing distance was 26 cm for subjects FK and PD and 40 cm for subject PB. The three different conditions succeeded each other at the rate of 2–3 min; each condition lasted about 1–2 min. Thus, we studied instantaneous changes of the orientation of Listing's planes in conditions simulating artificially close viewing. During each condition subjects made saccades at their natural rate.

2.3. Eye Movement Recording

Stimulus presentation and data collection were directed by a software developed under MS-DOS for real-time experiments (REX) and run on a PENTIUM PC. Three-dimensional eye movements were recorded from both eyes with the dual search-coil method (SKALAR two magnetic fields, Collewijn et al. 1975; Robinson 1963). The eye position signals were low-pass filtered with a cut-off frequency of 200 Hz and digitized with a 12-bit analog-to-digital converter. Each channel was sampled at 500 Hz. The data were stored on the disk for off-line analysis.

To determine the sensitivity of the search coils, an in-vitro calibration was performed with a Fick gimbal before each experiment. At the beginning of each experiment we did an in-vivo calibration during which the subject fixated monocularly a pair of nonius-lines (two parallel lines spaced by 2 min of arc); the lines stepped vertically in the mid-sagittal plane of the measured eye. The subjects were instructed to fixate as accurately as possible between these two lines. The same calibration procedure was repeated at the end of each experiment. For the data calibration we used the algorithm developed by Hess et al. (1992).

2.4. Data Analysis

Eye position data were expressed as rotation vectors (Haustein 1989). For the data representation, we used the commonly employed Cartesian head-fixed coordinate system with the positive x-, y-, and z-axis pointing forward, leftward, and upward, respectively. The x-component of the rotation vector indicates a torsional, the y-component a vertical, and the z-component a horizontal eye position; positive eye movements are leftward, downward and clockwise (CW). We calculated the best fit plane to the data, called "Displacement Plane", and its orientation. Due to the geometry of 3-dimensional rotations, the tilt of the primary position - and thus of Listing's plane - is twice the tilt of the displacement plane (Haslwanter 1995).

The vergence angle was calculated by subtracting the horizontal position of the right eye from the horizontal position of the left eye. The reference position was taken from the calibration data. The same data were used to calculate the vergence and to determine the displacement planes. The horizontal and vertical orientation of Listing's plane was determined by calculating the angle between the vector perpendicular to Listing's plane and the midsagittal plane and the horizontal plane, respectively. Since we want to investigate the effects of vergence on Listing's plane, we concentrate below on the horizontal orientation of Listing's plane.

To determine the LPVT, we subtracted the value of the orientation of the plane for each condition simulating close-viewing from the one in the far-control condition (1 m viewing distance). This was done for each eye individually. The change in vergence from the far condition was also measured. The gain of the tilt of Listing's plane was determined by

gain = (LPVT of the left eye + LPVT of the right eye) / change in vergence angle (1)

3. RESULTS

3.1. Thickness of Listing's Plane

Fig. 1 shows the thickness of Listing's plane for each individual eye in each condition, as well as the group means. The thickness of the Listing's planes was always below

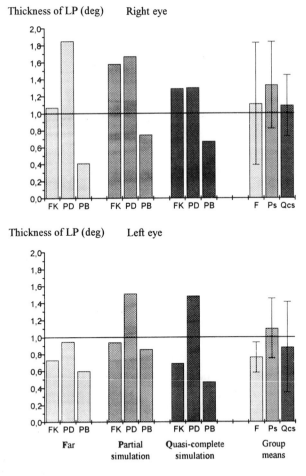

Figure 1. Thickness of Listing's plane for each individual eye and for each condition; the thickness is the standard deviation of eye position around the best fit plane. Group means show averages from our three subjects and the corresponding standard deviations (vertical lines).

2° (it varied from 0.41° to 1.85°). The group mean of thickness was close to 1° for all three conditions. These values are in agreement with prior studies (e.g. Mok et. al. 1992), and confirm Listing's law obedience as well as that our measuring and analysis algorithms were correct.

3.2. Vergence Gain

The measured vergence angle (in deg) is shown in Fig. 2. It was close to the expected value of vergence. The group mean vergence was also close to the expected value. Note that both the expected and the measured group mean vergence were almost the same for the two conditions simulating closeness.

3.3. Listing's Plane Orientation with Vergence

Fig. 3 shows data from subject FK for the three conditions in the order they were run. In Fig. 3A are shown top views of Listing's plane, i.e. torsion versus elevation for the left and for the right eye. Fig. 3B shows the corresponding planar fit to these data. The thin line is perpendicular to the best fit data-plane; the thick line P is the calculated primary position, which is perpendicular to Listing's plane, the horizontal tilt of the plane is indicated by the angle between P and the midsagittal plane, axis 1 (in Fig. 3B). At the control far viewing condition, the vergence angle was 3.3°. The planes were already temporally tilted by 8° in the left eye and 15° in the right eye. In the following 2 min during the close disparity condition, the vergence angle was 13.3°, and was symmetrically distributed in the two eyes (6.7° and 6.6° for the left and right eye, respectively). Listing's planes rotated temporally in both eyes; the left eye plane was tilted 16.3° left, the right eye plane was tilted 28° to right. The change from the far control condition was 8.02° in the left eye and 12.50° in the right eye; this corresponds to a gain (change in tilt of plane/change in vergence angle) of 1.54 and 2.60 for the left and right eye. Thus, disparity vergence alone caused temporal rotation of Listing's plane immediately and without prior adaptation to the disparity. The tilt was asymmetric in the two eyes even though vergence was symmetric.

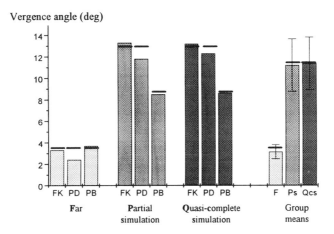

Figure 2. Measured vergence angle (left - right eye); horizontal line segments indicate the expected vergence angle.

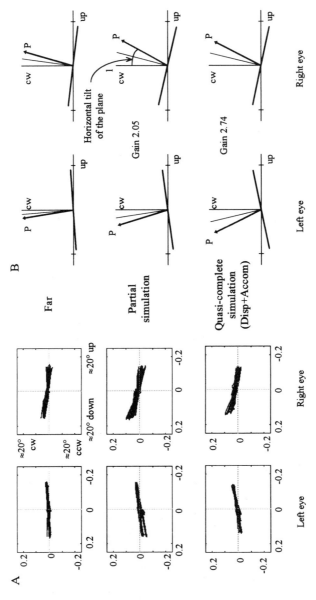

Figure 3. A) Torsion versus elevation of left and right eye position. B) Estimated best fit to the data, and the calculated primary position (P), and horizontal tilt of Listing's plane (see text).

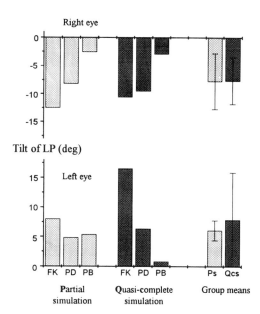

Figure 4. Tilt of Listing's plane in degrees (orientation of the plane in the far condition - orientation of the plane in the condition simulation of close). Temporal tilt is indicated by negative values for the right eye, positive values for the left eye.

In the subsequent, quasi-complete simulation condition (disparity+accommodation), the angle of convergence remained almost the same (6.2° and 7.0° for the left and right eye respectively). Insertion of a -3 D spherical lens in front of each eye in this condition aimed to bring accommodation from 1 m (distance of the screen) to 33 cm, that is close to the vergence angle and to the simulated viewing distance of 26 cm. The Listing's plane rotated more temporally in the left eye (from 16° to 25°) even though convergence of that eye was slightly reduced (from 6.7° to 6.2°); the gain of the tilt comparative to the far, control condition was now 3.51. In contrast, the plane of the right eye, shifted slightly nasally (became less temporal, from 28° to 26°) even though vergence of this eye increased (from 6.6° to 7.0°); relative to the control, in far condition the gain of the tilt of Listing's plane was 2.04. Thus, the addition of accommodative cue influenced the orientation of Listing's plane differently for the two eyes and regardless of the effect on the vergence itself.

Fig. 4 shows the tilt of Listing's plane for each individual eye. The planes were tilted temporally (to the left for the left eye, to the right for the right eye) for all subjects and conditions. For all subjects the tilt of the planes was largely asymmetric for the two eyes even though vergence was symmetric in the two eyes. The addition of accommodation in the condition quasi-complete simulation of close viewing modified the orientation of Listing's planes for all subjects relative to the partial simulation condition. The changes, however, were idiosyncratic and not consistent with the changes in the angle of convergence. The changes for subject FK were described above (see Fig. 3). For subject PD the planes of both eyes tilted more temporally relative to the partial simulation condition. This further tilt occurred even for the right eye for which the vergence angle remained unchanged. For subject PB the insertion of spherical lenses produced a drastic decrease of the temporal rotation of Listing's plane of the left eye, even though the vergence of this eye changed little (from 4.7° to 4.4° in the quasi-complete simulation condition). Thus, the accommodative cue combined with disparity-vergence influences the orientation of Listing's plane differently for different subjects.

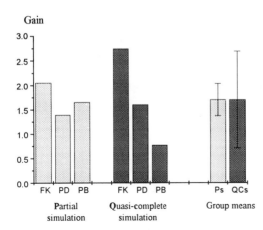

Figure 5. Individual gain of rotation of Listing's plane with vergence: (LPVT of the left eye + LPVT of the right eye)./ (change in vergence).

Fig. 5 shows the gain of Listing's plane rotation. Noteworthy is the large intersubject variability, particularly in the quasi-complete simulation condition. Individual gains ranged from 1.65 to 2.05 in the partial simulation condition; this range was even larger in the quasi-complete simulation condition (from 0.77 to 2.74). The gain in the quasi-complete simulation condition increased for two subjects (FK, PD) relative to the partial simulation, but decreased for the third subject (PB). The group mean gains are similar for the two conditions except the larger variability in the quasi-complete simulation condition.

In summary, disparity-vergence alone caused temporal rotation of Listing's planes immediately. Subsequent manipulation of accommodation influenced the orientation of Listing's plane in an idiosyncratic way.

4. DISCUSSION

This study confirms Listing's law obedience in normal subjects, since in all our conditions eye positions lay in a single plane. The thickness of Listing's planes (standard deviation of eye position around the best fit plane) averaged about 1 deg, comparable to that reported by Mok et al. (1992). The most important finding of our study is that temporal rotation of Listing's plane with convergence occurs immediately even in reduced-cue artificial situations, where vergence is driven by isolated cues. Mikhael et al. (1995) have shown that prism-induced disparity can cause tilt of the planes. In that study, however, subjects wore prisms for about 1 hr before eye movement recording, and adaptation may had been involved. Our study shows that disparity-driven vergence causes tilt of the planes instantaneously. Furthermore, it shows that subsequent manipulation of accommodation and the eventual conflict between accommodation and vergence can influence the orientation of Listing's plane. The ability of isolated visual cues to alter the tilt of Listing's plane instantaneously suggests that this is a robust phenomenon, regardless of whether its function is for motor efficiency, for visual perception, or for both.

4.1. Variability of LPVT and Dependency on Visual Conditions

The gain of the tilt of Listing's plane with convergence was highly variable between different subjects and for different testing conditions. The intersubject variability we observed contrasts with prior studies (e.g. Mikhael et al. 1995; Minken and Van Gisbergen 1994; Mok et al. 1992; Van Rijn and Van den Berg 1993), but is in agreement with the more recent study of Bruno and Van den Berg, (1997). Possible factors for the variability could be: a) the artificial nature of our conditions, i.e. our use of reduced cue situations; b) the high-rate at which the different condition succeeded each other; c) the relatively small range of vergence angle studied. The vergence in our different conditions varied from 3° to 13°; this range is smaller than the one investigated in most other studies (from infinity to 30°, Minken and Van Gisbergen 1994; Mok et al. 1992). It is possible that in the limited vergence range of 3°-13°, the orientation of Listing's plane and the vergence are more loosely linked.

Another intriguing observation is that the amount by which the plane tilted could be very different between the two eyes even when the vergence was symmetric for the two eyes (see Fig.4). The most important new finding is that LPVT is influenced instantaneously by individual cues related to vergence, accommodation, or their conflict. Bruno and Van den Berg (1997) suggested that the conflict between accommodation and disparity might influence the orientation of Listing's plane and that vergence and Listing's plane orientation can be decoupled. The present study provides evidence supporting these ideas. All our conditions were artificial and contained various degrees of conflict. In the partial simulation condition, disparity-driven vergence induced a consistent change in LPVT despite the conflict between disparity and accommodation. Subsequent addition of accommodation by inserting a lens, influenced LPVT for all subjects even though the vergence (L-R eye) remained on overall the same (see Fig. 2). The LPVT rotated more temporally for subjects FK and PD, but nasally for subject PB (see Fig. 5). This observation shows that vergence changes and changes in Listing's plane orientation can be decoupled. The idiosyncratic nature of changes in the quasi-complete simulation condition is most likely due to individual differences in the strength of mutual couplings between convergence and accommodation.For instance, the rotation of Listing's plane nasally for subject PB might had been caused by a strong CA/C ration, particularly in the left eye. Convergence driven by disparity might had modify the accommodation substantially; subsequent insertion of a negative lens lelaxed accommodation and created additional conflict with vergence rather than reducing the conflict.

In summary, our findings show, that the strength of the relationship between convergence and Listing's plane temporal rotation is subject-dependent and is influenced by the stimuli driving vergence. Binocular disparity alone drives vergence and Listing's plane orientation immediately and consistently over subjects. Accommodation and mutual interaction with vergence can influence the orientation of Listing's plane but they do so in an idiosyncratic way. These observations support the hypothesis that Listing's plane rotation with convergence is not exclusively a strategy for motor efficiency.

ACKNOWLEDGMENTS

Professor Marijus Bernotas was supported by the French Medical Research Foundation.

REFERENCES

Bruno P, Van den Berg AV (1997) Relative orientation of primary position of the two eyes. Vision Res 37:935–947.

Collewijn H, Van der Mark F, Jansen TC (1975) Precise recording of human eye movements. Vision Res 15:447–450.

Haslwanter T (1995) Mathematics of 3-dimensional eye rotations. Vision Res 35: 1727–1739

Haustein W (1989) Considerations on Listing's law and the primary position by means of a matrix description of eye position control. Biol Cybern 60:411–420

Helmholtz H (1867). Handbuch der Physiologischen Optik. Leipzig: Voss. English translation: Helmholtz' treatise on physiological optics. New York: Dover (1962).

Hess BJ, Van Opstal AJ, Straumann D, Hepp K (1992) Calibration of three-dimensional eye position using search coil signals in the rhesus monkey. Vision Res 32:1647–1654.

Kapoula Z, Eggert T, Bucci MP (1996) Disconjugate adaptation of the vertical oculomotor system. Vision Res 36:2735–2745.

Mays LE, Gamlin PDR (1995) Neural circuitry controlling the rear response. Current Opinion in Neurobiology 5(6):763–768.

Mikhael S, Nicole D, Vilis T (1995) Rotation of Listing's plane by horizontal, vertical and oblique prism-induced vergence. Vision Res 35:3243–3254.

Minken AWH, Van Gisbergen JAM (1994) Three-dimensional analysis of vergence movements at various level of elevation. Exp Brain Res 101:331–345.

Mok D, Ro A, Cadera W, Crawford JD, Vilis T (1992) Rotation of Listing's plane during vergence. Vision Res 32:2055–2064.

Robinson DA (1963) A method of measuring eye movement using a scleral search coil in a magnetic field. IEEE Trans Biomed Eng 10:137–145.

Ruete CGT (1853) Lehrbuch der Ophthalmologie. Braunschweig:36–37.

Semmlow JL, Hung G (1983). The near response. Theories of control. In Vergence eye movements: Basic and clinical aspects (ed. C. Schor and K. Ciuffreda), pp. 175–195, Boston, Butterworths.

Schor CM, Kotulak JC (1986) Dynamic interactions between accommodation and convergence are velocity sensitive. Vision Res 26: 927–942.

Tweed D (1997) Visual-motor optimization in binocular control. Vision Res 37:1939–1951.

Van Rijn LJ, Van den Berg AV (1993) Binocular eye orientation during fixations: Listing's law extended to include eye vergence. Vision Res 33:691–708.

Von Noorden GK (1990) Binocular vision and ocular motility. Theory and management of strabismus (4th edn.) St Louis, MO: Mosby.

25

INTRA- AND POSTSACCADIC DISPARITY-INDUCED VERGENCE CHANGES DURING REPEATED STIMULATIONS

A. Accardo,[1*] S. Pensiero,[2] and P. Perissutti[2]

[1]D.E.E.I. Universita' di Trieste
  via Valerio 10, I34100 Trieste, Italy
[2]I.R.C.S.S. Osp. Inf. "Burlo Garofolo"
  v. dell'Istria 65/1, I34100 Trieste, Italy

1. INTRODUCTION

The two primary stimuli eliciting disjunctive eye movements are disparity and blur, which lead to fusional and accomodative vergence movements, respectively. Accomodation and fusion work together to enable clear, single vision of objects, close or distant, because normally accomodative vergence alone is not sufficient being low the AC/A ratio (from 3 to 5), which leaves a divergence of visual axes during near fixation.

Vergence eye movements are necessary not only to bring the eyes to the right alignment, but also to maintain this alignment: if a patient has a heterophoria a compensatory vergence signal is sent to the extraocular muscles, causing fusional movements. To obtain a fusional movement, disparity of the two retinal images must exceed Panum's area size and be inferior to a maximum beyond which vergence is not produced. These two values delimit the motor fusion amplitude, varying conspicuously among the subjects and with subject (tired or rested, attention level) and neuromuscular conditions.

Disparity-induced vergence may be studied alone, or in combination with saccadic or smooth pursuit eye movements. Vergence speed is known to increase when a saccade is conjoined with vergence; this facilitation is greater for divergence. Disparity-induced vergence is under adaptive control: after a training period, the vergence response is adjusted to correct for the artificially induced dysmetria (Erkelens 1987). Adaptation to anisometropic spectacles is reached by preprogramming intrasaccadic and postsaccadic disconjugate movements (Erkelens et al. 1988).

---

* E-mail: accardo@gnbts.univ.trieste.it

Current Oculomotor Research, edited by Becker *et al.*
Plenum Press, New York, 1999.

Using pattern images (necessary for a correct stimulation of the motor fusion) we elicited a disparity-induced convergence joined to a horizontal saccade. We studied the variations of the saccadic and postsaccadic eye movements among different tests to evaluate the subject's capability to pre-program both version and vergence in order to reach a sensorial fusion of the target as fast as possible. Our stimuli were all placed at the same distance from the subject's eyes to prevent that accomodative vergence worked. Stimulus disparity was already present before the refixation eye movement start.

2. MATERIALS AND METHODS

On a colour monitor, placed at 40cm in front of a normal subject (male, 40 years old), who wore red-green glasses, three types of stimuli were presented: (1) A white circular image subtending 3.9deg alternated between the primary position and a 7.3deg position on the right, appearing for 2s at each position. (2) The white image was presented in front, while to the right two types of stimulations were alternatively presented, the white image and a couple of red and green images, identical to the white one, partially superimposed to realise a disparity of 1.4deg. (3) Only the couple of coloured images was alternated to the central white image.

Horizontal eye movements were measured by means of the limbus-tracking infrared technique and sampled at 500Hz. Version was calculated as the average of, and vergence as the difference between, the positions of the two eyes. Velocity criteria were used to identify the start and the end of saccades and vergence. Version and vergence parameters (amplitude, duration and peak velocity) were then calculated and compared among the three types of stimulation.

3. RESULTS AND DISCUSSION

As expected, during the first test, vergence eye movements were minimal and occurred within some tens of ms.

In the second test the same behaviour was found in cases of white stimulation to the right, while the haploscopic stimuli produced a large variability of the required convergence movements, which started from the end of the saccade up to about 600ms after, with a large range of durations.

During the third test (typical response in Figure 1) the postsaccadic convergence lasted from 80ms to about 250ms and an immediate vergence adaptation was evident already in the first movements. From the very beginning the intrasaccadic convergence increased (from about 10% in the second test to 22% in the third test in respect to the whole convergence duration). This was due to a more precocious start of the convergence, finalised to a faster achievement of the desired final eye position. So, in cases of simultaneous saccadic and vergence stimulations, a preprogramming of the vergence together with the saccade seems to immediately occur.

In Figure 2 the vergence components during the second and the third tests are shown. As pointed out, in the second test, two different kind of behaviour are present. In the first case, the response is similar to that of the third test in which the convergence starts during the saccadic movement, on the contrary, in the second case, the convergence starts well after the end of the saccade. In Figure 3 the peak velocity, duration and latency of convergence in the second and third tests are depicted, movement by movement. The

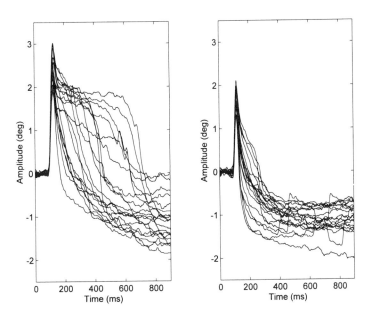

Figure 1. Example of ocular movement during the third test. Right (solid line) and left (dashed line) eye positions (top panel) and corresponding version and vergence amplitudes.

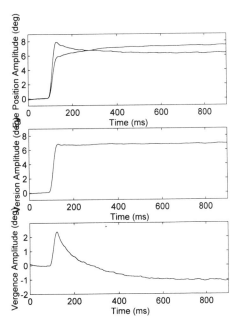

Figure 2. Saccadic responses (vergence component) during the second (left panel, only haploscopic stimulations) and the third (right panel) tests.

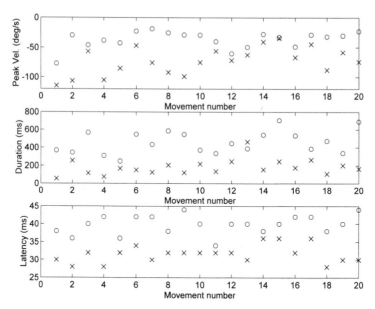

Figure 3. Characteristic parameters of the convergence component during the second (o) and the third (x) tests, movement by movement.

increase of peak velocity and the corresponding reduction of the duration in the third test support the hypothesis that a training with a repetitive stimulus decreases the time necessary to realise the disjunctive movement. Moreover a reduction of the convergence latency is evident.

Moreover, as can be seen in Figs. 2 and 3, during the second test the large variability of the convergence characteristics (in particular duration and peak velocity) as well as the occurrence of short disjunctive movements since the beginning of the test show that a pre-programming of the vergence component is immediately possible, even if repeated stimulations are not used.

ACKNOWLEDGMENTS

Work supported by the University of Trieste (MURST 60%) and by the Italian Ministry of Health.

REFERENCES

Erkelens CJ (1987) Adaptation of ocular vergence to stimulation with large disparity. Exp Brain Res, 66: 507–516
Erkelens CJ, Collewijn H, Steinman RM (1988) Asymmetrical adaptation of human saccades to anisometropic spectacles. Inv Ophth Vis Sci, 30, 1132–45

26

MODELLING VERGENCE EYE MOVEMENTS USING FUZZY LOGIC

A. S. Eadie, P. Carlin, and L. S. Gray

Glasgow Caledonian University
Glasgow G4 OBA, UK

1. INTRODUCTION

Target proximity has a significant effect on open loop accommodation and vergence. Proximal effects on accommodation and vergence are initiated by awareness of a near object. (Rosenfield et al, 1991; Rosenfield et al, 1993; Hung et al, 1996) A novel Fuzzy Logic controller has recently been used to model the effect of target proximity on the accommodation response under open and closed loop conditions. (Eadie and Carlin, 1996) The aim of the study described here was to extend the application of Fuzzy Logic to a dual interactive model of proximal accommodation and vergence.

Fuzzy logic allows the operations which govern a control system to be expressed linguistically, creating a more intuitive approach to model design and implementation. It has been shown that fuzzy logic can be used to describe any mathematical function no matter how complex. (Zadeh, 1965; Zadeh, 1994) This is especially useful in modelling natural control systems where the controller may be highly non-linear and may not be readily described by standard controllers. Thus, fuzzy logic control offers a simple, intuitive approach to modelling complex controllers.

2. METHODS

A Fuzzy Logic proximal vergence controller was developed using previously published experimental data. This controller, together with a previously developed Fuzzy Logic proximal accommodation controller, was incorporated into a dual interactive model of accommodation and vergence. The proximal input of each system was positioned after the controller and before the crosslinks (Figure 1).

The model was simulated over a range of stimuli between 0D and 6D and 0MA and 6MA. The simulations were performed for the various permutations of open and closed loop conditions in both the presence and absence of proximal inputs.

Current Oculomotor Research, edited by Becker *et al.*
Plenum Press, New York, 1999.

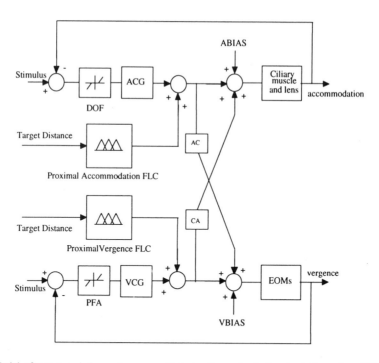

Figure 1. Model of accommodation and vergence featuring Fuzzy Logic Proximal Controllers (DOF - Depth of focus, ACG - Accommodative Controller Gain, ABIAS -Tonic Accommodation, PFA - Panum's Fusional Area, VCG - Vergence Controller Gain,VBIAS - Tonic Vergence, CA - Convergence Accommodation, AC - Accommodative Convergence EOMs - Extra Ocular Muscles).

2.1. Fuzzy Logic Proximal Controller

Fuzzy logic control is essentially a mapping procedure which relates the input of a system to the output using fuzzy sets. A list of if-then statements called rules, link the fuzzy input set to the fuzzy output set.

Here the input to the controller is target distance. This is fuzzified by the membership function to produce the fuzzy input set. Fuzzification defines the range of input values and the degree of membership is usually represented by geometrical shapes (e.g. triangular, trapezoidal, gaussian, sigmoid) arbitrarily chosen using expert knowledge. The fuzzy data value is passed to the rule evaluator which produces a fuzzy output set from a list of linguistic rules consisting of "If......then....." statements. For example: If distance is *far* then proximal accommodation is *low;* If distance is .... then proximal accommodation is ....; If distance is *near* then proximal accommodation is *high.* The fuzzy output set is passed to the response calculator (defuzzifier) which calculates the required control effort.

3. RESULTS

Steady state responses of model simulations were used to produce stimulus-response data and the contribution of proximity to the overall response was calculated from the difference between the "proximal present" and "proximal absent" model simulations (Figure 2).

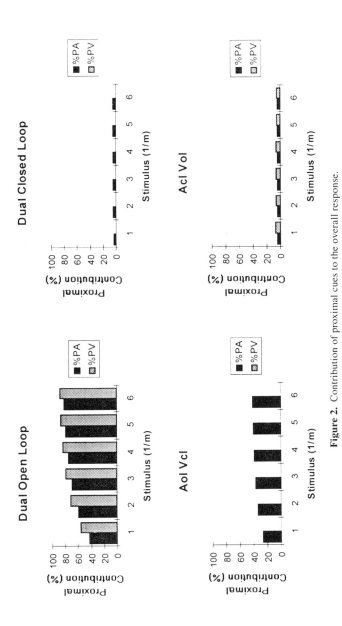

Figure 2. Contribution of proximal cues to the overall response.

3.1. Dual Open Loop Conditions

The effect of proximal cues produced a significant effect on accommodation and vergence responses (between ~ 40% and ~ 90%).

3.2. Dual Closed Loop Conditions

Closing both feedback loops produced a marked decrease in the contribution of proximity to the overall response with Proximal Accommodation (PA) and Proximal Vergence (PV) contributing approximately 4% and 0.04% respectively.

3.3. Accommodation Open Loop - Vergence Closed Loop (AOL VCL)

Proximal effects produced between 26% and 41% of the accommodation response. The vergence response is relatively unaffected by proximity with PV contributing less than 1% of the response (~0.25%).

3.4. Accommodation Closed Loop - Vergence Open Loop (ACL VOL)

Proximal effects have a very small effect on the overall response with PA 4% and PV ~6%.

4. CONCLUSIONS

The results of model simulations support previous experimental results obtained under open loop conditions and illustrate that under closed loop conditions the steady state accommodation and vergence responses are dominated by blur and disparity respectively. (Hung et al, 1996) The findings concur with a quantitative analysis of proximal accommodation and vergence and further support the use of fuzzy logic in models of oculomotor control. (Eadie and Carlin, 1996)

REFERENCES

Eadie, A S, Carlin, P and Gray, L S (1996). A New Approach in Control-Theory Modeling of Accommodation. Invest Ophthal Vis Sci 37(3):770.

Hung, G K, Ciuffreda, K J and Rosenfield, M (1996). Proximal contribution to a linear static model of accommodation and vergence. Ophthal Physiol Opt 16: 31–41.

Rosenfield, M, Ciuffreda, K J and Hung, G K (1991). The Linearity of Proximally Induced Accommodation and Vergence. Invest. Ophthal Vis Sci 32: 2985–2991.

Rosenfield, M, D'Amico, J L, Nowbotsing, S K and Ciuffreda, K J (1993). Temporal characteristics of proximally-induced accommodation. Ophthal Physiol Opt 13: 151–154.

Zadeh, L A (1965). Fuzzy Sets. Info Control 8: 338–353.

Zadeh, L A (1994). The role of fuzzy logic in modeling, identification and control. Modeling, Identification and Control 15: 191–203.

27

THE VARIATION OF CYCLOTORSION WITH VERGENCE AND ELEVATION

Jim Ivins, John Porrill, and John Frisby

A I Vision Research Unit
University of Sheffield, England S10 2TP

1. INTRODUCTION

Several recent studies of human eye movements have revealed systematic departures from Listing's law during changes in vergence. Two kinematic models of eye movements predict a vergence-dependent contribution to torsion T proportional to elevation E and vergence V (angles in radians):

$$T = kEV / 2 \tag{1}$$

The proposed value for k is either 1/2 according to Minken et al (1995) or 1 as suggested by Van Rijn and Van den Burg (1993); both values are supported by experimental evidence. These models do not obey Listing's law since the torsional state of each eye is not determined solely by its monocular fixation direction; however, they do obey a binocular generalisation of this law in which the state of the two eyes is completely determined by the fixation point.

2. METHOD

Vergence-dependent torsion was studied in five subjects by moving a fixation target inwards and outwards along the line-of-sight of the right eye at four different viewing elevations (-15°, 0°, +15° and +30°). The left eye moved to maintain binocular fixation; however, the right eye held a constant fixation direction, so any changes in its torsional state signalled departures from monocular Listing's law. This asymmetric vergence paradigm was originally used by Nakayama (1983). The torsional state of both eyes was recovered using a new video-based eye tracking system developed by Ivins et al (1997).

3. RESULTS

Monocular torsion measurements from two subjects (PD and SH) are shown in Figure 1; equivalent binocular results are shown in Figure 2.[*]

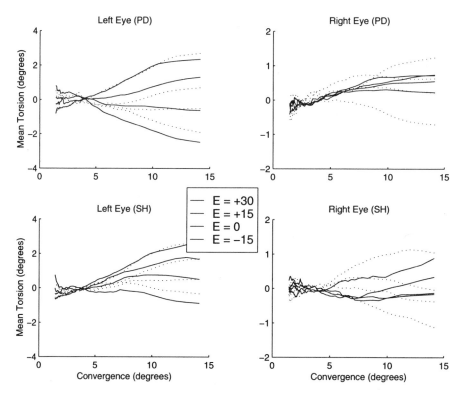

Figure 1. Variation of monocular torsion with vergence and elevation. These graphs show the monocular torsion response of two subjects during asymmetric vergence measured at four angles of right eye elevation. Graphs show mean results averaged over five trials. Solid lines indicate inward target motion, dotted lines indicate outward motion; intorsion is positive, extorsion is negative. Graph lines for different elevations of the left eye appear in the same order as the legend lines; however, this is not the case for the right eye.

3.1. Monocular

All five subjects exhibited torsion in the otherwise stationary right eye, as well as significant departures from Listing's law in the mobile left eye. These results differ from those previously reported in several ways. Firstly, although averaging over several runs revealed an underlying smooth trend, there were significant (seemingly random) variations in torsion during tracking, similar to those reported by Enright (1990). Secondly, the smooth component of torsion, though repeatable between experimental sessions, did not fit either of the proposed models.

The left eye shows torsion roughly in accordance with Listing's law, though there is some variation both between subjects and between inward and outward tracking conditons. The supposedly immobile right eye violates Listing's law by exhibiting up to a de-

---

* Distinguishing between all of the curves in Figures 1 and 2 would require eight different line styles (four each for the inward and outward conditions). Unfortunately, this makes the graphs very cluttered and hence difficult to interpret. The main point of the figures is to show the differences between convergence and divergence, and between cycloversion and cyclovergence; hence the use of just two line styles.

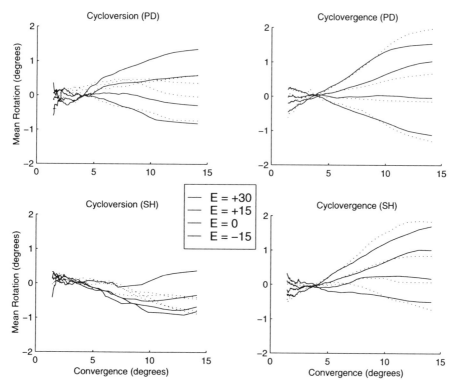

Figure 2. Variation of binocular torsion with vergence and elevation. These graphs show the binocular torsion response of two subjects during asymmetric vergence measured at four angles of right eye elevation. Graphs show mean results averaged over five trials; solid lines indicate inward target motion, dotted lines indicate outward motion. Graph lines for cyclovergence at different elevations appear in the same order as the legend lines; however, this is not the case for cycloversion.

gree of torsion; the exact form of this torsion varies between subjects and with the direction of target motion. A combination of these effects may explain the inconsistent experimental values for k, as suggested by Ivins et al (in press).

3.2. Binocular

When analysed in terms of cycloversion (mean of left and right eye torsion) and cyclovergence (difference in torsion) the results become much easier to interpret. Compared with cycloversion, the cyclovergence component is significantly less noisy, less variable between subjects, and less dependent on tracking history (inward versus outward motion). Cyclovergence is also consistently compatible with the model in Equation 1 taking a value of $k = 1/2$.

4. DISCUSSION

Although the results do not support the binocular Listing's law proposed above, they do support a weaker form: the relative torsional state (cyclovergence) of the two eyes is determined by binocular fixation. This gives a clue as to the functional significance of the observed eye movement control law. Control of cycloversion is not nearly so crucial to stereo vision as is the accurate maintenance of cyclovergence, which is important for the metric interpretation of stereo disparities. Furthermore, cyclovergence determines the slant of the vertical horopter and thus the 'working volume' for stereo. The better control of cyclovergence could thus be required for maintenance of metric stereo constancy, while the vertical horopter tilt implied by a combination of Listing and vergence-dependent torsion may be well-adapted to viewing both approximately horizontal surfaces below eye level, and nearby vertical objects at eye level.

REFERENCES

Enright J T (1990) Stereopsis, cyclotorsional "noise" and the apparent vertical. Vis Res 30: 1487–1497.

Ivins J, Porrill J, Frisby J (1997) A deformable model of the human iris driven by non-linear least-squares minimisation. Sixth International Conference on Image Processing and its Applications (IPA'97; Dublin, Ireland): vol 1, pp 234–238.

Ivins J, Porrill J, Frisby J (in press) Instability of torsion during smooth asymmetric vergence. Vis Res

Minken AWH, Gielen CCAM, Van Gisbergen JAM (1995) An alternative 3D interpretation of Hering's equal-innervation law for version and vergence eye movements. Vis Res 35: 93–102.

Nakayama K (1983) Kinematics of normal and strabismic eyes. In: Vergence Eye Movements: Basic and Clinical Aspects. Schur CM, Ciuffreda KJ (eds), Butterworths, Boston, pp 543–564

Van Rijn LJ, Van den Burg AV (1993) Binocular eye orientation during fixations: Listing's law extended to include eye vergence. Vis Res 33: 691–708

28

BLINKS AND ASSOCIATED EYE MOVEMENTS

L. J. Bour, B.W. Ongerboer de Visser, M. Hettema, A. Swaneveld, and
M. Aramideh

Department of Neurology, Clinical Neurophysiology
Academic Medical Centre, University of Amsterdam
The Netherlands

1. INTRODUCTION

Studies of blinks have revealed the reciprocal relationship between the innervation patterns of the levator palpebrae superioris (LP) and the orbicularis oculi (OO) muscles (Gordon 1951; Björk and Kugelberg 1953; Becker and Fuchs 1988; Evinger 1991; Aramideh et al. 1994a) resulting in a downward movement of the upper eyelid. Immediately prior to a blink, the discharge of the LP ceases whereas the OO motoneurons produce a short high-frequency burst of activity. At the end of a blink the OO actively turns off and the LP returns to its previous tonic activity either accompanied by an initial burst or not (Aramideh et al. 1994a). Concurrently the eye-globe makes a slight displacement of 1–2 millimeters back into the orbit (Evinger et al. 1984) and performs a horizontal, vertical (Collewijn et al. 1985; Riggs et al. 1987) and torsional rotation (Straumann et al. 1996). During blinks the rotation of the eye in straight-ahead position normally is directed nasally downward (Collewijn et al. 1985; Riggs et al. 1987). This rotation also depends on the initial eye position. Prolonged blinking or permanent closure of the eye may be accompanied by upward directed conjugate eye movements (Collewijn et al. 1985). To what extent the different extraocular muscles contribute to this combined translational and rotational movement is not yet known. Abnormalities of eye movements or eyelid movements or both have been reported in disorders of the basal ganglia and/or the midbrain. In essential blepharospasm occasionally eye movement disorders accompany the spasms of the eyelid closure (Aramideh et al. 1994b). This mutual interaction between some types of eye and eyelid movements may have a same origin. Earlier studies have established the relation between eye movements and the movement of the upper eyelid on the one hand (Riggs et al. 1987) and the relationship between upper eyelid movement and the electromyographic activity of the OO muscle during blinks on the other hand (Ongerboer de Visser and Kuypers 1978). However, simultaneous recording of EMG of the OO muscle and eye movements together with monitoring of the eyelid movement during various

Current Oculomotor Research, edited by Becker *et al.*
Plenum Press, New York, 1999.

blinks, including electrically elicited reflex blinks, to our knowledge, have not been investigated.

2. METHODS

Electromyographic recording (EMG) of the orbicularis oculi (OO) muscles was performed using surface electrodes. Concurrently, horizontal and vertical eye positions were recorded by means of the double magnetic induction (DMI) ring method (Bour et al. 1984). In addition, movement of the upper eyelid was measured by placing a specially designed search coil upon the upper eyelid. The reflex blink was elicited electrically by current stimulation of the supraorbital nerve either on the right or the left side (Ongerboer de Visser and Kuypers 1978).

3. RESULTS

It is found that disconjugate oblique eye movements accompany spontaneous, voluntary as well as reflex blinks. Depending on the gaze position prior to blinking, the amplitude of horizontal and vertical component of the eye movement during blinks varies in a systematic way. With adduction and downward gaze the amplitude is minimal. With abduction the horizontal amplitude increases, whereas with upward gaze the vertical amplitude increases. Unilateral electrical stimulation of the supra-orbital nerve elicits eye movements with an early ipsilateral and bilateral late component. At low stimulus intensities, the classical late bilateral blink reflex R_2 of the OO muscle appears to be accompanied by late bilateral eye movements. With increasing stimulus intensity, the amplitude of the corresponding eye movement increases from 2 to 6 degrees and the latency decreases from 70 to 40 ms. At stimulus intensities approximately 2–3 times above the threshold, the early ipsilateral blink reflex R_1 of the OO muscle can be observed together with an early ipsilateral eye movement component at a latency of 10–15 ms (Figure 1)

In addition, early ipsilateral and late bilateral components are also identified in the upper eyelid movement during electrically elicited blink reflexes. Ipsilateral to the side of stimulation, concurrent with the presence of the early eye movement component, the upper eyelid appears to open to a greater degree (arrows Figure 1). The latter component evinces prior to eyelid closure, coincides with the start of the R_1 blink reflex response and shortly appeared to open the eye to a slightly greater degree. Late components of the eye movements precede the late components of the eyelid movement (Figure 1). The difference latency between the latter two movements was found to be independent from the strength of the electric current and its mean value for 4 normal control subjects was lying between 7 to 8 milliseconds.

4. CONCLUSIONS

To inhibit the levator palpebrae superioris muscle during contraction of the orbicularis oculi, ascending pathways exist from the lower pons to the mesenchephalon (Büttner-Ennever JA and Holstege G 1986; Schmidtke K and Büttner-Ennever JA 1992). Our findings provide evidence for similar ascending pathways that project from the trigeminal complex in the pons to motoneurons of other auxiliary extra-ocular muscles. Synchroniza-

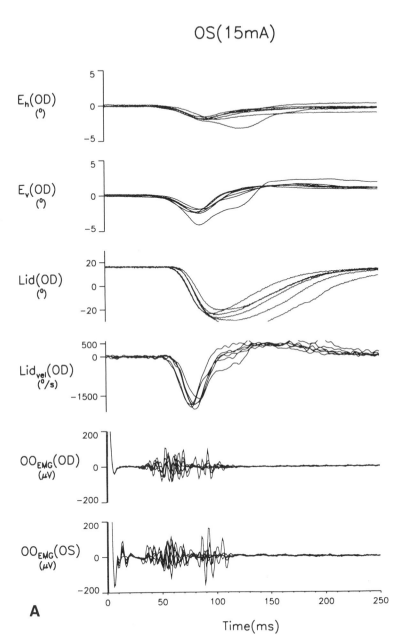

Figure 1. In a normal control subject is depicted from top to bottom; horizontal (E_h(OD)), vertical (E_v(OD)) eye movement of the right eye, upper eyelid movement (Lid(OD)) and upper eyelid velocity (Lid_{vel}(OD)) for the right eye and EMG of the orbicularis oculi of the right (OO_{EMG}(OD)) and the left eye (OO_{EMG}(OS)). Upward deflections relate to rightward eye movement for the horizontal component, upward eye movement for the vertical component and upward movement or upward velocity of the upper eyelid. Several responses after electrical stimulation with a 15 mA current of the supraorbital nerve above the left eye (A) and above the right eye (B) are superimposed. Note the early ipsilateral components both in the eye movement and the eyelid movement (arrows) with right side stimulation.

OD(15mA)

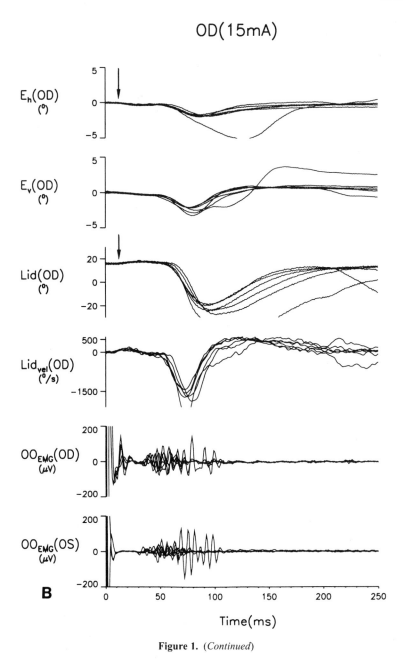

Figure 1. (*Continued*)

tion of EMG activity of the orbiclaris oculi, movements of eyelids and eyes, as well as constant latency differences between eyelid and eye movement components and in addition similarity of oblique eye movement components in different types of blinks suggest a common neural origin. The existence of a pre-motor neural "blinking centre" is hypothesized, acting as a generator that coordinates impulses to different motor nuclei during all types of blinks independent from the ocular saccadic and/or vergence system.

REFERENCES

Aramideh M, Ongerboer de Visser BW, Devriese PP, Bour LJ and Speelman JD (1994a) Electromyographic features of levator palpebrae superioris and orbicularis oculi muscles in blepharospasm. Brain 117: 27–38.

Aramideh M, Bour LJ, Koelman JHTM, Speelman JD and Ongerboer de Visser BW (1994b) Abnormal eye movements in blepharospasm and involuntary levator palpebrae inhibition: clinical and pathophysiological considerations. Brain 117: 1457–1474.

Becker W, Fuchs AF (1988) Lid-eye coordination during vertical gaze changes in man and monkey. J Neurophysiology, 60: 1227–1252.

Björk A, Kugelberg E (1953) The electrical activity of the muscles of the eyes and eyelids in various positions and during movements. Electroencephalography and Clinical Neurophysiology 5: 595–602.

Bour LJ, Van Gisbergen JAM, Bruijns J and Ottes FP (1984) The double magnetic induction method for measuring eye movements - results in monkey and man. IEEE Trans Biomed Eng BME-31: 419–427.

Büttner-Ennever JA and Holstege G (1986) Anatomy of premotor centers in the reticular formation controlling oculomotor, skeletomotor and autonomic motor systems. Progress in Brain Research 64: 89–98.

Collewijn H, Van der Steen J and Steinman RM (1985) Human eye movements associated with blinks and prolonged eyelid closure. J Neurophysiol 54: 11–27.

Evinger C, Shaw MD, Peck CK, Manning KA and Baker K (1984) Blinking and associated eye movements in human, guinea pigs and rabbits. J Neurophysiol 52: 323–339.

Evinger C, Manning KA and Sibony PA (1991) Eyelid movements. Investigative Ophthalmology and Visual Science 32: 387–400.

Gordon G (1951) Observation upon the movements of the eyelids. British Journal of Ophthalmology 35: 339–351.

Ongerboer de Visser BW and Kuypers HGJM (1978) Late blink reflex changes in lateral medullary lesions. An electrophysiological and neuroanatomical study of Wallenberg's syndrome. Brain 101: 285–294.

Riggs LA, Kelly JP, Manning KA and Moore RK (1987) Blink-related eye movements. Investigative Ophthalmology and Visual Sciences 28: 334–342.

Schmidtke K and Büttner-Ennever JA (1992) Nervous control of eyelid function. A review of clinical, experimental and pathological data. Brain 115: 227–247.

Straumann D, Zee DS, Solomon D and Kramer PD (1996) Validity of Listing's law during fixations, saccades, smooth pursuit eye movements, and blinks. Exp Brain Res 112: 135–146.

29

OPPOSING RESISTANCE TO THE HEAD MOVEMENT DOES NOT AFFECT SPACE PERCEPTION DURING HEAD ROTATIONS

Jean Blouin, Nicolas Amade, Jean-Louis Vercher, and Gabriel Gauthier

Movement and Perception, CNRS and Université de la Méditerranée
163 Avenue de Luminy, 13288 Marseille, France

1. INTRODUCTION

The neural encoding of the visual space is still a central issue in the general field of neurophysiology and psychophysiology. Many questions tickle the curiosity of the researchers in the face of spectacular daily spatial performance. Among the current questions that authors attempt to solve is how the central nervous system (CNS) updates the egocentric position of objects from the environment during self-motion? What is the nature of the cues that individuals rely on to determine the new position of objects with respect to the body after such displacements? How is the heterogeneous sensory information centrally processed to provide an uniformed and coherent representation of the extracorporeal world?

Signaling changes in head position is fundamental in spatial processes because the head carries essential sensory organs (e.g. nose, ears, eyes) that provide exteroceptive information about the environment. Hence, to determine the location of visual, olfactory or auditory sources, the CNS must be informed about head-in-space position and motion. Over the years, the contribution of two distinct sources of signals to spatial processes during head movements has been predominantly studied: neck muscle proprioception and vestibular signals.

1.1. Neck Muscle Proprioception

The cervical muscles are rich in proprioceptors such as muscle spindles, joint and tendon receptors (Abrahams and Richmond 1988). These receptors can provide the CNS with reliable information about head position and motion on the trunk (Mergner et al. 1991, 1992; Nakamura and Bronstein 1995; Taylor and McCloskey 1988).

Current Oculomotor Research, edited by Becker *et al.*
Plenum Press, New York, 1999.

Proprioception is likely to play a more general role in body orientation function than only referring body parts with respect to each others and providing feedback about unfolding movements. In 1960, Leonard Cohen reported that monkeys with dorsal laminectomies of the first three pairs of dorsal cervical roots lose balance and are greatly inaccurate in their spatially oriented motor behaviors. Later, Deecke and colleagues (1977) while discussing the role of proprioception suggested that: "exclusive vestibular information would be of no use for the purpose of body orientation" (p. 229). With this hypothesis, the authors gave a functional reason to the massive convergence of proprioceptive and vestibular cues found at different areas within the CNS. The results from a recent experiment conducted with a deafferented patient corroborated this hypothesis (Blouin et al. 1995b). The patient, who suffered a permanent and selective loss of the large myelinated fibers from the body including the neck, was largely inaccurate in estimating passive whole-body rotations about the yaw axis, despite an otherwise normal vestibular function (normal vestibulo-ocular reflex). Proprioception is then likely to provide the static and dynamic information about body elements necessary to build an egocentric reference system which allows encoding of spatial information (Blouin et al. 1993; Jeannerod 1991; Paillard 1987).

1.2. Vestibular Signals

To successfully produce spatially oriented actions, individuals cannot rely solely on neck proprioception because they also need information about head-in-space. The vestibular apparatus appears as a good candidate for participating to space updating during self-motion because it is based on sensors (semi-circular canals and otolith organs) which are sensitive to angular and linear acceleration/deceleration of the head in space. However, the results from a series of recent studies which were designed to specifically test this possibility showed that subjects (Ss) are unable to retrieve with accuracy the position of a memorized peripheral earth-fixed target positions after passive whole-body rotations (or a combination of active and passive head rotations) about the yaw axis (Blouin et al. 1995a, 1997; Blouin et al. in press a,b). Then, it appears that, despite Ss can determine with a relatively good accuracy the magnitude of whole-body rotations and translations in the dark (Berthoz et al. 1987, 1996; Bloomberg et al. 1991; Blouin et al. 1995a, 1997; Israël et al. 1995, 1996; Maurer et al. 1997; Mergner et al. 1991) they cannot rely on the vestibular signal to accurately update the visual space during these movements. Based on these results we have hypothesized that determining the magnitude of head-in-space motion in the dark and coding a target position after such movements correspond to different cognitive tasks involving different neural substrates (see Blouin et al. 1997 and Blouin et al. in press b, for more details about this issue).

1.3. Efference Copy

A third source of cues has been somewhat overlooked in the study of space perception during head movements: the feedforward motor command sent to the cervical muscles, known as 'efference copy'. Indeed, since activation of the neck muscles generates head movements, some information about head-on-trunk position, hence target-to-head position, could be extracted from efference copy mechanisms. The perception of the head position after active or passive rotations is known to be similar (Nakamura and Bronstein, 1995) but we cannot conclude from this that the efference copy is not involved in spatial processes. For instance, the greater precision in arm movements when Ss produce head rotations towards the goal targets (Biguer et al. 1984; Roll et al. 1986), may suggest some efference copy contribution.

In a recent experiment, Ss were asked to point at a memorized visual target after their trunk was passively rotated about the vertical axis in conditions in which Ss, with the head immobilized in space, were either relaxing or contracting their neck muscles (Blouin et al. in press b). Such conditions elicit a complex pattern of cervical and vestibular signals, each one providing different (sometimes contradictory) information about head position and/or motion. Yet, Ss showed similar pointing accuracy whether or not they contracted the cervical muscles during the trunk rotations. These results may suggest that the efference copy helped interpreting the afferent signals from the muscle spindles and the Golgi tendon organs whose discharge rates differ in conditions with or without neck muscle contraction (Gandevia et al. 1992). Indeed, the efference copy could provide a foreknowledge of the expected proprioceptive response given the voluntary neck muscle activation Ss are producing. This process would allow the Ss to distinguish the changes in proprioceptive input that result from the passive trunk rotation under the stationary head-in-space from those that result from neck muscle activation.

1.4. Goal of the Experiment

In the present study, we further examined the contribution of the efference copy in spatial processes. More specifically, we tested whether Ss perceive similarly the relative head-trunk position or the position of an extinguished visual target after head rotations when an increased neck muscle activation is required to reach and maintain a given head position.

2. METHODS

2.1. Experimental Set-Up

Figure 1 shows a schematic representation of the experimental set-up. The Ss (n = 5, mean age = 25.8 years) sat in a dark room at the center of a semi-circular cylinder with a radius of 1 m. Light emitting diodes (LEDs) were positioned at eye level straight-ahead (central light, CL) and 21° to the right of the Ss (target) on the cylinder. Ss used a laser diode to indicate the perceived position of either the extinguished 21° target or body midline after head rotations (see experimental conditions). The laser was mounted on the vertical axis of a motor that could be activated with a joystick fixed on the right armrest.

Head-on-trunk rotation was measured with a potentiometer fixed on a helmet worn by the Ss. A head-fixed light (HFL) was fixed to the tip of an 80-cm rigid light rod attached to the front of the helmet. In some conditions, a spring linking a bite bar to a sturdy earth-fixed rod was used to increase the resistance to the head movement. In this case, the magnitude of the torque to be exerted by the Ss was proportional to head angular rotation (460 g•cm/deg).

Horizontal eye movements were monitored by electro-oculography using silver-silver chloride electrodes fixed near the outer canthi of the eyes. All signals were sampled at 100 Hz through a 12-bit analog/digital converter. Hearing was masked with white noise played through headphones.

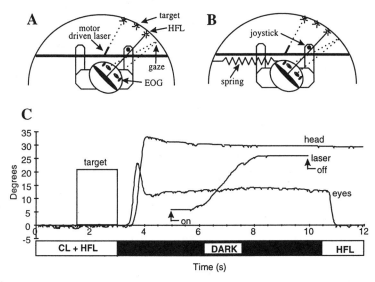

Figure 1. Schematic representation of the experimental set-up in the 'target, free movement' condition (A) and in the condition with increased resistance to the head movement (B). (C) Raw recordings in a typical trial in the 'target, free movement' condition. In this particular trial, the S perceived the extinguished visual target position at about 5° to the right of its actual position. The head restrained condition showed similar spatio-temporal organization. CL: central light, HFL: head-fixed light.

2.2. Experimental Conditions

'Target, free movement' Figure 1C shows raw recordings from a typical trial in 'the target, free movement' condition. At the start of a trial, the HFL and the CL were both illuminated. The Ss were instructed to gaze at the HFL and to align the head with the CL. After 1.5 s, the 21°-target was turned on for 1.5 s after which both the HFL and the CL were turned off. The Ss then produced a single head rotation to the right (i.e. same side as that of the target). The Ss self-selected the angular amplitude of the rotations and were instructed to cover a 5° to 60° range of rotations in 35 trials. In order to have Ss producing head movements as naturally as possible, no instructions about eye movements were given. The laser was turned on after the rotations and the Ss attempted to position it, using the joystick, on the perceived target position while maintaining the head and the eyes stationary at the reached positions. At the end of the trial, the HFL was turned on, and the Ss produced a saccade towards it without moving the head. This gave us a measure of the eye deviation in the orbit during Ss' estimation of the extinguished target position. Then the Ss moved the extinguished laser to a new (unknown) position by pushing the joystick back and forth several times.

'Target, resistance' This condition was in all aspects similar to the previous one except that the resistance to the head movement was increased using a spring that linked the bite bar to a sturdy earth-fixed rod. Therefore, compared to the 'target, free movement' condition, Ss had to produce a greater neck muscles activation to reach and to maitain a given head angular position.

'Target, no movement' We tested Ss' perception of the memorized target position without any previous head rotation. In these trials (n = 8), Ss were instructed to keep the head (and gaze) in the central position after the extinction of the target and to direct the laser towards it when the laser was turned on.

'Body midline, free movement' At the start of a trial, the HFL and the CL were both illuminated for 1.5 s after which the Ss rotated the head to the right with different magnitudes. After the rotations, the laser was turned on and the Ss attempted to position it in the direction of the body midline. Therefore, in this condition Ss had to precisely determine the relative head (or gaze)-trunk position because the body midline was estimated through visual modality.

'Body midline, resistance' This condition was identical to the previous one except that the resistance to the head rotations was increased using the spring.

3. RESULTS

3.1. Perception of the Target Position

Figure 2 shows the perceived target positions of one S in the different experimental conditions. The analysis of variance revealed that Ss' accuracy in retrieving the 21° visual target was similar whether or not they rotated the head after its extinction and whether or not resistance to the head movement was experimentally applied [$F(2,12) = 0.68, p > .05$; global mean = 21.39°]. However, the experimental conditions significantly affected the variability in the perception of the target position [$F(2,12) = 9.70, p < .05$]. Posthoc analyses (Tukey test, $p < .06$) showed that the Ss were less variable in the condition without head movement (mean = 1.38°) than when they produced head rotations after the target extinction (mean = 2.73°).

Linear regressions were used to determine, for each S, whether the perceived target position was proportional to the head rotation magnitudes in both head movement conditions. We also verified whether the perceived target position was a function of the total gaze shift. Indeed, in most of the trials, head movements were preceded by saccadic eye

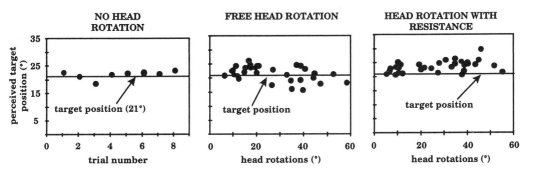

Figure 2. Examples of the perceived positions of the extinguished visual target in a S in the conditions without head movement (left), with head free rotations (middle) and with increased resistance to the head movement (right).

movements as shown in Fig. 1C. During the head rotations, the eyes tended to return towards the center of the orbit through the effect of the vestibulo-ocular reflex, but most frequently remained deviated in the same direction as the head movements (i.e. to the right). All fit equations were characterized by extremely low r^2 values indicating that the perceived target position was neither a function of the corresponding head rotation or gaze shift magnitudes (r^2 varied from 0.002 to 0.35, mean between Ss = 0.09) nor a function of whether or not head rotations unfolded against increased movement resistance (r^2 varied from 0.006 to 0.34, mean between Ss = 0.08). On the other hand, in both head conditions, the errors in the perceived target position was not correlated with the magnitude of the eye deviation in the orbit after the head rotations (r^2 varied from 0.01 to 0.34, mean between Ss = 0.05).

3.2. Perception of Head-on-Trunk Position

T-test analyses showed that Ss similarly perceived head-on-trunk position after the head rotations whether or not the torque necessary to reach and maintain a given head position was increased by an external resistance to the movement ($p > .05$). On average, Ss perceived body midline slightly deviated in the opposite direction to the head motion (mean = 2.74°). The variability in the Ss' estimates of body midline was not affected by the condition in which head movements unfolded ($p > .05$, mean = 3.05°).

In both the free and restrained head movement conditions, the perceived body midline was not affected by neither the magnitude of the head movements (r^2 varied from 0.01 to 0.38, mean between Ss = 0.14) nor by the extent of gaze shifts (r^2 varied from 0.001 to 0.40, mean between Ss = 0.14).

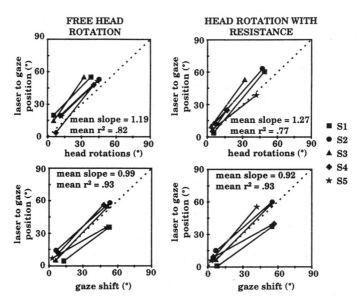

Figure 3. Regression lines for each S in each experimental condition computed when the angle between the perceived target position and gaze is plotted against either the head rotation or gaze shift magnitudes. For each S, minimum and maximum head rotation and gaze shift magnitudes are represented by the values of the extremities of the lines. Between Ss' mean slope and r^2 values of the regression lines obtained for each experimental condition are given in the corresponding panel.

Finally, the angle between the perceived target position and gaze was measured and plotted against both head rotation and gaze shift magnitudes. As shown in Fig. 3, the computed regression lines were similar in the conditions with and without increased resistance to the head rotations. However, the slope of the regression lines was close to unity when the laser to gaze position was plotted against gaze shift magnitudes and larger than unity when it was plotted against head rotation magnitudes. On the other hand, the strength of the correlation was greater when the laser-to-gaze position was plotted against gaze position than against head rotation magnitudes. These results suggest that the Ss did take into account eye deviation in the orbit after the head rotations to provide their estimates of the extinguished visual target position.

4. DISCUSSION

Ss were similarly accurate in estimating the position of the extinguished visual target in conditions with and without head rotations. Opposing external resistance to the head rotation did not affect this precision. However, the variability in Ss' estimate of the target position was larger when Ss rotated the head but again, no difference was found between the head free and the increased resistance conditions. The larger variability observed in the conditions where Ss rotated the head likely resulted from an accumulation of errors in perceiving and memorizing the target position, in producing the head movements and in updating the target position during the head motions. On the other hand, the perception of body midline after the voluntary head rotations was similar whether or not Ss produced head rotations against an external resistance.

Increasing the external resistance to the head movement elicited a complex pattern of cervical and vestibular signals that provided complementary (sometimes contradictory) cues about head position and/or motion. Compared to the (normal) head free condition, a greater activity in the neck muscles was necessary to reach and to maintain a given angle with the head when a resistance to the movement was added. This increased neck muscle activity likely modified the afferent message from the neck muscles as compared to that elicited in the head free condition. Indeed, for a given head-on-trunk deviation, the muscle spindles and the Golgi tendon organs discharge differently in conditions with and without neck muscles contraction (Gandevia et al 1992) and therefore in conditions with or without additional resistance to the head movement. Then, if Ss were to determine the change in the head position purely on the basis of neck muscle proprioception, the perception of both the target position and the head-trunk relative position would likely differ in conditions with and without augmented resistance to the head movement.

Results of a recent experiment (Blouin et al. in press a) showed that Ss are similarly accurate when pointing without visual feedback of the arm towards an extinguished visual target after passive trunk rotations in conditions where Ss are either relaxing or contracting their neck muscles while their head is maintained fixed in space. Because proprioceptively induced perception of target-trunk relative position could result in large pointing errors when contracting the neck muscles in a head-fixed condition, it is possible that the efference copy helps interpreting the cervical afferent message. Indeed, the efference copy could participate in building a foreknowledge of the expected proprioceptive input given the voluntary neck muscle activation the Ss are producing. Then, the change in head-trunk relative position during the passive trunk rotations could be computed from the comparison between expected and actual afferent cervical message.

In the present experiment, similar processes may have taken place in the determination of the head-target relative position following the head rotations. According to this hypothesis, the position of the head would not be derived directly from the afferent cervical message, but rather with respect to the motor commands sent to the neck muscles (efference copy contribution).

Furthermore, the discharge of the muscle spindles and Golgi organs in the antagonist muscles might also have provided cues about head-on-trunk relative position (hence relative head-target position). Because joint receptors are not very sensitive at the head positions used in the present experiment (Grigg and Greenspan 1977), their contribution was probably modest. On the other hand, based on the results from numerous studies showing that visual space cannot be updated accurately through vestibular signals (see the introduction), it is unlikely that the vestibular cues were much contributive in the precision with which Ss determined the position of the target position after the head rotations. However, some participation of the vestibular signals in the determination of the head position with respect to the trunk (body midline conditions) is more probable because this task does not imply updating of visual space as in the target condition but only requires computation of the magnitude of the head displacement in space. This process can successfully used vestibular cues (Blouin et al. 1995a,b, 1997; Israël et al. 1995; Maurer et al. 1997).

After the experiment session, most Ss mentioned that they did not expect their eyes to be deviated to that extent when the central light was turned on after their head rotations. Despite this erroneous introspective determination of the eye positions in the orbits, Ss did take into consideration the position of the eyes in their estimates of both the memorized target position and body midline. This is suggested, for the target conditions, by the fact that the magnitude of the eye deviation had no effect on the errors in perceiving the target position. On the other hand, for the body midline conditions, the fact that the distance between the perceived target position and gaze was better correlated with the gaze shift than with the magnitude of the head rotations confirms that Ss took into account eye positions in the orbits when determining the target position after the head movements.

ACKNOWLEDGMENTS

This work was supported by CNRS UMR 6559 grants. We would like to thank Alain Donneaud for helping in building the apparatus used for the experiment.

REFERENCES

Abrahams, VC, Richmond, FJR (1988) Specialization of sensorimotor organization in the neck muscle system. Prog Brain Res 76: 125–135

Berthoz A, Israel I, Georges-Francois P, Grasso R, Tsuzuku T (1996)!Spatial memory of body linear displacement: what is being stored? Science 269: 95–98

Berthoz A, Israël I,Vieville T, Zee D (1987) Linear head displacement measured by the otoliths can be reproduced through the saccadic system. Neurosci Lett 82: 285–290

Biguer B, Prablanc C, Jeannerod M (1984) The contribution of coordinated eye and head movements in hand ponting accuracy. Exp Brain Res 55: 462–469

Bloomberg J, Melvill Jones G, Segal B (1991) Adaptive modification of vestibularly perceived rotation. Exp Brain Res 84: 47–56

Blouin J, Bard C, Teasdale N, Paillard J, Fleury M, Forget R, Lamarre Y (1993) Reference systems for coding spatial information in normal subjects and a deafferented patient. Exp Brain Res 93: 324–331

Blouin J, Gauthier GM, van Donkelaar P, Vercher J-L (1995a) Encoding the position of a flashed visual target after passive body rotations. Neuroreport 6: 1165–1168

Blouin J, Gauthier GM, Vercher J-L (1997) Visual object localization through vestibular and neck inputs. 2: Updating off-mid-sagital-plane target positions. J Vest Res 7: 137–143

Blouin J, Labrousse L, Simoneau M, Vercher J-L, Gauthier GM (in press b) Updating visual space during passive and voluntary head-in-space movements. Exp Brain Res

Blouin J, Okada T, Wolsley C, Bronstein A (in press a) Encoding target-trunk relative position: cervical vs. vestibular contribution. Exp Brain Res

Blouin J, Vercher J-L, Gauthier GM, Paillard J, Bard C, Lamarre Y (1995b) Perception of passive whole-body rotation in the absence of neck and body proprioception. J Neurophysiol 74: 2216–2219

Cohen LA (1960) Role of eye and neck proprioceptive mechanisms in body orientation and motor coordination. J Neurophysiol 24: 1–11

Deecke L, Schwartz DWF, Fredrickson JM (1977) Vestibular responses in the rhesus monkey ventroposterior thalamus. II. Vestibulo-proprioceptive convergence at thalamic neurons. Exp Brain Res 30: 219–232

Gandevia SC, McCloskey DI, Burke D (1992) Kinaesthetic signals and muscle contraction. Trends Neurosci 15: 62–65

Grigg P, Greenspan BJ (1977) Response of primate joint afferent neurons to mechanical stimulation of kee joint. J Neurophysiol 40: 1–8

Israël I, Bronstein AM, Kanayama R, Faldon M, Gresty M (1996) Exp Brain Res 112: 411–419

Israel I, Sievering D, Koenig E (1995) Self-rotation estimate about the vertical axis. Acta Oto-laryngol 115: 3–8

Jeannerod M (1991) The interaction of visual and proprioceptive cues in controlling reaching movements. In: Humphrey DR, Freund HJ (eds) Motor control: concepts and issues. John Wiley & Sons, New York, pp 277–291

Maurer C, Kimmig H, Trefzer A, Mergner T (1997) Visual object localization through vestibular and neck inputs. 1 : Localization in space and relative to the head and trunk mid-sagittal planes. J Vestib Res 7 : 119–135

Mergner T, Rottler G, Kimmig H, Becker W (1992) Role of vestibular and neck inputs for the perception of object motion in space. Exp Brain Res 89: 655–668

Mergner T, Siebold C, Schweigart G, Becker W (1991) Human perception of horizontal and head rotation in space. Exp Brain Res 85: 389–404

Nakamura T, Bronstein AM (1995) The perception of head and neck angular displacement in normal and labyrinthine-defective subjects. A quantitative study using a 'remembered saccade' technique. Brain 118: 1157–1168

Paillard J (1987) Cognitive versus sensorimotor encoding of spatial information. In: Ellen P, Thinus-Blanc C (eds) Cognitive processes and spatial orientation in animal and man. Martinus Nijhoff, Dordrecht, pp 1–34

Roll R, Bard C, Paillard J (1986) Head orienting contributes to the directional accuracy of aiming at distant targets. Hum Movement Sci 5: 359–371

Taylor JL, McCloskey DI (1988) Proprioception in the neck. Exp Brain Res 70: 351–360

30

UPDATING THE LOCATION OF VISUAL OBJECTS IN SPACE FOLLOWING VESTIBULAR STIMULATION

G. Nasios, A. Rumberger, C. Maurer, and T. Mergner[*]

Neurological Clinic
Ioannina University, Ioannina, Greece
Neurologische Klinik
Universität Freiburg, Freiburg, Germany

1. INTRODUCTION

When updating the location of a visual object in space while moving around, we have to rely on sensory information from different modalities. Retinal signals provide us with a notion of the object's position on the retina, but we also have to take into account eye position in the head and head position in space. In other words, we perform a coordinate transformation from a retinotopic reference frame via a craniotopic to a spatiotopic reference frame (e.g. Andersen et al. 1993). Human psychophysical studies indicate that these transformations show specific errors under certain conditions, from which we may learn how the brain performs these complex neuronal computations.

It has repeatedly been shown that the transformation of the visual signal into space coordinates is performed with the help of vestibular input; subjects are able to perform rather accurate saccades towards the location of a previously presented target in space following horizontal whole-body rotation (Bloomberg et al. 1988; Israel and Berthoz 1989; Nakamura and Bronstein 1995). However, we observed in a number of studies that the vestibular contribution falls short, if rotational frequency (using sinusoidal stimulation) or angular velocity are low, due to the known high-pass frequency characteristics of the semicircular canal system (Fernandez and Goldberg 1971) and a rather high detection threshold (see Mergner et al. 1991). This observation applied to human self-motion perception (Mergner et al. 1991) and related tasks, like object motion perception (Mergner et al. 1992) as well as updating the location of a visual target in space by a reproduction pro-

---

[*] Supported by DFG Me 715

Current Oculomotor Research, edited by Becker *et al.*
Plenum Press, New York, 1999.

cedure (Maurer et al, 1997) or by performing saccades towards the remembered location (Mergner et al. 1998).

In the latter studies we have shown that the vestibular transformation is performed by means of neck, trunk and leg proprioceptive inputs, which link head and body to the haptically perceived ground support (overview, Mergner et al. 1997). These proprioceptive inputs improve performance; head or body rotations relative to stationary body support (combination of vestibular and proprioceptive inputs) yielded veridical results, unlike the vestibular input alone. In our studies (overview, Mergner et al. 1997) the vestibular-proprioceptive interactions could be described by linear summations (given that the axes of rotation of the eye, the head and the trunk are approximately collinear).

Less is known to date about visual-vestibular interaction. In our study on object motion perception (Mergner et al. 1992) the interaction between visuo-oculomotor and vestibular-proprioceptive inputs also could be described by linear summation. However, in our previous studies on the vestibular role for updating the location of the visual target in space the mode of visual-vestibular interaction remained open, because only the vestibular stimulus was varied and the visual stimulus was kept constant (Maurer et al. 1997; Mergner et al. 1998). In these studies the target presentation prior to body rotation always was centric with respect to the retina and to the head, similar as in previous studies of other authors (Bloomberg et al. 1988; Israel and Berthoz 1989; Nakamura and Bronstein 1995). In particular, the target always was presented close to the head mid-sagittal plane and subjects fixated the target, so that the visual input stemmed mainly from eye eccentricity in the orbit (i.e. from an ocular motor efference copy and/or an eye muscle proprioceptive signal) rather than from retinal eccentricity which was close to zero.

The present study was undertaken to extend the latter studies on vestibular updating of target location in space by varying target eccentricity. This issue is of particular interest because previous work by Blouin et al. (1995a,b 1996) indicates that subjects make considerable errors when reproducing the location of an eccentrically presented visual target following vestibular stimulation. These authors showed that the errors can be attributed, in part, to an underestimation of the vestibular stimulus, but that they are enlarged, in addition, by a pronounced non-linearity of visual-vestibular interaction.

Our present study on the visual-vestibular interaction was performed in two steps. In the first step we assessed the updating of target location following visual stimulation alone. In this part we presented different target eccentricities relative to the stationary head and varied the retinal and oculomotor contributions to the visual input by using two viewing conditions. In one condition subjects looked straight ahead and visual stimulation thus was in retinal coordinates. In the other condition subjects gazed at the target, so that the visual input was approximately identical to the oculomotor signal. In the second part of the study we added a vestibular stimulus and varied its spectral component.

2. METHODS

Six healthy subjects (Ss) participated in the study (4 males and 2 females; mean age, 34.3 ±6.3 yrs). All Ss gave their informed written consent. The study was approved by the local Ethics Committee. The methods we used were similar to the ones applied in a previous study and are described here in abbreviated form (for details, see Maurer et al. 1997).

2.1. Experimental Setup, Stimuli, and Procedures

Subjects were seated on a Bárány chair which allowed horizontal body rotation in space. The chair rotations we used consisted of angular displacements of 18° to either the left or right side with bell-shaped velocity profile ('raised cosine' velocity function) containing either a predominant frequency of 0.8 Hz or 0.1 Hz (stimulus durations, 1.25 s and 10 s; peak angular velocities, 28.8°/s and 3.6°/s, respectively).

Subjects' heads were kept in the primary position with respect to the trunk with the help of a chair-fixed bite board. The chair was surrounded by a cylindrical screen (radius, 1 m) onto which a red spot (target; luminance, approximately 20 cd/cm^2; diameter, 0.5° of visual angle) was projected at Ss' eye level. The target was projected via a mirror galvanometer positioned above Ss' heads, with the rotation axis of galvanometer and chair being collinear.

The galvanometer received three input signals:

a. A computer generated signal which stepped the target by a given amount (0, 4, 8, 12, 16 or 20°) to the right or left side. This input was used to generate the eccentric visual stimuli.

b. Another computer generated signal stepped the target, after Ss had adjusted it to a given direction (see below) by 8° to either the right or left side (three times to each side in a pseudo-random order; inter-step interval, 2.5 s). This 'probe stimulus sequence', as we call it, forced Ss to repeat their indication six times. It served to balance a directional bias introduced by the visual stimulus itself.

c. The third signal stemmed from a hand-held potentiometer (joystick) which Ss adjusted such that they perceived the target at the direction predesignated by instruction (straight ahead, remembered target location in space; see below). As shown before, the remote control prevented that Ss' responses were 'distorted' by the motor performance in the conditions investigated.

During each jump the target was extinguished for 100 ms. Because luminance was low and because the target was moving most of the time no afterimages occurred.

Each experimental trial consisted of five parts (compare example in Fig. 1):

i. Indication of the subjective straight ahead direction. At the beginning of each trial the room lights were extinguished and Ss were presented with the target at a random position in space. By means of the joystick they brought the target in the subjective straight ahead (SSA) direction (6 times).

ii. Presentation of visual target location in space. Two seconds after its extinction the target reappeared for 3 s at a predesignated eccentricity relative to SSA.

iii. Vestibular stimulus. During the subsequent 12 s Ss remained in complete darkness. During this time the chair was kept either stationary (first series, no vestibular stimulus), or was rotated to the right or left side (second series). Ss were instructed to keep gaze straight in their heads (the instruction was given to minimize lasting eye deviations which are known to produce shifts of the SSA.

iv. Reproduction of target location in space. The target reappeared at a random position. Subjects' tried to restore its remembered position in space (6 times).

v. Final interval. After extinction of the target the chair was rotated back to its primary position in the series with vestibular stimulation. Thereafter the room was illuminated, Ss reoriented in space, released their heads from the bite board and performed moderate head shaking.

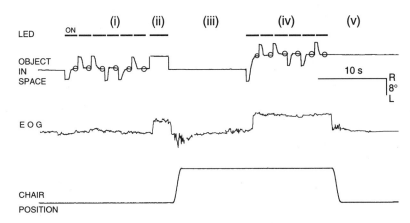

Figure 1. Example of stimulus trial (viewing condition: RET+OM; vestibular stimulus: 18° to the right, dominant frequency of 0.8 Hz). Subdivisions of trial indicated on top (see text). The circles on the object in space position curve indicate where response values were sampled. The object was visible only when the light emitting diode (LED) was on (thick horizontal lines). The electro-oculogram trace (EOG) gives eye-in-orbit position. The vestibular stimulus is shown in bottom trace (chair position). R: right, L: left.

As mentioned in the Introduction, target presentation was performed with two different viewing conditions:

a. Retinal (RET) condition. Subjects kept gaze in the direction into which they previously had brought the target to indicate SSA.

b. Retinal-plus-oculomotor (RET+OM) condition. Subjects shifted gaze on the target and fixated it during its presentation.

During reproduction of the target location Ss were to gaze at the target (compare Fig. 1), because pilot experiments had indicated that this reduced data scatter as compared to a condition in which Ss performed the task with the target viewed peripherally. Compliance to the viewing instruction was controlled by recording Ss' eye movements (bitemporal conventional DC EOG; compare Fig. 1).

Two experimental series were performed:

A. 'Visual-only series'. The tests were performed without vestibular stimulation. Each run consisted of 10 trials (target eccentricities: ±4, ±8, ±12, ±16 and ±20°). For each of the two viewing conditions the run was repeated eight times.

B. 'Visual-plus-vestibular series'. In this series the vestibular stimulus (see above) was applied. Each run comprised 10 trials, covering the 5 target eccentricities (0°, ±8, and ±16°) and the two directions of body rotation. There were three runs for each of the four different conditions: 2 dominant frequencies of the vestibular stimulus (0.4 Hz and 0.1 Hz) and 2 viewing conditions. Note that the trial with target eccentricity 0° was the same in the two viewing conditions; we instructed Ss to actively foveate the target in the RET+OM condition and to avoid foveation in the RET condition.

2.2. Data Analysis and Statistics

The potentiometer readings of the remote control device (joystick) and the EOG-signal were fed into a laboratory computer (sampling rate 50 Hz) together with the position readings of the Bárány chair and the galvanometer. Data were displayed on a computer screen and stored simultaneously on hard disk. Data analysis was performed off-line.

As a measure of Ss' indication of SSA or remembered target location in space in a given trial (compare samples in Fig. 1) we took the mean value across the indication repeats, dismissing the first and the sixth of the six indications. The S.D. across these four values were taken as a measure of indication precision. Furthermore, each S's mean values across runs in a given experiment were calculated and the corresponding S.D. value was taken as a measure of intra-subject variability. In addition, the average values across all Ss were calculated (statistics for mean and median values yielded very similar results; only the former are presented). By comparing each S's indication of SSA with an initial SSA indications in the fully illuminated laboratory we obtained a measure of SSA bias in dark. At the present stage of analysis we concentrated on comparisons between viewing conditions, vestibular stimulus conditions (stimulus present or not) and the two frequencies of the vestibular stimulus (criterion for similarity: overlap of 95% confidence intervals).

3. RESULTS

3.1. Comparison between Retinal and Retinal-Plus-Oculomotor Stimulation (Visual-Only Series)

Figure 2 gives the reproduction of target location in space as a function of target eccentricity, separately for the two viewing conditions (A: RET= retinal, B: RET+OM= retinal-plus-oculomotor). The two conditions yielded similar results. The slope of the curves derived from a linear regression analysis are close to unity (RET: $y= 1.02x + 0.35$, $r^2= 0.97$; RET+OM: $y= 1.03x + 0.08$, $r^2= 0.97$). Responses for right and left target eccentricities are virtually identical. Data scatter increased with target eccentricity in both conditions; in terms of standard deviation (S.D.) of the individual subjects ('intra-subject variability'), it amounted to approximately ±1° at 4° eccentricity and to ±2° when eccentricity reached 20°, on average (not shown). Response precision within trials amounted to approximately 0.5°, with only a slight tendency to increase by about 0.2° at 20° eccentricity in both conditions.

The data in Fig. 2 are referred to subjects' SSA which they had adjusted prior to each trial. On average, SSA bias was similar in both conditions; it was shifted to the right by 3.7 ±2.8° (S.D.) in the RET condition and by 3.9 ±3.0° in the RET+OM condition.

3.2. Effects of Vestibular Stimulation (Visual-Plus-Vestibular Series)

The results are shown in Fig. 3, separately for the two stimulus frequencies (A: 0.8 Hz, B: 0.1 Hz). Results obtained with rightward and leftward chair displacement were essentially the same and were therefore pooled together, such that positive values on the abscissas give target eccentricities in the same direction as chair displacement and negative values give eccentricities counter to chair displacement.

The results for the two viewing conditions resemble each other closely, both for the 0.8 Hz and the 0.1 Hz stimulus, and therefore will be described together. At 0.8 Hz (A) the slopes of the regression lines clearly exceed unity (RET: $y= 1.21x + 3.79$, $r^2= 0.88$; RET+OM: $y= 1.23x + 3.44$, $r^2= 0.88$). Note, however, that the data for 0° target eccentricity clearly deviate from the calculated intercepts of the regression lines. Because of considerable data scatter and the limited number of eccentricities tested, it is not clear at the

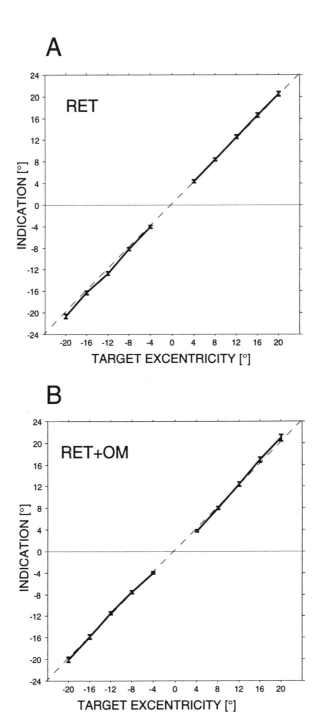

Figure 2. Reproduction of target location in space upon visual stimulation for the two viewing conditions used (A: RET= retinal, B: RET+OM= retinal-plus-oculomotor). Indicated locations are plotted as a function of actual locations (positive and negative values give target eccentricity in head coordinates on right and left side, respectively). Mean values together with their 95% confidence intervals across all subjects and trial repeats. Note that the response curves are close to veridical (dashed 45° lines).

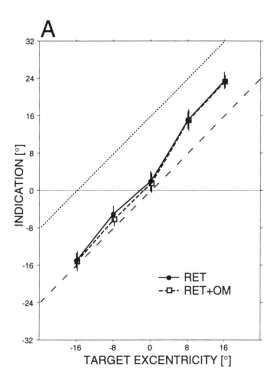

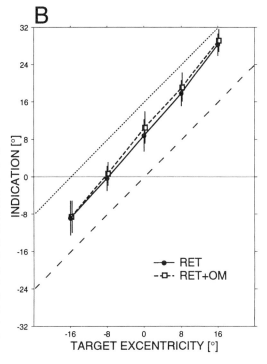

Figure 3. Reproduction of target location in space following vestibular stimulation (dominant frequency, A: 0.8 Hz, B: 0.1 Hz; angular displacement, 18°). Results for the two viewing conditions (RET, RET+OM) are given in terms of mean values and 95% confidence ranges. Dashed 45° lines give ideal correct response curves in space coordinates and the dotted 45° lines give the erroneous responses which a (hypothetical) subject without vestibular function would produce. Positive (negative) values indicating that body displacement was oriented towards (counter to) the target. Target eccentricity is overestimated with body rotation towards the target in A. In B there is an additional shift of the response curves due to an underestimation of the vestibular stimulus.

present stage of data analysis whether these values at 0° eccentricity are particular in that they reflect a qualitatively different response behavior with target presentation at the subjects' mid-sagittal plane, or whether we are dealing here with an asymmetry that, in the form presented here, shows a steeper rise in the direction of chair displacement than in the opposite direction.

At 0.1 Hz (B) the response curves show a pronounced shift towards the dotted 45° line, which gives the hypothetical response curve for a subject without vestibular function. The shift of our Ss' response curves indicates an underestimation of body displacement. An additional finding is that the slope of the regression lines is again clearly above unity (RET: y= 1.16x + 9.15, r^2= 0.73; RET+OM: y= 1.18x + 10.18, r^2= 0.74), similar as in A. Yet, unlike in A, all mean values are close to, or on the regression lines. The latter findings suggest that the asymmetry observed with the 0.8 Hz stimulus is absent or less pronounced at 0.1 Hz. However, a considerable increase in data scatter limits the validity of this finding (compare lower r^2 values at 0.1 Hz as compared to 0.8 Hz and see below).

Both at 0.8 Hz and 0.1 Hz there was a pronounced increase in data scatter in the experiments in which the chair was rotated (compare 95% confidence ranges in Fig. 3 with those in Fig. 2). Furthermore, the amount of data scatter depended on stimulus frequency; it was clearly larger at 0.1 Hz as compared to 0.8 Hz. In terms of intra-subject variability the values amounted to ±3,5° at 0.8 Hz and to ±6.2° at 0.1 Hz, on average. Indication precision, in contrast, was only marginally affected (RET: 0.85°, RET+OM: 0.81). Also the mean values for the SSA bias were similar to those in the visual-only series.

4. DISCUSSION

With visual stimulation alone, our Ss' target reproduction was veridical at all eccentricities tested. This is at variance to a number of previous studies. For instance Bock (1986, 1993), assessing retrospective manual pointing to eccentric targets, reported an overshoot error in the perifoveal region. Blouin et al. (1995b), using a verbal estimation, found a clear overestimation at 10° (factor of 1.26), which vanished at 18° (1.02). The discrepancies likely depend on differences in the experimental procedures. For instance, Ss in the latter studies viewed a central fixation point while being presented with the eccentric target. Possibly, they perceived not only the target's location in space in an egocentric reference frame, but also its location (or distance) relative to the fixation point (i.e. in a visual reference frame). We avoided this by presenting only one visual stimulus at a time. Whatever the reason for the discrepancy, however, we hold that the veridical visual updating of target location by our Ss represents an ideal basis for the investigation of visual-vestibular interaction, which was the main aim of our study.

Our results on visual-vestibular interaction appear to confirm previous findings by Blouin et al. (1995a,b, 1997). These authors found a clear non-linearity of the interaction with body displacements towards the side on which the target was presented (they apparently tested only this mode of stimulus combination). Their subjects, similar as ours, misplaced the target too far in the direction of body rotation, as if underestimating this rotation. In a series of experiments the authors showed that the error depended not only on a vestibular underestimation, but also on the fact that target presentation was eccentric.

Our results extend these previous findings in two ways. One additional observation is that the effect does not depend on the viewing condition used, i.e. whether subjects perceive the target with the peripheral retina or whether they make a saccade and thereby foveate it. Furthermore, we show that the effect of target eccentricity, which is quite pronounced with body rotation towards the side of target eccentricity, does not occur in the same way when the two stimuli are counter to each other. However, at present our data do not allow to characterize this asymmetry in more detail (see Results). An uneqivocal finding was the underestimation of the vestibular stimulus at 0.1 Hz (shift of response curves towards dotted line in Fig. 3B) which is similar to findings in our previous studies and is consistent with a linear summation of the two inputs (Maurer et al. 1997; Mergner et al. 1998).

Noticeably, the effect of target eccentricity on the slopes of the response curves was considerably weaker with the 0.1 Hz than with the 0.8 Hz stimulus (slopes of 1.16 and 1.23, respectively). We deem it unlikely that the attenuation stems primarily from the increase in data scatter observed at 0.1 Hz or from stimulus frequency. Rather we speculate that the effect depends on the intensity of the vestibular stimulus in terms of peak angular velocity, which was much higher at 0.8 Hz (28.8°/s) as compared to 0.1 Hz (3.6°/s). This notion is in agreement with the findings of Blouin et al. (1997) who varied amplitude (and thus velocity) rather than frequency. These authors noticed that overestimation was rather small or absent with body displacements <18° and quite pronounced with displacements of 18° or larger (dominant frequency in their experiments was kept close to 1 Hz).

Interestingly, the vestibular stimulus led to a pronounced increase in data scatter. We assume that the vestibular signal introduce considerable noise in conditions in which it is not complemented by the visual or somatosensory inputs that normally help to establish a space reference. This effect was more pronounced with the 0.1 Hz stimulus, which is underestimated, than with the 0.8 Hz stimulus, which almost yields veridical estimates.

We conceive that the observed non-linearity in the visual-vestibular transformation somehow is related to the fact that the full set of sensory information, which normally is available, was incomplete in the laboratory conditions we used. It is therefore of interest to repeat the experiments in conditions in which input from a visual background is added to the vestibular input. Furthermore, it would be of interest to know the effect of additional proprioceptive input, as it is present when the head or the trunk is rotated relative to a stationary body support.

REFERENCES

Andersen RA, Snyder LH, Li CS, Stricanne B (1993) Coordinate transformations in the representation of spatial information. Curr Opin Neurobiol 3: 171–6

Bloomberg J, Melvill Jones G, Segal B, McFarlane S, Soul J (1988) Vestibular-contingent voluntary saccades based on cognitive estimates of remembered vestibular information. Adv Oto-Rhino-Laryngology 41: 71–75

Blouin J, Gauthier GM, van Donkelaar P, Vercher JL (1995a) Encoding the position of a flashed visual target after passive body rotations. Neuroreport 6: 1165–1168

Blouin J, Gauthier GM, Vercher JL (1995b) Failure to update the egocentric representation of the visual space through labyrinthine signal. Brain & Cognition 29: 1–22

Blouin J, Gauthier GM, Vercher JL (1997) Visual object localization through vestibular and neck inputs. 2: Updating off-mid-sagittal-plane target positions. J Vestib Res 7: 137–43

Bock O (1986) Contribution of retinal versus extraretinal signals towards visual localization in goal-directed movements. Exp Brain Res 64: 467–481

Bock O (1993) Localization of objects in the peripheral visual field. Behav Brain Res 56: 77–84

Fernandez C, Goldberg JM (1971) Physiology of peripheral neurons innervating semicircular canals of the squirrel monkey. II. Response to sinusoidal stimulation and dynamics of peripheral vestibular system. J Neurophysiol 34: 661–75

Israel I, Berthoz A (1989) Contribution of the otoliths to the calculation of linear displacement. J Neurophysiol 62: 247–263

Maurer C, Kimmig H, Trefzer A, Mergner T. Visual object localization through vestibular and neck inputs. I. Localization with respect to space and relative to the head and trunk mid-saggital planes. J Vest Research 7:113–135, 1997.

Mergner T, Hlavacka F, Schweigart G (1993) Interaction of vestibular and proprioceptive inputs for human self-motion perception. J Vest Res, 3: 41–57

Mergner T, Huber W, Becker W (1997) Vestibular-neck interaction and transformation of sensory coordinates. J Vestib Res 7: 347–367

Mergner T, Nasios G, Anastasopoulos D (1998) Vestibular memory-contingent saccades involve somatosensory input from the body support. NeuroReport 9: 1469–1473

Mergner T, Siebold C, Schweigart G, Becker W (1991) Human perception of horizontal trunk and head rotation in space during vestibular and neck stimulation. Exp Brain Res, 85: 389–404

Mergner T, Rottler G, Kimmig H, Becker W (1992) Role of vestibular and neck inputs for the perception of object motion in space. Exp Brain Res 89: 655–668

Nakamura T, Bronstein AM (1995) The perception of head and neck angular displacement in normal and labyrinthine-defective subjects. A quantitative study using a 'remembered saccade' technique. Brain 118: 1157–1168

31

SENSORY AND MOTOR COMPONENTS OF SMOOTH PURSUIT EYE MOVEMENTS IN EXTRASTRIATE CORTEX

An fMRI Study

S. A. Brandt,[1] T. Takahashi,[2] J. B. Reppas,[2] R. Wenzel,[1] A. Villringer,[1] A. M. Dale,[2] and R. B. H. Tootell[2]

[1]Department of Neurology, Charité
10098 Berlin, Germany
[2]Massachusetts General Hospital, NMR-Center
Charlestown, Massachusettes

1. INTRODUCTION

Ample evidence from monkey electrophysiology suggests that eye movements are controlled by two parallel cortico-cortical networks, including a frontal eye field (FEF) and a parietal eye field (PEF). Each cortical eye field contains largely separate groups of neurons devoted to either saccadic eye movements, or visual pursuit eye movements (Tian and Lynch 1996). Both eye fields are directly connected to the brain stem oculomotor system. The posterior eye movement network has strong [anatomical and functional] links to the visual "dorsal stream", and especially to motion perception. Experimental studies in non-human primates suggest that areas MT/MST are intimately involved in pursuit tracking (Newsome et al. 1985; Dursteler et al. 1987). If a given motion is misperceived or not seen at all, the target cannot be pursued faithfully (Baloh et al. 1980). This implies that information about an ongoing eye movement must be incorporated at some level(s) of the visual motion processing hierarchy. Here we ask at a systems level how analoguous regions in human cortex are interrelated. Human neuroimaging studies have clarified the localization of saccade-related activity (for a review see Carter and Zee 1997). However, only few imaging studies have addressed the functional anatomy of smooth pursuit eye movement in extrastriate visual cortex (Petit and Clark 1997; Barton et al. 1996). Previous human brain imaging experiments have also examined cortical responses to stimulus motion (e.g. Watson et al. 1993; Dupont et al. 1994; Tootell et al. 1995b; Tootell et al. 1997). Less is known about how

Current Oculomotor Research, edited by Becker *et al.*
Plenum Press, New York, 1999.

the activity in specific motion areas is related to different components of an ongoing pursuit eye movement. Here, by using fMRI of intrinsic hemodynamics, we measured activities during smooth pursuit and motion stimuli in specific areas of the human extrastriate cortex. Improved controls for eye movement related activity include measuring eye movements during the actual scans, and reducing visual stimulation during tracking tasks to an absolute minimum, or (in other tests) eliminating it entirely. To functionally dissect the nature of this activity further, we analyzed it in the same subjects, in comparison to: 1) the location of retinotopic visual areas (e.g. V1, V2, V3, V3A, V4v), 2) the location of visual motion areas (e.g. MT, V3A), 3) to areas activated by pursuit eye movement in the absence of retinal slip and 4) areas activated during passively moving the eyeball. In contrast to earlier studies these experiments revealed which human cortical areas carry an extraretinal signal enabling them to differentiate between equivalent retinal motion signals generated either by eye movements or by real stimulus motion. Specifically we were interested in distinguishing the differential contribution of sensory (retinal slip) and motor related activation in areas MT/MST, V3a, SPO and LIP induced by smooth pursuit eye movements.

2. METHODS

2.1. Protocol

The study consisted of three main parts.

2.1.1. Retinotopic and Full Field Motion Stimuli. In part 1, a standard battery of retinotopic and full-field motion stimuli was presented to the subject to localize pursuit related activation within the context of previously mapped visual areas. Retinotopic stimulations were undertaken to define the borders of visual areas V1, V2, V3, VP, V3A and V4v (Sereno et al. 1995). Motion areas MT/MST were identified on the basis of their selective response to low contrast (~ 1%) visual motion and V3A by its characteristic relationship to the representation of the vertical and horizontal meridia (Tootell et al. 1997). The criteria for defining the retinotopic and motion areas in this paper are described elsewhere (Sereno et al. 1995; Tootell et al. 1995b). For simplicity, we retain the macaque nomenclature for visual areas when describing apparently homologous areas in the human brain, but only when multiple topographic or functional similarities pertain; these similarities are summarized in the discussion. In such cases a "p" is added as a prefix to the name to indicate that this identification is presumptive/preliminary.

2.1.2. Smooth Pursuit Stimuli. In Part II, smooth pursuit tracking experiments were performed. Subjects followed a single dot, 0.2 degrees in size, moving sinusoidaly across the horizontal axis with a constant speed of 20°/sec. and with a maximum amplitude of 15° on both sides. During the tracking experiments the dot was tracked in front of a black background and made as dim as possible using neutral density filters (2–3 log units) and a Kodak wratten filter (#29) to reduce the maximum display luminance to just above threshold. Subjects verified that there were no visible stimulus borders except for the target itself.

2.1.3. Control Conditions. In Part III, two control experiments were undertaken in an attempt to differentiate between sensory and motor components of eye movement related activity. In one experiment subjects were asked to manually move one eye by poking the eyeball (the other eye was covered). Passive eye movement led to apparent motion of the stationary fixation point and textured background in the direction opposite to the eye displacement. In another control experiment subjects observed two stationary parafoveal afterimages (placed horizontally at 0.25 degrees eccentricity to the left and right side of the fovea center) in complete darkness. Intentional fixation of one afterimage led to smooth pursuit eye movements. Intentional shifting of attention and fixation to the left and right afterimage respectively led to horizontal, pendular eye movements and, correspondingly, to an apparent horizontal sinewave motion for the afterimage (Grüsser and Landis 1991). The latter experiment was used to imprint a long-lasting (~16 seconds) retinal afterimage produced by two bright parafoveal strips (0.2 degrees in size). For each other experiment, activation in response to a particular kind of tracking was compared to central fixation of the same visual target. In a subset of subjects experiments were repeated with "blank stare" in the baseline condition and did not produce significantly different results. 10 normal volunteers (ages 25–45) with normal or corrected-to-normal vision participated in parts 1 and 2. Three of these subjects also participated in control conditions of part 3. All subjects gave their informed consent.

2.2. Eye Movement Recording during fMRI

To ensure subjects compliance with the experimental task, eye movements were recorded with a binocular infra-red pupiltracker (Ober2, Permobil) during fMRI. Pulsed infra-red light emitting diodes illuminated the orbital fields of the eyes and eye movement induced changes in distribution of infra-red light reflected to an array of photo diode detectors were recorded. Sampling frequency was 250 Hz. The spatial resolution was 0.5 degrees. Artefacts in the eye movements recorded during fMRI were due to radiofrequency pulses (RF) and gradient (Gx) changes. We developed a two step filter algorithm that reliably eliminated non-physiological signal changes in the eye movement recordings on the basis of the unphysiological amplitude and velocity changes without affecting the physiological signal (Brandt et al. 1997).

2.3. Functional Magnetic Resonance Imaging

Functional magnetic resonance images were acquired in a 1.5 Tesla MRI scanner (General Electric Signa, Milwaukee,Wi) equipped with echo-planar imaging (Instascan, ANMR Systems, Wilmington, MA), using a bilateral quadrature surface coil (made by Patrick Ledden, Massachusetts General Hospital NMR Center) with the head immobilized by a bite bar. This coil was positioned over the subjects parietal and occipital lobes and provided excellent signal strength in the posterior brain regions, with lower signal strength in more anterior regions. We imaged brain activity in 16 contiguous 4 mm slices parallel to the calcarine fissure to cover the main areas of interest: early visual areas, motion areas and parietal cortex. Functional MRI acquisition used asymmetric spin echo pulse sequences (TR = 2 sec, TE = 70 msec, flip angle = 90°, 180° offset = 25 msec) to minimize the contribution of large blood vessels in a multi-slice (16 slices) mode at a resolution of 3.125 x 3.125 x 4 mm. Cortical surface reconstruction and flattening techniques were used to clarify the cortical topography. These techniques render activation on the 2-D cortical surface of the "inflated" brain which has been unfolded with little distortion (~ 15%) to show both the gyri and the sulci on a contiguous surface (Dale and Sereno 1993). Such data can be shown in either inflated views, showing a whole cortical hemisphere, or in a flattened view in which the posterior cortex is "cut" into a flat sheet to facilitate comparison with retinotopic areas (see

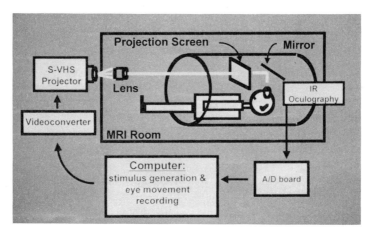

Figure 1. Subjects lay on their back within the bore of the magnet and viewed the stimuli via a mirror that reflected the images displayed on a rear projection screen placed perpendicular to the subject's body at neck level. Eye movements were recorded with a binocular infra-red pupiltracker (Ober2, Permobil) during fMRI. Visual pursuit stimuli were generated with custom software (Permobil, Ober 2) on a PC and presented with a LCD projector (Sony, LCD 2000). Motion stimuli were generated by a Silicon Graphics Onyx computer.

Figure 3). These techniques provide an intuitive presentation of activated regions and help disambiguate the localization of activation related to sulcus landmarks, which are more reliable functional localizers than standard coordinate systems. Statistical analysis required the cyclic alteration between two conditions. Runs lasted 256 seconds, composed of eight cycles of alternating 16 sec eye movements and fixation. Two or three runs were obtained and averaged to provide greater statistical power and more reliable activation patterns. Statistical significance of the activation was determined with a Fourier based analysis of the time

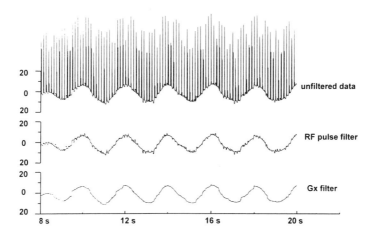

Figure 2. Eye movements are identified on the basis of typical amplitude and velocity characteristics, which were distinct from the artefacts induced by fMRI. A two step filter algorithm that reliably identified non-physiological signal changes in the eye movement recordings was developed. RF-pulse filter: by comparing trend and local slope, RF pulse artefacts were identified as outliers with unphysiological amplitudes and velocities. Outliers were then deleted and missing data filled by extrapolation. Gx filter: Square wave shaped discontinuities were identified and rated as outliers if their total duration was shorter then 40 ms. This criterion avoids confusion with small saccades or square wave jerks.

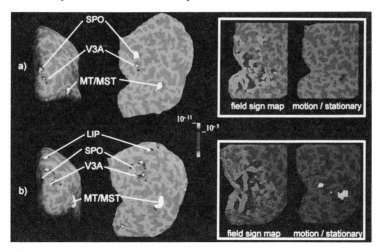

Figure 3. Location of smooth pursuit related activation (left panels) to the location of retinotopic visual areas and visual motion areas (right panels) in two representative subjects (a and b). Posterior views of inflated right hemispheres and patches of flattened occipital cortex showing selective activation in the labelled areas.

series from each voxel. F-statistics compared the ratio of the signal power at the stimulus frequency to the power at all other frequencies (excluding the harmonics). The resulting p-value were smoothed with ten iterations of a box car filter, leading to spatial smearing on the order of 2–4 mm. Thresholds were set at p≤ 0.001 (dim red) making a linear transition to red (p≤ 10^{-5}) then white (p≤ 10^{-11}). A more detailed description of data analysis is given elsewhere (Sereno et al. 1995; Tootell et al. 1995b).

3. RESULTS

The overall pattern of activation qualitatively resembles in part that seen in previous PET and fMRI imaging studies (see Carter and Zee 1997 for a review), although motion areas were not simultaneously identified in those earlier experiments. Our fMRI maps of pursuit-activated cortical areas also overlap human brain regions where lesions are known to compromise smooth pursuit eye movements (Sharpe and Morrow 1991; Barnes et al. 1991). First, individual retinotopic areas were mapped to better identify the functional anatomy of eye movement related activation. As in previous studies (DeYoe et al. 1994; Sereno et al. 1995) we mapped the retinotopy using slowly moving phase-encoded stimuli filled with flickering checks (Figure 3, right panels).

3.1. Smooth Pursuit Related Activation

Then we explored the overlap between the representation of visual motion and smooth pursuit eye movements in primary and extrastriate visual cortex. In all subjects the fMRI response was significantly elevated during smooth pursuit relative to fixation in motion areas V3A and MT/pMST (Figure 3). Furthermore, an area adjacent to the medial margin of V3A, not being activated by the motion stimulus alone and not showing significant retinotopic organization was activated in all subjects. According to its anatomical localization we refer to this area as SPO for superior parietal occipital (Figure 3). In most subjects (8/10) the dorsal portion of the lateral intraparietal sulcus (dLIP) showed significant stimulus related signal intensity changes. During smooth pursuit we did not observe significant positive activation in areas V1, V2, or V3/VP, either in the foveal representation or outside of it. One would logically expect a few single units to respond in foveal V1 due to the retinal slip during pursuit. Evidently the very small and dim stimulus dot did not produce sufficient activation exceeding the fMRI threshold in V1 with the present level of averaging in the same way that low contrast gratings do not produce significant fMRI activity in V1 at similar levels of averaging (Tootell et al. 1995a). The gain and phase of the standard 20°/sec smooth pursuit were calculated from the eye movement recordings. The subjects pursued the dot almost perfectly, with gains of 0.97 and 0.95 and phase delays of 30 and 50 ms, respectively.

3.2. Contribution of Sensory and Motor Related Activation

In the previous tracking experiments, we attempted to reduce the visual components of the tracking task as much as possible. The failure of a given area's pursuit-related fMRI activity to covary with the amount of retinal slip suggested an extraretinal component to pursuit. In this final set of experiments, we tried to completely exclude retinal slip by asking the subject to pursue an apparently moving but retinally imprinted afterimage. We then compared these results with activation patterns obtained when subjects passively move an eye and thus inducing retinal slip without producing an oculomotor command. Any cortical motion area showing a differential fMRI response to these stimuli must have access to an extraretinal pursuit signal.

Figure 4 reviews the results of one representative subject for a) smooth pursuit eye movements, b) pursuit eye movement to an apparent moving afterimage, and c) passive movement of the eye ball. Interestingly pursuit eye movements to a stabilized retinal image (Figure 4b) induces the same pattern of activation as smooth pursuit eye movements to a moving stimulus (Figure 4a). In both tasks motion areas V3A, MT/pMST as well as SPO and dLIP are being activated. The lower level of significance indicates that smooth pursuit to real stimulus motion is better suited to activate these areas, but the qualitative pattern remains the same. However, passive movement of the eye ball (Figure 4c) leads to a completely different pattern of activation. While primary and secondary visual cortices and a subportion of MT/pMST show significant activation, areas SPO and LIP are not being activated.

4. DISCUSSION

We explored the role of human motion areas during the sensorimotor processing that accompany eye movements. We found that two areas which responded selectively to wide field visual motions - V3A and MT/MST - were also active when the eyes track a small, moving target. The pursuit-related activity in MT/pMST, SPO and dLIP is distinguishable from that in V3A by an apparently extraretinal pursuit signal in the former.

4.1. V3A and MT/MST

In the macaque, area V3A is connected with LIP and MT and receives input from V1. Its neurons have activity influenced by angle of gaze (Galletti and Battaglini 1989). The responses of monkey V3A neurons during smooth pursuit have not been systemati-

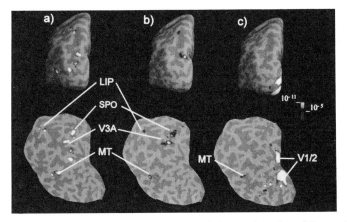

Figure 4. Dorsal views (upper panel) of the inflated left hemisphere and patches of flattened occipital cortex (lower panels) of one representative subject. Panel a) shows areas responding to smooth pursuit eye movements, b) pursuit to an apparent moving but retinally stabilized afterimage, and c) areas responding to passive movement of the eyeball while looking at a textured background.

cally explored to our knowledge. In the present experiments, V3A responded non-specifically during all kinds of eye movements and the full field motion. Therefore results a predominantly visual component in V3A response during eye movements. In the monkey, smooth pursuit modulates the responses of single units in MT and MST (Komatsu and Wurtz 1988a,b; Newsome et al. 1988). MSTl neurons are distinguished from those in MT and MSTd by their preferential role in the initiation and maintenance of smooth pursuit eye movements (Dursteler and Wurtz 1988; Komatsu and Wurtz 1989) and their sluggish visual responses to full-field motions (Saito et al. 1986). In some subjects, the eye movement related activation centred on the MT focus was of greater spatial extent than the selective response to high contrast radial motion (see Figure 3 and 4). This is probably due to the recruitment of a small region (3–6 mm wide) which is activated during pursuit eye movements but not labelled by wide-field visual motion. This small region is typically located dorsal to MT and was selectively activated under conditions eliciting smooth pursuit, but not during viewing of full-field motions reflecting the properties resembling the physiological responses of macaque MST lateral (MSTl) neurons. As these findings lie close to the spatial resolution of the functional images collected, we prefer to refer to these motion areas as the MT/MST complex. The present experiments do not reveal whether this is a command signal that directs pursuit, or a re-afference signal that apprises the motion system of ongoing eye movements. However, the latter is more likely, given that phase delays of human pursuit are too short to be supported by a cortical loop.

4.2. SPO and LIP

The response of SPO and dLIP, which were activated by voluntary eye movements (both with and without retinal slip, see Figure 4 a,b) but not by passive eye movements (Figure 4 c), suggests that their sensorimotor roles are distinguishable from the motion areas (i.e. V3A and MT respond different from SPO). It also implies that the retinal stimulation occurring during tracking does not account for the entire response of MT/MST, since the visual stimulation is largest during passive eye moving, when these areas show their weakest activation. An extraretinal influence specific to the process of registering eye motions, and/or the process of executing a predominantly smooth eye movement, must therefore underlie the responses of MT/MST, SPO and dLIP in experiments of voluntary smooth pursuit. Macaque LIP has strong cortico-cortical and subcortical connections with established saccade and smooth pursuit subregions separated from areas MT and MST by area 7a (Andersen et al. 1990; Blatt et al. 1990; Baizer et al. 1991, Tian and Lynch 1996). Macaque LIP neurons have visual receptive fields that are largely confined to the contralateral visual field and motor fields that participate in the planning and execution of visually guided saccades (Blatt et al. 1990; Barash et al. 1991a,b). This area is typically located in the posterior portion of the lateral intraparietal sulcus. We consider it a candidate for the human "posterior eye field" which may correspond to LIP in the macaque monkey (Barash et al. 1991a,b). The localization of this area is similar to LIP candidates previously identified using PET (Fox et al. 1985; Paus et al. 1993; Petit et al. 1993; Anderson et al. 1994), lesion studies (Pierrot-Deseilligny et al. 1991) and transcranial magnetic stimulation (Elkington et al. 1992; Oyachi and Ohtsuka 1995). We showed for the first time, that it is possible to dissect sensory and motor components of smooth pursuit related activation in the human visual "dorsal stream" using functional MR. Even with its limited spatial and temporal resolution, the fMRI technique can be expected to make a real and complementary contribution to understanding primate visual cortex. The fMRI allows unlimited sampling of neuronal activity throughout a single brain, and sophisticated behavioural paradigms involving fixation, eye movements, or attention are certainly easier to arrange in humans than in animals. With such an approach, it may eventually be possible to construct an objective hierarchy of dorsal stream visual areas on the basis of functional criteria (e.g. Friston et al. 1993), similar to previous approaches using anatomical criteria (Felleman and Van Essen 1991; Young 1992).

REFERENCES

Andersen RA, Asanuma C, Essick G, Siegel RM (1990) Cortico-cortical connections of anatomically and physiologically defined subdivisions within the inferior parietal lobule. J Comp Neurol 296: 65–113
Anderson TJ, Jenkins IH, Brooks DJ, Hawken MB, Frackowiak RS, Kennard C (1994) Cortical control of saccades and fixation in man. A PET study. Brain 117:1073–1084
Baizer JS, Ungerleider LG, Desimone R (1991) Organization of visual inputs to the inferior temporal and posterior parietal cortex in macaques. J Neurosci 11:168–190
Baloh RW, Yee RD, Honrubia V (1980) Optokinetic nystagmus and parietal lobe lesions. Ann Neurol 7: 269–276
Barash S, Bracewell RM, Fogassi L, Gnadt JW, Andersen RA (1991a) Saccade-related activity in the lateral intraparietal area. I. Temporal properties; comparison with area 7a. J Neurophysiol 66: 1095–1108
Barash S, Bracewell RM, Fogassi L, Gnadt JW, Andersen RA (1991b) Saccade-related activity in the lateral intraparietal area. II. Spatial properties. J Neurophysiol 66: 1109–1124
Barton JJ, Simpson T, Kiriakopoulos E, Stewart C, Crawley A, Guthrie B, Wood M, Mikulis D (1996) Functional MRI of lateral occipitotemporal cortex during pursuit and motion perception. Ann Neurol 40: 387–398
Barnes GR, Asselman PT (1991) The mechanism of prediction in human smooth pursuit eye movements. J Physiol 439: 439–461
Blatt GJ, Andersen RA, Stoner GR (1990) Visual receptive field organization and cortico-cortical connections of the lateral intraparietal area (area LIP) in the macaque. J Comp Neurol 299: 421–445
Brandt SA, Reppas JB, Dale AM, Wenzel R, Savoy RL, Tootell RBH (1997) Simultaneous infra-red oculography and fMRI. Proc ISNMR Vancouver 3: 1978
Carter N and Zee DS (1997) The anatomical localization of saccades using functional imaging studies and transcranial magnetic stimulation. Curr Opin Neurol 10: 10–7
Dale AM, Sereno MI (1993) Improved localization of cortical activity by combining EEG and MEG with MRI cortical surface reconstruction: a linear approach. J Cog Neurosci 5:162–176
DeYoe EA, Bandettini P, Neitz J, Miller D, Winans P (1994) Functional magnetic resonance imaging (FMRI) of the human brain. J Neurosci Methods 54: 171–187
Dupont P, Orban GA, De Bruyn B, Verbruggen A, Mortelmans L (1994) Many areas in the human brain respond to visual motion. J Neurophysiol 72: 1420–1424

Dursteler MR, Wurtz RH, Newsome WT (1987) Directional pursuit deficits following lesions of the foveal representation within the superior temporal sulcus of the macaque monkey. J Neurophysiol 57: 1262–1287

Dursteler MR, Wurtz RH (1988) Pursuit and optokinetic deficits following chemical lesions of cortical areas MT and MST. J Neurophysiol 60: 940–965

Elkington PT, Kerr GK, Stein JS (1992) The effect of electromagnetic stimulation of the posterior parietal cortex on eye movements. Eye 6: 510–514

Felleman DJ, Van Essen DC (1991) Distributed hierarchical processing in the primate cerebral cortex. Cereb Cortex 1: 1–47

Friston KJ, Frith CD, Dolan RJ, Liddle PF, Frackowiak RS (1993) Functional connectivity: the principal components analysis of large PET data findings. J Cereb Blood Flow Metab 13: 5–14

Fox PT, Fox JM, Raichle ME (1985) The role of cerebral cortex in the generation of voluntary saccades: a positron emission tomographic study. J Neurophysiol 54: 348–369

Galletti C, Battaglini PP (1989) Gaze-dependent neurons in area V3A of monkey prestriate cortex. J Neurosci 9: 1112–1125

Grüsser OJ, Landis T (1991) Visual movement agnosias, or motion blindness: A rare clinical syndrom. In: Grüsser OJ and Landis T (eds) Visual agnosias and other disturbances of visual perception and cognition. The Macmillan Press, London, pp 359–384

Komatsu H, Wurtz RH (1988a) Relation of cortical areas MT and MST to pursuit eye movements. I. Localization and visual properties of neurons. J Neurophysiol 60: 580–603

Komatsu H, Wurtz RH (1988b) Relation of cortical areas MT and MST to pursuit eye movements. III. Interaction with full-field visual stimulation. J Neurophysiol 60: 621–644

Komatsu H, Wurtz RH (1989) Modulation of pursuit eye movements by stimulation of cortical areas MT and MST. J Neurophysiol 62: 31–47

Newsome WT, Wurtz RH, Dursteler MR, Mikami A (1985) Deficits in visual motion processing following ibotenic acid lesions of the middle temporal visual area of the macaque monkey. J Neurosci 5: 825–840

Newsome WT, Wurtz RH, Komatsu H (1988) Relation of cortical areas MT and MST to pursuit eye movements. II. Differentiation of retinal from extraretinal inputs. J Neurophysiol 60: 604–620

Oyachi H, Ohtsuka K (1995) Transcranial magnetic stimulation of the posterior parietal cortex degrades accuracy of memory-guided saccades in human. Invest Ophthalmol Vis Sci 36: 1441–1449

Paus T, Petrides M, Evans AC, Meyer E (1993) Role of the human anterior cingulate cortex in the control of oculomotor, manual and speech responses: a positron emmision tomography study. J Neurophysiol 70: 453–469

Petit L, Orssaud C, Tzourio N, Salamon G, Mazoyer B, Berthoz A (1993) PET study of voluntary saccadic eye movements in humans: basal ganglia-thalamocortical system and cingulate cortex involvement. J Neurophysiol 69: 1009–1017

Petit L, Clark VP, Ingeholm J, Haxby JV (1997) Dissociation of saccade-related and pursuit-related activation in human frontal eye fields as revealed by fMRI. J Neurophysiol 77: 3386–3390

Pierrot-Deseilligny C, Rivaud S, Gaymard B, Agid Y (1991) Cortical control of reflexive visually-guided saccades. Brain 114: 1473–1485

Saito H, Yukie M, Tanaka K, Hikosaka K, Fukada Y, Iwai E (1986) Integration of direction signals of image motion in the superior temporal sulcus of the macaque monkey. J Neurosci 6: 145–157

Sereno MI, Dale AM, Reppas JB, Kwong KK, Belliveau JW, Brady TJ, Rosen BR, Tootell RB (1995) Borders of multiple visual areas in humans revealed by functional magnetic resonance imaging. Science 268: 889–893

Sharpe JA, Morrow MJ (1991) Cerebral hemispheric smooth pursuit disorders. Acta Neurol Belg 91: 81–96

Tian JR, Lynch JC (1996) Functionally defined smooth and saccadic eye movement subregions in the frontal eye field of Cebus monkeys. J Neurophysiol 76: 2740–2753

Tootell RB, Reppas JB, Dale AM, Look RB, Sereno MI, Malach R, Brady TJ, Rosen BR (1995a) Visual motion aftereffect in human cortical area MT revealed by functional magnetic resonance imaging. Nature 375: 139–141

Tootell RB, Reppas JB, Kwong KK, Malach R, Born RT, Brady TJ, Rosen BR, Belliveau JW (1995b) Functional analysis of human MT and related visual cortical areas using magnetic resonance imaging. J Neurosci 15: 3215–3230

Tootell RB, Mendola JD, Hadjikhani NK, Ledden PJ, Liu AK, Reppas JB, Sereno MI, Dale AM (1997) Functional analysis of V3A and related areas in human visual cortex. J Neurosci 17: 7060–7078

Watson JD, Myers R, Frackowiak RS, Hajnal JV, Woods RP, Mazziotta JC, Shipp S, Zeki S (1993) Area V5 of the human brain: evidence from a combined study using positron emission tomograpy and magnetic resonance imaging. Cereb Cortex 3: 79–94

Young MP (1992) Objective analysis of the topological organization of the primate cortical visual system. Nature 358: 152–155

CORTICAL CONTROL OF SEQUENCES OF MEMORY-GUIDED SACCADES

W. Heide,[1] F. Binkofski, S. Posse,[3] R. J. Seitz,[2] D. Kömpf,[1] and H-J. Freund[2]

[1]Department of Neurology
Medical University
D-23538 Lübeck, Germany
[2]Department of Neurology
Heinrich-Heine-University
Moorenstr. 5, D-40225 Düsseldorf, Germany
[3]Institute of Medicine
Research Center Jülich
D-52428 Jülich, Germany

1. ABSTRACT

To determine the role of frontal and parietal cortical areas for sequences of memory-guided saccades, we performed functional magnetic resonance imaging (fMRI) in 6 healthy adults, using echoplanar sequences, alternating between activation and control conditions. After realignment, spatial normalization and smoothing, individual and group analysis was performed (SPM96b). We applied a triple-step stimulus consisting of 3 successively flashed laser targets that had to be memorized and fixated in darkness. Control conditions included fixation, visually-guided saccades, single memory-guided saccades, and a spatial working memory task (SWM). Triple-step saccades and the SWM task activated both frontal eye fields (FEF), the premotor cortex (PMC), the supplementary eye field (SEF), the anterior cingulate (AC) gyrus, and 3 areas around the medial and posterior portion of the intraparietal sulcus, the probable location of the human parietal eye field. Comparison of the activation patterns in the different task-control conditions permitted the following conclusions: The FEF is important for the initiation of voluntary saccades, the SEF for the triggering of saccadic sequences, the AC for sustained attention, the parietal and PMC areas for spatially-directed attention, spatial cueing, and spatial working memory. The dorsolateral prefrontal cortex was activated only in the SWM task.

Current Oculomotor Research, edited by Becker *et al.*
Plenum Press, New York, 1999.

2. INTRODUCTION

2.1. Cortical Areas Involved in Saccadic Eye Movements

Although the main neural generators for saccadic eye movements are located in the brainstem, the cerebral cortex plays an important role in controlling the initiation and spatial accuracy of various types of saccades. The respective cortical areas were first identified in the cerebral cortex of monkeys (Goldberg and Segraves 1989, Andersen and Gnadt 1989, Funahashi et al. 1993), e.g. the frontal eye field (FEF), the supplementary eye field in the anterior portion of the supplementary motor area (SMA), the dorsolateral prefrontal cortex (PFC), and the parietal eye field, the so-called lateral intraparietal area (LIP), located on the lateral bank of the intraparietal sulcus (IPS). These areas are distributed as a network over the frontal and posterior parietal lobes of both hemispheres. The probable location of their homologous counterparts in human cerebral cortex has been inferred from lesion (Pierrot-Deseilligny et al. 1995; Heide et al. 1995) and activation studies (Anderson et al. 1994, Petit et al. 1993 and 1996, Sweeney et al. 1996), the latter with positron emission tomography (PET). Thus there is considerable evidence that the human FEF is located in the middle portion of the precentral sulcus and gyrus, the PFC anterior to it, extending into Brodmann's area 46, the SMA in the dorsomedial superior frontal gyrus, and the parietal eye field in the posterior parietal cortex (PPC), around the middle and posterior portion of the IPS. However, the exact localization and homology of these areas is still a matter of discussion. Since a more exact mapping has become possible with functional magnetic resonance imaging (fMRI), activated areas in humans have been reported to show some anatomical differences from the macaque monkey in both frontal and parietal cortex (Müri et al. 1996, Luna et al. 1998). In the present study, we investigated the functional significance of these activations by performing different saccadic eye movement tasks during fMRI.

2.2. Saccade Tasks Appropriate for the Analysis of Cortical Functions

Primate studies have yielded evidence that the specific function of each of the cortical areas involved in saccades is related to its role in spatial cognition and must be investigated in a specific behavioural context of the saccadic paradigm. So it has become important to record not only classical visually-guided saccades, triggered externally by a suddenly appearing peripheral visual target, but also memory-guided saccades, which are triggered externally by a go-signal (e.g. extinction of the fixation point), but executed towards an internally-represented memorized location of a visual target that had been flashed previously. Further, internal (self-paced) triggering of saccades to internally-represented targets as well as the use of extraretinal spatial information is required during the performance of sequences of memory-guided saccades.

The shortest possible sequence is performed in the double-step task (Hallett and Lightstone 1976), where two saccades have to be executed to the location of two extrafoveal targets that had been flashed previously in rapid succession. As the second target is seen before the first saccade, a spatial dissonance arises between the retinal coordinates of the 2nd target and the motor coordinates of the necessary 2nd saccade. Spatial accuracy of the 2nd saccade requires updating of the 2nd target's spatial representation by subtracting extraretinal information about the motor vector of the 1st saccade (most probably the efference copy signal). Single neuron studies in monkeys have demonstrated the particular importance of posterior parietal neurons in area LIP for the this spatial updating, which seems to be achieved by a remapping of their receptive fields prior to an impending saccade, thus anticipating the retinal image shift according to the information provided by efference copy (Goldberg et al. 1990, Duhamel et al. 1992). Neural correlates of the efference copy signal have also been found in the superior colliculus, the central thalamus, the FEF, and the SMA (Goldberg and Bruce 1990, Schlag-Rey et al. 1990, review in Heide and Kömpf 1997).

2.3. Functional Specialization of Cortical Saccade Areas

According to the results of clinical lesion studies, each of the cortical saccade areas is critical for the control of certain saccadic subfunctions (Heide and Kömpf 1994, Pierrot-Deseilligny et al. 1995): the FEF more for the initiation of internally-triggered intentional saccades and - together with the PFC - for the suppression of inappropriate reflexive saccades, the SMA for the initiation of learned saccadic sequences, the PFC for short-term memorization of the saccade goal's spatial location, and the PPC for the initiation of visually-triggered reflexive saccades and for saccade-related spatial transformations. In the double-step paradigm (Heide et al. 1995) specifically patients with PPC lesions showed a significant dysmetria or even a complete failure of the second saccade, whenever the first saccade had been directed into the contralesional hemifield. In contrast, frontal lesions left this function intact, but impaired temporal properties of double-step saccades, such as the correct temporal order (FEF, PFC, and SMA lesions), the timing of the 2nd saccade (SMA lesions), and the spatial working memory for the 2nd target (PFC lesions). Thus the PPC (with right hemispheric dominance) seems to be essential for the spatial programming of saccades that require the use of extraretinal information (efference copy), and for the maintenance of spatial constancy across saccades (Heide and Kömpf 1997).

It was the the main objective of the present study to delineate specific cortical activation patterns reflecting this functional specialization, e.g. spatial working memory, or the use of the efference copy signal by PPC neurons for the spatial programming of saccades in the presence of retino-spatial dissonance. Thus we performed fMRI in normal subjects during the execution of triple-step sequences of memory-guided saccades. However, in contrast to the results of lesion studies, previous studies with functional brain imaging have shown that the whole network of cortical saccade areas is active in almost any saccade task (Sweeney et al. 1996, Petit et al. 1996). Therefore we aimed at identifying specific task-related activations by choosing various combinations of the different saccadic paradigms as task-control comparisons and by averaging image sets across subjects to obtain group activation maps.

3. METHODS

3.1. Subjects and Scanning Procedures

In 6 naive healthy right-handed subjects, aged 27 to 41 years, we performed functional magnetic resonance imaging (fMRI) measurements on a Siemens Vision system at 1.5 Tesla, using a standard head coil and echoplanar sequences (EPI), sensitive to blood oxygen level dependent (BOLD) effects. Acquisition parameters were: TR = 3 s; TE = 66 ms; a = 90°; acquisition matrix of 64 x 64 with a voxel size of 3 x 3 x 4 mm. The imaged volume included 16 axial slices of 3 mm thickness, covering the dorsal part of the brain down to the internal capsule, but not including the whole primary visual cortex. For each experiment, the protocol consisted of 6 cycles, alternating between activation and control conditions. Each condition lasted for 24 s, thus each cycle for 48 s, and one complete experiment for 288 s (almost 5 min). All subjects gave their informed consent in written form.

3.2. Data Analysis

After realignment, spatial normalization, and smoothing with a radius of 2 pixels, individual and group analysis was performed using SPM 96b (Wellcome Department of Cognitive Neurology, London, UK) and thus aligning all images into Talairach space. Categorial task-control comparisons were thresholded at $P < 0.01$ for each voxel and at $P < 0.05$ for spatial extent. For intertask-comparisons (e.g. sequences of memory-guided saccades versus visually-guided saccades) the threshold was set to $P < 0.05$ for each voxel. In the results section, we will further present the t-values as calculated by SPM96b. They reflect the degree of increase in MR signal intensity for the respective voxel during the activation condition relative to the control condition, for the entire group of subjects.

3.3. Visual Stimuli and Behavioral Tasks

For visual stimulation, a red laser spot was projected to a screen that was shown to the subjects on a mirror, positioned within the head coil 15 cm above the eyes. The critical task was a triple-step stimulus (analogous to the double-step stimulus) consisting of 3 successively flashed targets (for 265 ms, 235 ms, and 200 ms, respectively) of different horizontal eccentricities ($5°$, $7°$, $8°$, or $10°$), presented in a pseudo-randomized order. Subjects were instructed to maintain central fixation during target presentation and to memorize the locations of the 3 targets. After a delay of 500 ms, 3 saccades had to be performed in total darkness towards these remembered locations in the correct order. After 3.3 s, the central fixation point reappeared to start the next trial. Each triple-step trial lasted for 6 s, thus one activation cycle (24 s) consisted of 4 triple-step sequences.

Five other tasks served as control conditions: fixation of central laser spot; central fixation during triple-step stimulation, requiring the suppression of visually-triggered reflexive saccades to the targets; further a spatial working memory (SWM) task, visually-guided saccades, and single memory-guided saccades. The latter two saccade tasks consisted of the same number and the same sequences of saccades as the triple-step stimulus. In the SWM task subjects had to maintain fixation and to memorize the triple-step stimulus, just as in the triple-step task. However, after a delay of 2.5 s, the laser jumped to a peripheral location, which was either identical to one of the triple-step targets presented previously, or it was different. Only when it was identical, it had to be foveated by a visually-guided saccade. Before each measurement, at least one cycle of the respective task was presented to the subjects for practice. Subjects's performance was controlled by electrooculography.

4. RESULTS

4.1. Visually-Guided Saccades

The performance of visually-guided saccades, controlled against central fixation, yielded significant activations of almost the entire network of cortical saccade areas (Fig. 1A): in the FEF of both hemispheres, in the left SMA, and in 2 distinct regions of the

PPC, further in the right lateral premotor cortex (PMC), located ventral and slightly ante-rior to the FEF (Talairach coordinates [in mm] of the voxel with peak activation: x/y/z = 52/0/36; t-value: 5.64). In the region of the FEF itself, there were two peaks of ac-tivation in each hemisphere: one was centered around the superior portion of the precen-tral sulcus, extending posteriorly into the adjacent part of the precentral gyrus and dorsally towards the superior frontal sulcus (Talairach coordinates 32/-8/56 in the right and -28/-8/52 in the left hemisphere; t = 6.69), and the other more ventrally around the middle por-tion of the precentral sulcus (48/-8/44, or -44/-8/44, respectively; t = 6.44). SMA activation was only moderate (t = 4.95) in this task, centered in the paramedian portion of the left superior frontal gyrus (peak voxel at -4/4/48). In the PPC, one peak of activation was located in the postero-lateral portion of the superior parietal lobule (SPL), medio-dor-sal of the IPS (coordinates 20/-60/68, or -28/-56/60; t-values 5.82 and 5.44, respectively). The other center of activation was only weak in this task (t = 3.12), but much stronger in the triple-step and memory-guided saccade tasks (t = 6.39); it was located in the parame-dian posterior portion of the right PPC, extending into the precuneus (8/-68/64).

If activation and control conditions were interchanged, there was one significant fo-cus of activation in the region of the left posterior cingulate cortex, extending into the pre-cuneus (at -4/-52/40; t = 4.52), which was even more pronounced when the triple-step paradigm was taken as control condition (t = 6.58). It might be a functional correlate of continuous visual fixation.

4.2. Single Memory-Guided Saccades

The performance of successive single memory-guided saccades, controlled against maintenance of central fixation despite visual stimulation (flashing of the saccade targets), activated a similar network of cortical areas, with slight differences with respect to visu-ally-guided saccades: The centers of bilateral FEF activation were restricted to the medial precentral sulcus and gyrus (44/-8/48), there was no significant SMA activity in the group data, and there were 3 distinct centers of activation in the right PPC. The strongest parietal activation was measured in the precuneus (12/-80/48; t = 6.08), another in the posterior SPL, medial to the IPS (24/-72/52; t = 5.54), and a third weak activation in the posterior portion of the inferior parietal lobule (IPL), ventro-lateral to the IPS (40/-76/36; t = 3.44). In the left PPC, significant activation was restricted to the SPL (-32/-56/60; t = 4.79).

4.3. Triple-Step Saccades

When triple-step saccades were controlled against central fixation (with or without peripheral visual stimulation), the following cortical regions were significantly activated (Fig. 1B): the FEF bilaterally, with the 2 peaks of activity located around the superior and the medial portion of the precentral sulcus, as outlined in section 4.1. (t-values ranging be-tween 7.11 and 7.39); the lateral PMC bilaterally (coordinates 48/4/28 and -48/4/28; t-val-ues 6.62 and 6.02, respectively); the SMA bilaterally, with left hemispheric dominance (peak activation at 8/0/52 and at -4/4/48, t-values 4.62 and 7.51, respectively); at least 3 regions of the PPC bilaterally, namely the antero-lateral SPL, adjacent to the middle por-tion of the IPS (at 36/-56/52 and -32/-56/56; t-values 4.03 and 6.24, respectively), the pos-tero-medial SPL (16/-68/56 and -20/-72/56; t-values 6.53 and 6.85, respectively), and the adjacent precuneus (at 12/-80/48 and -16/-76/60; t > 6.10).

Further, when the control condition was central fixation without visual stimulation, triple-step saccades activated also the right IPL in its anterior portion and the adjacent IPS

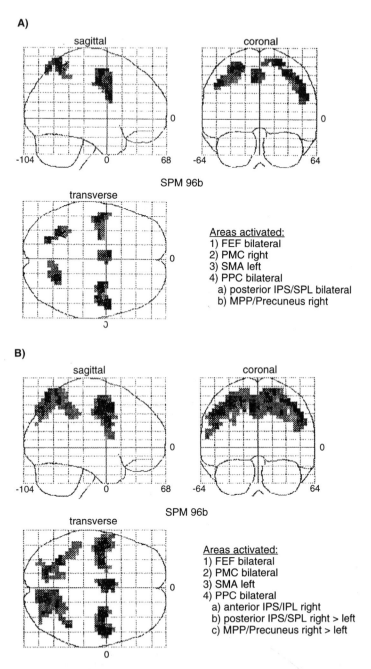

Figure 1. Statistical parametric mapping (SPM96b) in Talairach coordinates, showing the cortical regions that were significantly activated during the performance of visually-guided saccades (A), relative to central fixation, or during the performance of triple-step saccades, relative to central fixation (B), or relative to visually-guided saccades (C). FEF: frontal eye field; PMC: premotor cortex; SMA: supplementary motor area; PFC: prefrontal cortex; AC: anterior cingulate cortex; PPC: posterior parietal cortex; IPS: intraparietal sulcus; IPL: inferior parietal lobule; SPL: superior parietal lobule; MPP: medial posterior parietal region, extending into the precuneus.

c)

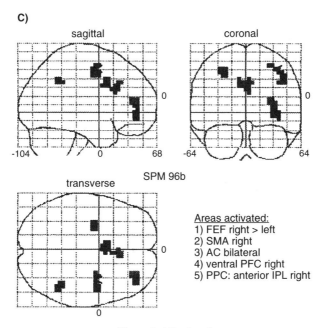

Areas activated:
1) FEF right > left
2) SMA right
3) AC bilateral
4) ventral PFC right
5) PPC: anterior IPL right

Figure 1. (*Continued*)

(at 44/-48/48; t = 4.78). As this activity was not present with central fixation during peripheral visual stimulation as control condition, it seems to be related either to the triple-step visual stimulus itself or to the suppression of reflexive visually-triggered saccades towards the flashed targets. In summary, during triple-step saccades activation of all these areas was stronger and spatially more extended than during visually-guided saccades, although the basic network of activated areas was almost identical. It may be noted, however, that there was no significant activation of the PFC in any of these tasks.

In order to evoke patterns of activaty that might be related specfically to the triple-step task, we used the other saccade tasks as control conditions. This reduced not only the number of activated regions, but also their spatial extent and their activation level. With triple-step saccades, controlled versus visually-guided saccades (Fig. 1C), significant activation (p < 0.05) was found in the FEF (its superior portion bilaterally and its right inferior portion, t-values ranging from 3.43 to 3.95), in the right IPL (t = 3.11), in the right ventral SMA (t = 3.85), in the adjacent right and left anterior cingulate gyrus (AC; peak activation at 4/20/28 and -4/12/32, t = 4.37), and in the right ventral PFC (32/48/0; t = 3.23). However, there was no activation in the PMC, the SPL, and the precuneus. If single memory-guided saccades were used as control condition, the triple-step task activated the FEF bilaterally (its right superior portion and its inferior portion bilaterally; t > 4.5), the left SMA (t = 5.17) , the right anterior cingulate cortex (4/12/32, t = 4.15), the right precuneus (12/-80/ 48; t = 5.1) as the only parietal region, and weakly the right PFC (4/12/32, t = 2.91). In summary, these intertask-comparisons revealed some activation of frontal areas, related to triple-step saccades, namely in the FEF, the SMA, the anterior cingulate gyrus, and weakly in the PFC. However, there was no consistent parietal activation left that might have been regarded as a functional correlate of the efference copy signal or the respective spatial transformations needed for the spatial accuracy of triple-step saccades.

4.4. Spatial Working Memory Task

To our surprise, the spatial working memory task (SWM), relative to central fixation, activated the same network of cortical areas as the triple-step task, some of them even at a higher level, suggesting greater intersubject homogenity (t-values ranging between 6.22 and 7.82). Also the clusters of activated voxels were larger. Active areas included the superior and inferior portions of both FEFs, the PMC and the PFC bilaterally, the left SMA, the right AC, and all the mentioned parietal regions (precuneus, anterior and posterior IPL and SPL, centered around the IPS) bilaterally, with a mild right hemispheric preponderance. If the triple-step task was controlled against the SWM task, significant activation was left in the postero-inferior portion of the right FEF (44/-16/48; t = 3.81) and in the right SMA (4/-8/48; t = 5.03), but nowhere else. In the reverse condition (SWM versus triple-step), activated regions were restricted to the PFC and the IPL of both hemispheres.

5. DISCUSSION AND CONCLUSIONS

All the different saccade tasks as well as the SWM task activated largely the same network of cortical areas, resembling the network for the control of visuo-spatial attention (Mesulam 1990, Nobre et al. 1997). Obviously all these areas are involved not only in the control of saccades, but also in spatial cognition, particularly in spatial working memory and in spatially-directed attention, needed for the performance of the SWM task. Task-re-

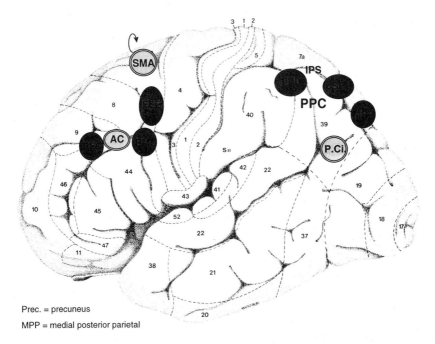

Figure 2. Schematic lateral surface of a human brain showing the network of cortical areas involved in the control of sequences of memory-guided saccades. The numbers indicate the Brodmann areas. The SMA, the AC, and the posterior cingulate cortex (P.Ci.) are located on the medial surface of the brain. For abbreviations see Fig. 1.

lated differences in the patterns of activation and the results of intertask-comparisons led us to the following assumptions, concerning the specific functional contribution of each area:

1. The *FEF* seems to be the the main cortical center for the initiation of intentional and internally-guided saccades, but it is also involved in the control of visually-guided saccades and of voluntary shifts of spatial attention, as needed in the SWM task. In accordance with recent fMRI studies (Petit et al. 1997, Luna et al. 1998), we presented evidence that the human FEF is centered around the pre-central sulcus and the adjacent portion of the precentral gyrus, but it does not extend into the primary motor cortex (area 4) itself. The FEF is composed of at least two foci of activation, one in the superior and one in the middle part of the precentral sulcus.

2. In close vicinity to the FEF, directly ventral and slightly anterior to it, parts of the lateral *PMC* were activated during the SWM task and the saccade tasks. To our knowledge, this has never been reported before. The activity in the right PMC (activated in each of the tasks) might reflect spatially directed attention for action, whereas the left PMC might be involved in spatial working memory, as it was active only when saccadic sequences had to be memorized.

3. As the supplementary eye field (*SEF*) in the *SMA* was not activated during single memory-guided saccades, it is obviously involved in the triggering and timing of saccadic sequences, particularly if they are memory-guided or self-paced. This is consistent with the results of a similar study with PET (Petit et al. 1996) as well as with previous human lesion studies (Gaymard et al. 1990, Heide et al. 1995) and single-neuron data in monkeys (Mushiake et al. 1990)

4. The *PFC* was activated almost exclusively in the SWM task, indicating its involvement in spatial working memory whenever the memorization time exceeds 1 s, like in non-human primates (Funahashi et al. 1993). However, we found no evidence in this study that the human PFC plays a specific role in saccade generation.

5. An activation of the *AC* during saccades has rarely been reported before, and its functional significance is unclear. We speculate that it might reflect the duration of sustained attention, as it occurred only in the SWM task, relative to fixation, and in the triple-step task, relative to other saccade tasks. Previous research has presented evidence that the AC is part of the cortical network controlling premotor attention (Mesulam 1990), further that it is involved in the preparation of motor responses (Paus et al. 1993) and in the initiation of intentional saccades (Gaymard et al. 1996).

6. In accordance with two recent studies using saccadic (Luna et al. 1998) and attentional paradigms (Nobre et al. 1997), we found at least 3 foci of activation in the *posterior parietal cortex*. Their homology with respect to the parietal eye fields of macaque monkeys is unclear. Functionally, parietal activation at least in the medial and posterior SPL and in the precuneus might reflect the spatial allocation of the attentional vector, even if the subject is just waiting for the appearance of the behaviorally relevant stimulus during the SWM task. This behavior resembles that of neurons in the primary parietal eye field (area LIP) of monkeys (Colby et al. 1996). Activation of the anterior IPL, however, might rather be related to the spatial coding of the stimulus trajectory, in accordance with the results of a recent PET study on parietal representations of graphomotor trajec-

tories (Seitz et al. 1997). Alternatively, IPL activation could reflect the suppression of inappropriate visually-triggered reflexive saccades, but this is not supported by lesion studies which attribute this function rather to the FEF (Heide and Kömpf 1994) or the PFC (Pierrot-Deseilligny et al. 1995). In summary, multiple foci of activation in human PPC have been confirmed in several recent functional imaging studies, indicating the existence of multiple parietal representations of saccades and other visuo-motor or visuo-spatial functions. However their functional role and their homology to the PPC of macaques requires further research. Our triple-step data provided no specific parietal correlate for the saccade-associated updating of spatial representations by the use of efference copy, probably because the efference copy signal is present in all types of saccades, no matter if it is essential for their spatial programming or not.

7. The *posterior cingulate cortex* might be involved in the maintenance of central fixation. There is evidence from a recent primate study that its neurons show gaze-dependent firing during periods of visual fixation between eye movements (Olson et al. 1996). They seem to monitor eye movements and eye position.

In conclusion, our fMRI study demonstrates the network character of cortical areas involved in the control of saccades, thus making it difficult to identify the specific function of each area. For this purpose, lesion studies are more appropriate. However, it must be taken into account that both approaches investigate different aspects of the same issue: Lesion studies identify the cerebral sites that are critical for the control of a certain function, whereas functional imaging identifies all cortical areas that are involved in a certain function. This might explain some of the discrepancies between the conclusions of this study and the results of previous lesion studies.

REFERENCES

Andersen RA, Gnadt JW (1989) Posterior parietal cortex. In: Wurtz RH, Goldberg ME (eds) The neurobiology of saccadic eye movements. Elsevier, Amsterdam 3: 315–336.

Anderson TJ, Jenkins IH, Brooks DL, Hawken MB, Frackowiak RSJ, Kennard C (1994) Cortical control of saccades and fixation in man. A PET study. Brain 117: 1073–1084.

Colby CL, Duhamel J-R, Goldberg ME (1996) Visual, presaccadic, and cognitive activation of single neurons in monkey lateral intraparietal area. J Neurophysiol 76: 2841–2852.

Duhamel J-R, Colby CL, Goldberg ME (1992) The updating of the representation of visual space in parietal cortex by intended eye movements. Science 255: 90–92.

Funahashi S, Bruce CJ, Goldman-Rakic PS (1993) Dorsolateral prefrontal lesions and oculomotor delayed-response performance: evidence for "mnemonic" scotomas. J Neurosci 13: 1479–1497.

Gaymard B, Rivaud S, Pierrot-Deseilligny C (1990) Impairment of sequences of memory-guided saccades after supplementary motor area lesions. Ann Neurol 28:622–626.

Gaymard B, Rivaud S, Cassarini JF, Vermersch A-I, Pierrot-Deseilligny C (1996) Involvement of the anterior cingulate cortex in eye movement control. Soc Neurosci Abstr 22: 1688.

Goldberg ME, Segraves MA (1989) The visual and frontal cortices. In: Wurtz RH, Goldberg ME (eds) The neurobiology of saccadic eye movements. Elsevier, Amsterdam 3: 283–314.

Goldberg ME, Bruce CJ (1990) Primate frontal eye fields. III. Maintainance of a spatially accurate saccade signal. J Neurophysiol 64: 489–508.

Goldberg ME, Colby CL, Duhamel J-R (1990) Representation of visuomotor space in the parietal lobe of the monkey. Cold Spring Harbor Symp 55: 729–739.

Hallett PE, Lightstone AD (1976) Saccadic eye movements to flashed targets. Vision Res 16: 107–114.

Heide W, Kömpf D (1994) Saccades after frontal and parietal lesions. In: Fuchs AF, Brandt T, Büttner U, Zee DS (eds) Contemporary Ocular Motor and Vestibular Research: A Tribute to David A. Robinson. Georg Thieme Verlag, Stuttgart, pp 225–227.

Heide W, Kömpf D (1997) Specific parietal lobe contribution to spatial constancy across saccades. In: Thier P, Karnath H-O (eds) Parietal Lobe Contributions to Orientation in 3D Space. Springer Verlag, Heidelberg, pp 149–172.

Heide W, Blankenburg M, Zimmermann E, Kömpf D (1995) Cortical control of double-step saccades - implications for spatial orientation. Ann Neurol 38: 739–748.

Luna B, Thulborn KR, Strojwas MH, McCurtain BJ, Berman RA, Genovese CR, Sweeney JA (1998) Dorsal regions subserving visually guided saccades in humans: An fMRI study. Cerbral Cortex 8: 40–47.

Mesulam M-M (1990) Large-scale neurocognitive networks and distributed processing for attention, language and memory. Ann Neurol 28: 597–613.

Müri RM, Iba-Zizen MT, Derosier C, Cabanis EA, Pierrot-Deseilligny C (1996) Location of the human posterior eye field with functional magnetic resonance imaging. J Neurol Neurosurg Psychiatry 60: 445–448.

Mushiake H, Inase M, Tanji J (1990) Selective coding of motor sequence in the supplementary motor area of monkey cerebral cortex. Exp Brain Res 82: 208–210.

Nobre AC, Sebestyen GN, Gitelman DR, Mesulam MM, Frackowiak RSJ, Frith CD (1997) Functional localization of the system for visuospatial attention using positron emission tomography. Brain 120: 515–533.

Olson CR, Musil SY, Goldberg ME (1996) Single neurons in posterior cingulate cortex of behaving macaque: eye movement signals. J Neurophysiol 76: 3285–3300.

Paus T, Petrides M, Evans AC, Meyer E (1993) Role of the human anterior cingulate cortex in the control of oculomotor, manual, and speech responses: a positron emission tomography study. J Neurophysiol 70: 453–469.

Petit L, Orssaud C, Tzourio N, Salamon G, Mazoyer B, Berthoz A (1993) PET study of voluntary saccadic eye movements in humans: basal ganglia-thalamocortical system and cingulate cortex involvement. J Neurophysiol 69: 1009–1017.

Petit L, Orssaud C, Tzourio N, Crivello F, Berthoz A, Mazoyer B (1996) Functional anatomy of a prelearned sequence of horizontal saccades in humans. J Neurosci 16: 3714–3726.

Petit L, Clark VP, Ingeholm J, Haxby JV (1997) Dissociation of saccade-related and pursuit-related activation in human frontal eye fields as revealed by fMRI. J Neurophysiol 77: 3386–3390.

Pierrot-Deseilligny C, Rivaud S, Gaymard B, Müri R, Vermersch A-I (1995) Cortical control of saccades. Ann Neurol 37: 557–567.

Schlag J, Schlag-Rey M, Pigarev I (1990) Supplementary eye field - influence of eye position on neural signals of fixation. Exp Brain Res 90: 302–306.

Seitz RJ, Canavan AGM, Herzog H, Tellmann L, Knorr U, Huang Y, Hömberg V (1997) Representation of graphomotor trajectories in the human parietal cortex: evidence for controlled processing and automatic performance. Eur J Neurosci 9: 378–389.

Sweeney JA, Mintun MA, Kwee S, Wiseman MB, Brown DL, Rosenberg DR, Carl JR (1996) Positron emission tomography study of voluntary saccadic eye movements and spatial working memory. J Neurophysiol 75: 454–468.

33

FUNCTIONAL MRI OF DOUBLE STEP SACCADES

The Role of Cingulate Cortex

R. M. Müri, A. C. Nirkko, C. Ozdoba, P. Tobler, O. Heid, G. Schroth, and C. W. Hess

Departments of Neurology and Neuroradiology
University of Bern, Inselspital
CH-3010 Bern, Switzerland

1. INTRODUCTION

The medial surface of the hemispheres including the cingulate cortex shows an important functional heterogeneity (Vogt et al. 1992). Experimental studies in animals and studies in humans provided evidence that the medial wall is involved in motor control, in attentional and emotional processes, and in eye movements. Furthermore, there is a fundamental dichotomy between functions of the anterior part of the cingulate cortex which serves primarily executive function and the posterior cingulate cortex controlling evaluative functions such as spatial orientation and memory (Vogt et al. 1992). For eye movement control, the role of the cingulate cortex is not fully understood. Most of the functional studies in humans described activity in the anterior (Paus et al. 1993; O'Sullivan et al. 1995; Sweeney et al. 1996; Doricchi et al. 1997) or median cingulum (Petit et al. 1993; 1996; Lang et al. 1994) during eye movements or fixation (Anderson et al. 1994; Petit et al. 1995). However, the observed activity in different studies was not always consistent, and activity seems to be dependent on the ocular motor paradigm. On the other hand, single cell recordings in animals suggest that the posterior cingulate region plays an important role in eye movement control: Olson et al. (1996) found neurons in the posterior cingulate that fired during periods of ocular fixation, dependent on eye position in the orbita and of the size and direction of the preceding eye movement. Furthermore, discharging rate changed during saccadic eye movements, and many neurons exhibited significant excitation after saccades. Similar results were found in the posterior cingulate cortex of the cat (Olson and Musil 1992). They concluded that the posterior cingulate cortex may assess spatial coordinates relative to retinal images. The aim of our study was to examine

Current Oculomotor Research, edited by Becker *et al.*
Plenum Press, New York, 1999.

235

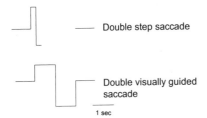

Double step saccade

Double visually guided
saccade

1 sec

Figure 1. Ocular motor paradigm used in this study. The activation patterns of two paradigms were compared: 1) double step saccades in which the first saccade can be programmed in retinotopic coordinates; for the second saccade, extraretinal information (or a craniotopic coordinate system) is needed to calculate the amplitude. 2) Control paradigm with two consecutive visually guided saccades, each amplitude can be calculated in retinotopic coordinates.

the posterior cingulate functions by using fMRI. The eye movement paradigm we applied was the double step paradigm: two visual targets were consecutively flashed for 70 ms, and both targets were switched off before the first saccade was performed by the subject. Consequently, the brain can calculate only the amplitude of the first saccade with retinotopic coordinates. The second saccade has to be calculated in a craniotopic coordinate system which integrates information about the orbital position of the eye after the first saccade (Figure 1). In the control experiment, a paradigm with presentation of two consecutive visual targets with the same amplitude for 1 second each, was used. Therefore, both saccades were visually guided, i.e. the amplitude of both saccades could be calculated in retinotopic coordinates.

2. SUBJECTS AND METHODS

Five healthy subjects, 1 woman and 4 men with a mean age of 36 years (range: 25 to 45 years) were examined. They were all right-handed and gave their informed consent to the study. The study was approved by the local ethical committee. Eye movements were elicited by projecting the visual target with a video- projection system onto a screen in front of the magnet. The performance of eye movements was controlled by an adapted electrooculography system (Felblinger et al. 1996) which allows on-line registration of eye movements during fMRI acquisition.

In each subject, T_2 weighted spin-echo images and T1 weighted MPR (magnetisation prepared rapid gradient echo) volume data of the brain were acquired for individual anatomical registration of the regions of interest. fMRI was performed with a 1.5 Tesla MR system (Magnetom VISION, Siemens, Medical Systems, Erlangen, Germany) using a single shot 2D multislice gradient echo planar imaging (EPI) technique. The axial slices were acquired with an angulation along a line between genu corporis callosi and torcular Herophili to minimise EPI-typical artefacts. Thirty slices covering the whole brain with an acquisition time of 5.6 seconds, were acquired, the pixel size was 1.56 x 1.56 mm with a slice thickness of 5mm and a slice distance of 4 mm. The field of view was 200 x 200 mm (Matrix 90 x 128, TE = 62ms, flip angle 90 degrees). The images were acquired during 8 cycles of alternating double step saccades or visually guided saccades, with a duration of 24 seconds each and a total duration of 6.4 minutes. Z-score maps with z-score values of > 3.0 were generated and overlaid on the anatomic echo planar images. To reduce movement artefacts, head restraints were used to immobilise the volunteer's head with lateral foam pads and a velcro stretch across the forehead. Furthermore, sagittal reconstructions of the images for each subject were calculated for localising the activated region on the medial surface of the hemispheres.

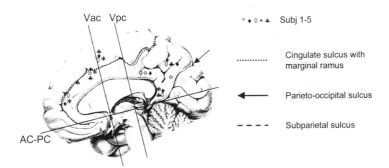

Figure 2. Summary of significant individual activation on the medial wall of the hemispheres. Results for each subject are marked by different symbols. In the anterior cingulate cortex, activity was observed near the Vac line and close to the genu of the corpus callosum. In the posterior cingulate cortex, activity was centred around the isthmus of the cingulate gyrus and the region between the subparietal sulcus and the parietooccipital sulcus. AC-PC: bicommissural (anterior commissure – posterior commissure) line; Vac: anterior vertical to the AC-PC line; Vpc: posterior vertical to the AC-PC line.

3. RESULTS

In all subjects activation on the medial wall of the hemisphere, mainly associated with or adjacent to the sulci, was found (Figure 2). Although the activation was bihemispherical, a dominance of activation in the right hemisphere was generally observed. Three regions in the anterior cingulate were activated: 1) a region in the cingulum close nearby the genu of the corpus callosum, and 2) a region anterior to the Vac line close to the sulcus cinguli, and 3) a region posterior the Vac line in the superior frontal gyrus corresponding to the supplementary motor area (SMA). In the posterior part of the cingulum, activation was located around subparietal sulcus which forms the inferior boundary of the precuneus. Another center of activity in the posterior cingulum was identified at the posterior end of the splenium of the corpus callosum, near the isthmus of the cingular gyrus. Finally, a further center of activity was found in the precuneus near the parieto-occipital sulcus. Activity in the primary visual cortex was inconstantly found.

4. DISCUSSION

The performance of double step saccades compared with that of visually guided saccades resulted in an extensive activation of the medial wall of the hemisphere. Mainly on the right hemisphere, the anterior cingulate showed activation at two regions, a center of activity close to the genu of the corpus callosum and a second center at the Vac line. The latter region is confirmed in PET studies dealing with eye movements. Several studies using memory-guided saccades (Paus et al. 1993; Anderson et al. 1994; O'Sullivan et al. 1995) could significantly activate this region. On the other hand, the study of Sweeney et al. (1996) was not able to show activity of this region in memory-guided saccades. The second region adjacent to the Vac line, located posteriorly and on the superior frontal gyrus reflects SMA activation during the saccade paradigm. Fox and colleagues were among the first showing SMA activity during saccades (Fox et al. 1985), and successively other studies confirmed such eye movement related activity (Paus et al. 1993; Anderson et al. 1994; Lang et al. 1994; Petit et al. 1993, 1996; Doricchi et al. 1997) using different saccade paradigms. The more anteriorly located activity near the genu of the corpus callosum, mostly found on the right hemisphere, probably reflects activity not exclusively related to eye movements. Although activity of this region has been shown in other functional studies of eye movements (Paus et al. 1993; Doricchi et al. 1997), it is well known that this region is essential for behaviour, attention, and exploratory movements (Paus et al. 1993.; Devinsky et al. 1995; Gitelman et al. 1996). Such exploratory or attentional activation could be the reason for the activity found in our subjects since in our experiment we compared activity related to a visually-guided task (low attentional demand) with activity correlated to the double step task that requires more attentional effort. Furthermore, our experimental design was to eliminate pure motor effects of eye movements since the subject performed the same number of saccades in both conditions. It is, therefore, not very probable that the observed activity simply reflects eye movement activity.

As far as we are aware, systematical analysis of activation in the posterior cingulate cortex in human functional studies has not been described. PET has low spatial resolution compared to fMRI, and the close vicinity of the primary visual cortex, the cuneus, and precuneus in the region of the posterior cingulate cortex near the isthmus of the cingulate gyrus probably does not allow a detailed separation of these regions. fMRI on the other hand has a high spatial resolution and the functional activation information can be overlaid on the anatomic echo planar images allowing exact anatomical correlation with the activated region. In our subjects we found activation in the posterior cingulate cortex near the subparietal sulcus which is set apart from the cingulate sulcus and, by the way, not always easy to identify anatomically. Another center of activity was localised in the isthmus of the cingulate gyrus, clearly separated from the primary visual cortex. Finally, precuneus activation near the parieto-occipital sulcus was found.

Does the observed activity reflect postulated transformation of coordinates during visuospatial processing, or is its activity related to the visual stimuli? There are good arguments against the last interpretation: It is known from single cell studies in the monkey (Olson et al. 1996), that many cells have phasic responses to visual stimulation arising only from large textured patterns, and are influenced by the background illumination. In our experiment, however, we used a small dim target for eliciting visually-guided saccades or double step saccade, which was not able in monkeys to elicit phasic responses (Olson et al. 1996). Furthermore, visual presentation was similar in the double step and visually-guided saccades condition (with exception of the short visual presentation of the lateral targets in the double step condition) and the background illumination was identical in both conditions. Finally, the primary visual cortex was not regularly activated in our subjects. In monkeys, the posterior cingulate cortex has strong anatomical connections to the posterior parietal areas including area 7a and lateral intraparietal area (LIP) in the intraparietal sulcus, regions involved in visuospatial processing and in the control of double step saccades. Patients with lesions of the posterior parietal cortex are severely impaired in double step saccades, especially for the second saccade (Heide et al. 1995). Moreover, neurons in the posterior cingulate cortex encode the angle of the eyes in the orbit and the size and direction of the preceding saccade. Therefore, the posterior cingulate cortex is indeed a good candidate for participating in the cortical network involved in visuospatial processing and in transformation of coordinates.

In conclusion, the results of our study show the importance of the medial wall of the hemisphere in the control of complex oculomotor behaviour. Parts of both the anterior and posterior cingulate cortex are significantly activated during double step saccades compared with visually guided saccades. In the anterior cingulate, regions near the Vac and close to the genu of the corpus callosum are activated, the posterior cingulate cortex shows activation near the subparietal sulcus and the isthmus of the cingulate gyrus.

REFERENCES

Anderson TJ, Jenkins IH, Brooks DJ, Hawken MB, Frackowiak RSJ, Kennard C (1994). Cortical control of saccades and fixation in man. A PET study. Brain 117: 1073–1084

Devinsky O, Morrell M, Vogt B (1995). Contributions of anterior cingulate cortex to behaviour. Brain 118: 279–306

Doricchi F, Perani D, Incoccia C, Grassi F, Cappa S, Bettinardi V, Galati G, Pizzamiglio L, Fazio F (1997). Neural control of fast-regular saccades and antisaccades: an investigation using positron emission tomography. Experimental Brain Research 116: 50–62

Felblinger J, Müri RM, Ozdoba C, Schroth G, Hess CW, Boesch C (1996) Recordings of eye movements for stimulus control during fMRI by means of electro-oculographic methods. Magn Reson Med 36: 410–414

Fox PT, Fox JM, Raichle ME, Burde RM (1985). The role of cerebral cortex in the generation of voluntary saccades: A positron emission tomographic study. J Neurophysiol 54(2): 348–369

Gitelman D, Alpert N, Kosslyn S, Daffner K, Scinto L, Thompson W, Mesulam M (1996). Functional imaging of human right hemispheric activation for exploratory movements. Ann Neurol 39: 174–179

Heide W, Blankenburg M, Zimmermann E, Kömpf D (1995). Cortical control of double-step saccades: implications for spatial orientation. Ann Neurol 38(5): 739–48

Lang W, Petit L, Hollinger P, Pietrzyk U, Tzourio N, Mazoyer B, Berthoz A (1994). A positron emission tomography study of oculomotor imagery. Neuroreport 5(8): 921–4

Olson C, Musil, S (1992). Posterior cingulate cortex: sensory and oculomotor properties of single neurons in behaving cat. Cereb Cortex 2: 485–502

Olson C, Musil,S, Goldberg ME (1996). Single neurons in posterior cingulate cortex of behaving macaque: eye movement signals. J Neurophysiol 76: 3285–3300

O'Sullivan EP, Jenkins IH, Henderson L, Kennard C, Brooks DJ (1995). The functional anatomy of remembered saccades: a PET study. Neuroreport 6(16): 2141–2144

Owen A, Evans A, Petrides M (1996). Evidence for a two-stage model of spatial working memory processing within the lateral frontal cortex: a positron emission tomography study. Cereb Cortex 6: 31–38

Paus T, Petrides M, Evans AC, Meyer E (1993). Role of the human anterior cingulate cortex in the control of oculomotor, manual, and speech responses: a positron emission tomography study. J Neurophysiol 70: 453–69

Petit L, Orssaud C, Tzourio N, Crivello F, Berthoz A, Mazoyer B (1996). Functional anatomy of a prelearned sequence of horizontal saccades in humans. J Neurosci 16(11): 3714–26

Petit L, Orssaud C, Tzourio N, Salamon G, Mazoyer B, Berthoz A (1993). PET study of voluntary saccadic eye movements in humans: Basal ganglia- thalamocortical system and cingulate cortex involvement. J Neurophysiol 69(4): 1009–1017

Petit L, Tzourio N, Orssaud C, Pietrzyk U, Berthoz A, Mazoyer B (1995). Functional neuroanatomy of the human visual fixation system. Eur J Neurosci 7: 169–174

Sweeney J, Mintun M, Kwee S, Wiseman M, Brown D, Rosenberg D, Carl J (1996). Positron emission tomography study of voluntary saccadic eye movements and spatial working memory. J Neurophysiol 75: 454–468

Vogt BA, Finch DM, Olson CR (1992) Functional heterogeneity in cingulate cortex: the anterior executive and posterior evaluative regions. Cereb Cortex 2. 435–443

34

OBJECT RECOGNITION AND GOAL-DIRECTED EYE OR HAND MOVEMENTS ARE COUPLED BY VISUAL ATTENTION

Ingo Paprotta, Heiner Deubel, and Werner X. Schneider

Department of Experimental Psychology
Ludwig Maximilians University
Munich, Germany

1. ABSTRACT

A dual-task paradigm required the preparation of a goal-directed movement (hand or eye) concurrently with a letter discrimination task. In the first experiment a hand movement to a location on a virtual circle was required and indicated by a central cue. Simultaneously, the ability to discriminate between the symbols "E" and "∃", presented tachioscopically with various delays on a circular position within surrounding distractors, was taken as a measure of selective perceptual performance. The location of discrimination target remained constant within blocks and was known to the subjects. In the second experiment a saccadic eye movement was required instead of a pointing movement. The data in both experiments clearly demonstrate that discrimination performance is superior when the discrimination target location (DT) is identical to the location of the movement target (MT). When DT and MT refer to different objects, performance deteriorates drastically. We conclude that it is not possible to maintain attention on a stimulus for the purpose of discrimination while preparing a movement to a spatially separate object. This holds, in a quantitatively similar way, for both saccades and manual pointing.

2. INTRODUCTION

The primate visual system can be divided into a ventral stream for perception and recognition and a dorsal stream for computing spatial information for motor action (e.g. Goodale and Millner, 1992). For a goal-directed movement towards an object two types of selection processes are required: dorsal selection to calculate the object position for motor reaction and ventral selection to recognize the specific object (Schneider, 1995). How are

Current Oculomotor Research, edited by Becker *et al.*
Plenum Press, New York, 1999.

these mechanisms in both processing streams coordinated ? The results of early experiments on this issue were controversal (e.g. Klein, 1980; Posner, 1980), partly due to methodological problems (see, Shepard et al.,1986). More recent work (Hoffman and Subramaniam, 1995; Kowler et al., 1995; Deubel and Schneider, 1996; Schneider and Deubel, 1995) demonstrated a strict link between ventral selection-for-perception and dorsal saccade target selection. In the experiments of Deubel and Schneider (1996), subjects had to saccade to locations within horizontal letter strings left or right from a fixation cross. The data showed that discrimination performance is best when discrimination target and saccade target referred to the same object. These findings argued for an obligatory and selective coupling of dorsal processing for saccade programming and ventral processing for perception and discrimination; this coupling is restricted to one common target object at a time.

Using a similar experimental paradigm, we recently demonstrated that the strict coupling also holds for the execution of other goal-directed movements such as pointing (Deubel et al., in press). The data from these experiments showed that the execution of a pointing movement leads to an improved performance of target object identification, independent of the preknowledge of the discrimination targets position. But, in this paradigm only the eccentricities of the target objects was varied.

In the first experiment we investigated whether this coupling also holds for manual pointing movements to target locations in different directions. As in our previous experiments a dual-task paradigm was used which required the preparation of pointing movements concurrently with a letter discrimination task. The position of the discrimination target was constant and known to the subjects. DT was displayed either before, during or after movement execution, such that the discrimination performance during the preparation and during the execution of the pointing movement could be determined. The second experiment required the execution of a saccadic eye movement instead of a pointing movement, using the same experimental setup. Control conditions were the corresponding single task situations for movement and discrimination performance. A further aim of the study was to directly compare perceptual performance in both types of goal-directed movements: pointing and saccades.

3. METHODS

3.1. Participants

Six subjects (4 women, 2 men, aged 22–28) participated in the experiments. They were students of psychology, had normal vision and normal motor behavior. All subjects had experience in a variety of experiments in oculomotor research. One subject was one of the authors, the others were naive with respect to the aim of the study.

3.2. Apparatus

Figure 1 shows a sketch of the experimental setup. The subjects were seated in front of a table in a dimly lit room. The visual stimuli that were presented on a fast 21" monitor were visible through a one-way mirror. The monitor provided a frame frequency of 100 Hz at a spatial resolution of 1024 x 768 pixels. Active screen size was 40 x 30 cm; the viewing distance was 57,7 cm. The stimuli appeared on a gray background which was adjusted to a mean luminance of 2,2 cd/m^2. The luminance of the stimuli was 23 cd/m^2.

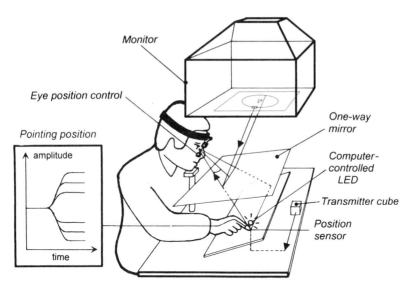

Figure 1. Experimental set-up.

The subjects hand laid behind the mirror, so pointing movements were executed to the projected position of the stimuli without visual feedback about the hand. Hand movements were recorded with a FASTRAK electro-magnetical position and orientation measuring system (Polhemus Inc., 1993) and sampled at 400 Hz. Connected to the receiver that was mounted on the subjects fingertip was a red LED (5 mm diameter), controlled by the PC. The LED allowed to provide controlled visual feedback about the spatial position of the fingertip.

In the first experiment, eye movements were measured by an IRIS infrared eyetracker (Skalar medical) for the purpose of fixation control. Head movements were restricted by an adjustable chin rest.

In the second experiment a Dual-Purkinje-eyetracker was used. For a detailed description see Deubel and Schneider (1996).

The experiments were completely under control of a 486 Personal Computer. The PC also served for the automatic off-line analysis of the eye and pointing movement data in which movement parameters were determined.

3.3. Calibration and Data Analysis

Each session of Experiment 1 started with a calibration procedure of the eyetracker in which the subject had to sequentially fixate 3 positions arranged on a horizontal line at distances of 8,5 deg of visual angle. Further, the origin and coordinate alignment frame of the position sensor were set relative to the projected position of the monitor center. The position sensor behaved linearly within 30 cm around the center position. The overall accuracy was better than 2 mm.

For each of the parameters landing position, amplitude, latency and movement duration a analysis of variance (repeated measures ANOVA) between test- and control condition (repeated measures) was calculated. Further, a contrast analysis was used.

For data analysis only trials with movement latencies between 200 ms and 600 ms and movement durations between 100 ms and 400 ms were accepted. For experiment 1, all trials where eye fixation was not maintained were rejected; this led to the exclusion of 6 % of all trials.

3.4. Procedure

Experiment 1 required the execution of a pointing movement to a location indicated by a central cue. Moreover, the subjects had to report the identity of a discrimination target, that was displayed either before, during or after movement onset. For each block, the position of DT was constant and known to the subjects. The first control task served to discern movement reaction times in a single task situation. For this purpose, the subjects were asked to point to the indicated position, but were not required to discriminate. The second control task served to test the discrimination performance without a movement reaction. Here the subject was only asked to indicate the identity of the DT, but no movement reaction was required.

Each subject participated in 4 sessions with 3 blocks each of each of the experiments. First, 2 blocks of the control condition "movement only" were run. After that, 6 blocks of the dual-task were required. The sequence of these blocks were counterbalanced between the subjects. Finally, 60 trials of the single-task "discrimination only" were run. Together there were 1080 trials in the double-task and 864 trials in the single-task conditions per subject in each of the experiments.

Experiment 2 was identical to experiment 1 except that a saccadic eye movement was required instead of a pointing movement. The discrimination target was always displayed with a delay of 100 ms after cue appearence, that is, well before movement onset.

Figure 2 shows a sequence of the visual stimuli in a single trial of experiment 1. First a small fixation cross (0,25 deg) was displayed in the center of the screen, surrounded by 12 mask items resembling the number "8", that were arranged on a circle like numbers on a clock (radius 7,2 deg). The width of each item was 0,9 deg of visual angle, its height was 1,4 deg. Subjects were asked to keep the eyes fixed to the center during the whole trial. Fixation was controlled by the infrared eyetracker. First, the pointing finger was also kept on the center of the screen. The LED was switched on, aiding the precise positioning. After a delay of 1000 to 1600 ms the fixation cross was replaced by a triangle of 0,7 deg that indicated the movement target location (MT). The primary task was to "point to this target as fast and precisely as possible". Simultaneous with the cue onset the LED was switched off to disable any further visual feedback of hand or pointing position. Before, during, or after movement onset (i.e., with a stimulus onset asynchrony – SOA- of 100 ms, 300 ms or 600 ms after cue onset), the premask characters changed into 11 distractors and one discrimination target (DT). The distractors were randomly selected and similar to the characters "2" and "S", the discrimination target was resembling the letter "E" or a mirror-symetrical version of this letter ("Ǝ", see Figure 1). Possible target locations were the clock positions 1,3,5,7,9, or 11. The position of the DT was constant during each block and known to the subject. The movement target positions, however, were varied independently within the possible clock positions. Target and distractors were presented for 80 ms, and again replaced by mask items. Feedback about the reached movement position and latency was given. After pointing the identity of DT had to be reported by pressing one of two buttons (2AFC-task). The ability to identify DT was taken as a measure of selective perceptual performance. Finally the next trial was initiated by the computer without time pressure.

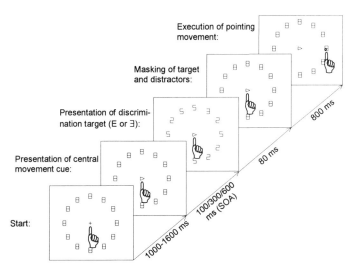

Figure 2. Stimuli sequence of a single trial.

4. RESULTS

4.1. Experiment 1: Movement Performance

A central rationale of the experimental approach was that the discrimination task should not interfere with the movement task, implying that the movement execution should be independent of discrimination target position. The ANOVA makes sure that this is the case. The trials with different SOAs were pooled for movement performance because the SOA showed no significant effect. For all movement parameters only the factor MT shows a significant effect, while for the factor DT and DT-MT interaction no differences were found.

The reaching movements were very precise: mean amplitude was 7,25 deg and thus differed by only 0,05 deg from the target position. ANOVA confirms a significant main effect of MT position, and no differences were found for DT position and DT-MT interaction ($F(5,25)=11.39$; $p=0.001$; $F(5,25)=1.14$; $p=0.365$; $F(25,125)=1.4$; $p=0.118$).

4.2. Experiment 1: Discrimination Performance

The subjects reported that they had no difficulties to point quickly to the indicated target item. After the experiment the subjects were asked about their subjective impression and how they solved the task. They reported that the peripheral items that were indicated as movement target seemed to "light up" in a circle of almost unstructured items. For some trials they reported to see the DT item at the different MT location. This could be an "illusionary conjunction" of the positions of DT and MT.

Our indicator for the momentary allocation of attention in the ventral stream (selective perceptual performance) was the accuracy with which the DT can be identified. Discrimination performance can be expressed as the percentage of correct decisions upon target identity; chance level is 50% correct. Figure 3 presents the discrimination performance of experimental- and control condition in percent as a function of DT-MT interaction.

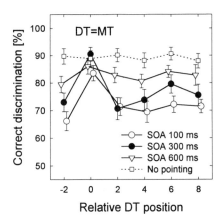

Figure 3. Discrimination performance depending on DT-MT interaction.

Valid position means that the randomized movement cue was indicating the known discrimination position (DT=MT). For invalid positions DT and MT location differ. The dotted graph shows the pooled performance of the control condition ("discrimination only – no pointing").

In the single-task control condition subjects show very high performance because the DT location was known. This is independent of the SOA. In the experimental condition the data analysis reveals 2 main effects:

First, for coincidence of DT and MT the discrimination performance is clearly improved, especially before and during the pointing movement (100 and 300 ms SOA). If the discrimination target was displayed after the movement execution (600 ms SOA) the discrimination performance comes close to the single-task condition. ANOVA shows a significant effect for the interaction between DT and MT for all SOAs ($F(25,125)=3,81$; $p=0,001$). The contrast analysis confirms the superiority of discrimination performance for valid positions compared to all other combinations which did not differ significantly ($F(1,175)=6,97$; $p=0,009$). These results are similar to the findings of our former experiments, in which the subjects didn´t have the information about the DT position. As expected, there was no influence of DT position in the control condition (discrimination only).

Second, the discrimination performance was best under all conditions when DT was presented on a horizontal position (3 and 9 o´clock). This is confirmed by ANOVA and contrast analysis, which shows a highly significant advantage of horizontal DT positions compared to all others ($F(5,25)=2,75$; $p=0,041$; $F(1,175)=36,69$; $p<0,000$). The discrimination performance for invalid pointing movements is very similar to the control condition.

The location of MT shows no significant effect, neither for experimental condition, nor for the control condition ($F(5,25)=1,71$; $p=0,171$). For a separation of valid and invalid locations there was a clear difference at horizontal positions: DT was easy to identify if the movement cue was valid, while an invalid cue led to a discrimination performance close to chance level. As mentioned before, discrimination performance is independent of the MT location – the presentation of the movement cue has no effect on the discrimination task.

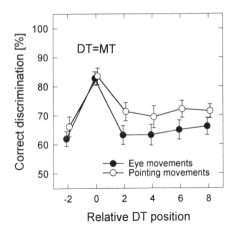

Figure 4. Comparison of discrimination performance between eye and pointing movements.

4.3. Experiment 2: Discrimination Performance

The selection coupling is not limited to pointing movements only. We ran the identical experiment using eye movements instead of pointing movements. DT was displayed with a SOA of 100 ms, that is, before movement onset (Figure 4). Nearly identical to the pointing experiment performance is best for the coincidence of discrimination and movement target and is close to chance level at all other positions. The performance at invalid positions is slightly improved for the execution of pointing movements.

5. DISCUSSION

In summary, the results show best perceptual performance when discrimination target and movement target refer to the same object. This holds independent of the subject's preknowledge of DT position, and for DT presentation before and during the movement. Nearly identical results were found for the programming of goal-directed saccades.

The results are consistent with our previous work (Deubel et al., in press). They indicate that the direction of movement execution has no influence on the coupling between ventral and dorsal selection. We conclude that a unitary selection mechanism selects one target at a time for object recognition and provides the spatial coordinates for all kind of goal-directed movements (Schneider, 1995).

The object specificity of the coupling is in line with the findings of Castiello (1996). This author asked whether the kinematics of the target movement are influenced by non-target objects. The results indeed demonstrated interactions when the distractor object has to be used also for carrying out a simultaneous, secondary task. This suggests that preparing and executing a reaching movement cannot be done simultaneously with attentional selection in the ventral stream when the two selection processes refer to different objects. When both tasks referred to the same object parallel selection was possible.

In line with Rizzolatti et al. (1987) we assume that the strict coupling holds for the preparation and programming of the movement but does not necessarily require, or entail, its overt initiation. Therefore, in cases where visual attention moves but not the hand, we assume that the spatial parameters for the potential movement are available and provided by the attentional mechanism, but that the movement is prevented from being converted into overt action due to the missing release of a "Go"-signal.

ACKNOWLEDGMENT

This research was supported by the Deutsche Forschungsgemeinschaft, SFB 462 "Sensomotorik".

REFERENCES

Castiello U (1996) Grasping a Fruit: Selection for Action. J Exp Psychol: Hum Percept Perform 22: 582–603

Deubel H, Schneider WX (1996) Saccade target selection and object recognition: Evidence for a common attentional mechanism. Vision Res 36, 1827–1837

Deubel H., Schneider WX, Paprotta I (in press) Selective dorsal and ventral processing: Evidence for a common attentional mechanism in reaching and perception. Visual Cognition

Goodale MA, Millner AD (1992) Separate visual pathways for perception and action. TINS 15: 20–25

Hoffman JE, Subramaniam B (1995) The role of visual attention in saccadic eye movements. Percept Psychophys 57: 787–795

Jeannerod M (1981) Intersegmental coordination during reaching at natural visual objects. In J. Long and A. Baddeley (Eds.) Attention and Performance IX. Hillsdale, NJ: Erlbaum, pp 153–169

Klein R (1980) Does oculomotor readiness mediate cognitive control of visual attention ? In R. Nickerson (Ed.), Attention and Performance VIII. Hillsdale, NJ: Erlbaum, pp 259–276

Kowler E, Anderson E, Dosher B, Blaser E (1995) The role of attention in the programming of saccades. Vision Res 35: 1897–1916

Posner MI (1980) Orienting of attention. Q J Exp Psychol 32: 3–25

Rizzolatti G, Riggio L, Dascola I, Umilta C (1987) Reorienting attention across the horizontal and vertical meridians: Evidence in favor of a premotor theory of attention. Neuropsychologia 25: 31–40

Rizzolatti G, Riggio L, Sheliga BM (1994) Space and selective attention. In C. Umilta and M. Moscovitch (Eds.), Attention and Performance XV. Conscious and nonconscious information processing). Cambridge, MA: MIT Press, pp 231–265

Schneider WX (1995) A neuro-cognitive model for visual attention control of segmentation, object recognition, and space-based motor action. Visual Cognition 2: 331–375

Schneider WX, Deubel H (1995) Visual attention and saccadic eye movements: Evidence for obligatory and selective spatial coupling. In Findlay JM, Walker R, Kentridge RW (Eds.) Eye movement research. Amsterdam: Elsevier, pp 317–324

Shepherd M, Findlay JM, Hockey RJ (1986) The relationship between eye movements and spatial attention. Q J Exp Psychol 38A, 475–491

SACCADIC INHIBITION IN COMPLEX VISUAL TASKS

Eyal M. Reingold and Dave M. Stampe

Department of Psychology
University of Toronto
100 St. George Street
Toronto, Ontario, Canada M5S 3G3

1. INTRODUCTION

Several gaze contingent studies that used a fixed delay between physical eye movements and a display change documented a dip in the fixation duration distributions (e.g., Blanchard et al. 1984; McConkie et al. 1985; van Diepen et al. 1995). In a study by van Diepen et al. (1995), a moving mask paradigm was employed in which subjects searched line drawings of everyday scenes for non-objects. The appearance of the mask was delayed relative to the end of a saccade (beginning of fixation) by 17, 46, 76 or 121 msec. All fixation duration distributions in the masking conditions exhibited a dip with longer masking delays resulting in the dip occurring at longer fixation durations. In contrast, a no-mask condition did not produce a dip. Similar effects in reading were reported by Blanchard et al. (1984), and McConkie et al. (1985). In both these studies the text was masked at a fixed delay from the end of the saccade, and the fixation duration distributions exhibited dips. McConkie et al. (1992) interpreted these dips as reflecting a disruption to automatic, parallel encoding or registration processes that are time locked to the onset of the visual pattern on the retina. Processing disruption causes an eye movement disruption after a constant transmission delay in the neural system.

An alternative explanation to the processing disruption hypothesis is that the display change produced saccadic inhibition with maximum inhibition occurring at a constant latency following the onset of the display change. We will refer to this as the saccadic inhibition hypothesis. There are several differences between these two contrasting interpretations. The saccadic inhibition hypothesis postulates a low-level effect that should occur in any task involving saccadic eye movements, and regardless of the relevance of the display change to the task being performed. In addition, the profile of saccadic inhibition should be identical regardless of the delay between the end of saccade and the appearance of the display change. In contrast, the process disruption hypothesis predicts differences across tasks because different tasks are likely to involve different encoding

Current Oculomotor Research, edited by Becker *et al.*
Plenum Press, New York, 1999.

processes. According to this model, processes are likely to differ during the time course of fixations, and consequently, a display change earlier in a fixation should result in a different amount of disruption relative to a display change which occurs later during the fixation.

The purpose of the present paper was to disentangle these two alternative explanations. We recorded eye movements from subjects performing a visual search task or a reading comprehension task. In each of these tasks we employed two paradigms. In the first paradigm, the display change occurred at a fixed delay following the end of a saccade (beginning of fixation). We will refer to this as the Fixed Delay Paradigm (henceforth FDP). The FDP is in essence a gaze contingent paradigm. Two fixed delays of 110 msec and 158 msec were used. In addition, we developed another paradigm which will be referred to as the Random Delay Paradigm (henceforth RDP) in which the display change could occur at any point in time, thus at a random delay from the end of saccade (beginning of fixation). To summarize, three experimental conditions were used in each task: FDP 110 msec, FDP 158 msec and RDP. The saccadic inhibition hypothesis predicts an identical inhibition profile across these three conditions in each task whereas the processing disruption hypothesis predicts differences across conditions.

2. METHOD

2.1. Subjects

Two groups of 10 subjects were tested. One group participated in the visual search experiment and one group in the reading comprehension experiment. All subjects had normal or corrected to normal vision, and were paid $10.00 for a single one hour session.

2.2. Apparatus and Display Generation

The eyetracker employed in this research was the SR Research Ltd. EyeLink system. This system has high spatial resolution (0.005°), and a sampling rate of 250 Hz (4 msec temporal resolution). The EyeLink headband has three cameras, allowing simultaneous tracking of both eyes and of head position for head-motion compensation. By default, only the subject's dominant eye was tracked in our studies. The EyeLink system uses an Ethernet link between the eyetracker and display computers for real-time saccade and gaze position data transfer. The system also performs saccade and blink detection on-line for the FDP paradigm. In the present study the configurable acceleration and velocity thresholds were set to detect saccades of 0.5° or greater.

Displays were generated using an S3 VGA card and a 17" ViewSonic 17PS monitor. The display had a resolution of 360 by 240 pixels, with a frame rate of 120 Hz. At the 60 centimeter viewing distance the display subtended a visual angle of 30° horizontally and 22.5° vertically.

A 9-point calibration was performed at the start of each block of trials, followed by 9-point calibration accuracy test. Calibration was repeated if any point was in error by more than 1°, or if the average error for all points was greater than 0.5°. Before each trial, a black fixation target was displayed at the center of the display. The subject fixated this target and the reported gaze position was used to correct any post-calibration drift errors. The background of the target display had the same luminance as the image to be displayed during the trial, to minimize pupil size changes.

Display changes were generated by displaying a transient image beginning at a vertical retrace, and restoring the normal display 4 retraces (33 msec) later. The transient image for the visual search study was a gray field matched in luminance to the picture presented during the trial. In the reading experiment the transient image was a black screen.

In the FDP condition, a display change was generated at a fixed delay of either 110 or 158 msec after the end of each saccade made by the subject. These delays were verified using an artificial eye and an optical sensor. In the RDP condition the interval between consecutive display changes varied randomly between 250 to 350 msec in the visual search task and between 300 to 400 msec in the reading task. Subjectively it was very difficult to distinguish between the three experimental conditions.

2.3. The Visual Search Task

In this task subjects searched for 4 targets embedded in grayscale images of residential interiors. Average brightness across images was 27 cd/m^2. Targets were 0.5° by 0.5° checkerboard patterns with 35% contrast, and were locally matched in luminance to the picture background in order to make search difficult and generate numerous saccades per trial. Subjects were allowed up to 30 seconds for the search. If subjects located all the targets before the deadline they terminated the trial with a button press. A total of 64, 64 and 128 trials were used in the FDP 110 msec, FDP 158 msec, and RDP conditions respectively. Trial order and the pairing of stimuli to conditions were randomly determined for every subject.

2.4. The Reading Comprehension Task

Subjects read a short story for comprehension and enjoyment. The text was presented in black (brightness = 4 cd/m^2) on a white background (brightness = 68 cd/m^2). Proportional spaced fonts were used with an average of 2.2 characters per degree of visual angle and an average of 10 lines per screen. A total of 12, 12 and 24 screens were read in the FDP 110 msec, FDP 158 msec, and RDP conditions respectively. The pairing of screens to conditions was determined randomly for every subject. Screens were pages of text in the story, and were presented in the same order to all subjects. When subjects finished reading a screen they pressed a button to proceed to the next screen.

3. RESULTS

Histograms of fixation duration distributions collapsed across all subjects in a given condition are plotted in Figure 1. These show that the FDP conditions in both the visual search task and reading comprehension task replicated the results obtained in previous gaze contingent studies. In particular, the fixation duration distributions for the FDP conditions exhibited a dip. In both tasks the location of the dip across the two delay conditions (i.e., 110 vs. 158 msec) was displaced by approximately the difference between the delays (48 msec). In contrast, no dip was seen in the histograms of fixation duration distributions for the RDP condition in either task.

Whereas the fixation duration distributions for the RDP versus the FDP conditions appear on the surface to be very different, a re-plotting of the results reveals a striking similarity. This is shown in Figure 2 which plot the proportion of saccades by latency after

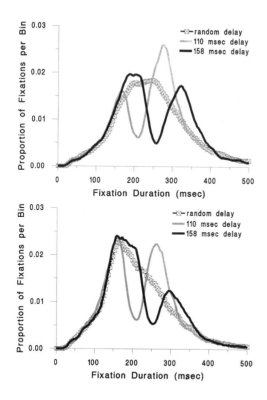

Figure 1. Histogram of fixation duration distribution by experimental condition and task. Top panel = visual search. Bottom panel = reading comprehension. Bin size = 4 msec.

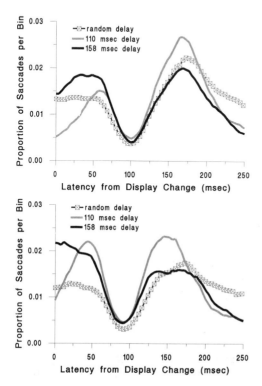

Figure 2. Proportion of saccades as a function of the latency from display change by experimental condition and task. Top panel = visual search. Bottom panel = reading comprehension. Bin size = 4 msec.

Table 1.   Mean Latency (msec) to the center of the dip by
experimental condition and task.

	Latency to dip (in msec)	
Condition	Visual search	Reading
Fixed delay, 110 msec	91.6 (4.3)	98.4 (5.1)
Fixed delay, 158 msec	89.2 (4.1)	99.2 (4.9)
Random delay	91.2 (5.7)	99.6 (5.2)

These correspond to the center of the dips in Figure 2. Standard deviations are
shown in parentheses.

the display change, using saccades and display change data from the eye movement file and collapsing across all subjects in a given condition. For the two FDP conditions this is equivalent to aligning the fixation duration distributions by subtracting the value of the delay from each fixation duration and plotting values greater than zero. As can be seen in Figure 2 the dip is present and appears to be similar in shape and latency for all of the FDP and RDP conditions in both tasks.

Although the dip is quite similar across all three conditions, the pattern before and after the dip differs. This occurs because the two FDP conditions depend on the underlying shape of the fixation duration distribution. That is, a fixed delay causes the dip to occur at a particular point along the continuum of fixation durations. In contrast, the RDP pattern reflects a condition in which the saccade to display change delay varies continuously, and consequently a wide range of fixation durations are affected (hence the absence of a dip in the fixation duration distributions in this condition). Accordingly, only the RDP condition reveals the true nature of the saccadic interference effect. An inspection of this condition in Figure 2 indicates that for the first 50 msec following the display change the proportion of saccades remains flat. In all likelihood these saccades are unaffected by the display change and therefore may serve as a baseline. At a later point the proportion of saccades decreases below baseline constituting the dip and then increases above baseline constituting the peak. Finally, following the peak the proportion of saccades returns to baseline levels.

To perform statistical tests on the latencies to the center of the dip, histograms of saccadic frequency by latency from display change were produced for each subject and condition, and the latency of the center of the dip was measured for each histogram. The results are given in Table 1, which shows the average latency and standard deviation across subjects for each condition in each task. Comparisons between the two FDP conditions and the RDP condition using t-tests indicated no significant differences across all conditions within the same task.

4. DISCUSSION

The results of the present study are consistent with the saccadic inhibition hypothesis and are difficult to reconcile with the processing disruption hypothesis. In both the visual search and reading comprehension tasks, and across the FDP and RDP conditions, a specific pattern of saccadic frequency is produced following a display change. This was independent of the precise timing of the display change during fixations. The pattern is clearly visible in the RDP condition in Figure 2, and can be decomposed into three intervals. Immediately following the display change, saccadic frequency is stable and is probably unaffected by the display change. This interval can serve as an estimate of baseline saccadic frequency. The second interval (the dip) indicates saccadic inhibition (i.e., saccadic rates below baseline). The third interval (the peak), reflects recovery from saccadic inhibition (i.e., saccadic rates above baseline).

The RDP methodology introduced here has several advantages over traditional gaze contingent paradigms (i.e., FDP) for studying the saccadic inhibition phenomena. First, the technical implementation of gaze contingent methodology is challenging and expensive in terms of both software and hardware, and consequently may not be widely available to researchers. Second, the RDP reflects a continuous rather than a discrete manipulation of saccade to display change delay. Consequently the RDP reveals the pattern of saccadic inhibition independent of the shape of the fixation duration distribution. Finally, the RDP allows estimation of the baseline saccadic frequency, which enables the computation of additional measures such as the magnitude and duration of the dip and the peak. We are currently evaluating a variety of dip and peak measures. In addition, research employing the RDP is being conducted in our lab to assess the influence of stimulus factors (i.e., the nature of displays and transient images) as well as observer factors (e.g., attentional and strategic factors) on the pattern of saccadic inhibition.

The current findings of saccadic inhibition in complex visual tasks must be compared with findings from previous psychophysical and neurophysiological studies. Several psychophysical studies reported inhibition or slowing of saccades following the presentation of a visual event which was displayed at the same time or after the presentation of the saccadic target (e.g., Ross and Ross 1980, 1981; Walker et al. 1997). Walker et al. (1997) suggested that the neurophysiological locus of the saccadic inhibition they observed may be related to inhibitory processes in the superior colliculus (e.g., Dorris and Munoz 1995; Munoz and Wurtz 1993). Further studies employing a variety of psychophysical and neurophysiological paradigms are required to converge on an adequate theory of saccadic inhibition.

ACKNOWLEDGMENTS

Preparation of this paper was supported by a grant to Eyal M. Reingold from the Natural Science and Engineering Research Council of Canada. We wish to thank Elizabeth Bosman her helpful comments on an earlier version of this paper. We also thank Esther Meisels for testing the subjects.

REFERENCES

Blanchard HE, McConkie GW, Zola D, Wolverton GS (1984) Time course of visual information utilization during fixations in reading. J Exp Psychol Hum Percept Perform, 10:75–89

Dorris MC, Munoz DP (1995) A neural correlate for the gap effect on saccadic reaction times in monkeys. J Neurophysiol 73:2558–2562

McConkie GW, Underwood NR, Zola D, Wolverton GS (1985) Some temporal characteristics of processing during reading. J Exp Psychol Hum Percept Perform, 11:168–186

McConkie GW, Reddix MD, Zola D (1992) Perception and cognition in reading: Where is the meeting point? In: Rayner K (ed) Eye movements and visual cognition: Scene perception and reading. Springer Verlag, NY, pp 293–303

Munoz DP, Wurtz RH (1993) Fixation cells in monkey superior colliculus. I. Characteristics of cell discharge. J Neurophysiol 70:559–575.

Ross LE, Ross SM (1980) Saccade latency and warning signals: Stimulus onset, offset, and change as warning events. Percept Psychophys 27:251–257

Ross SM, Ross LE (1981) Saccade latency and warning signals: Effects of auditory and visual stimulus onset and offset. Percept Psychophys 29:429–437

van Diepen PMJ, De Graef P, d'Ydewalle G (1995) Chronometry of foveal information extraction during scene perception. In: Findlay JM, Walker R, Kentridge RW (eds) Eye movement research: Mechanisms, processes and applications. Elsevier, Amsterdam, pp 349–362

Walker R, Deubel H, Schneider WX, Findlay JM (1997) Effect of remote distractors on saccade programming: Evidence for an extended fixation zone. J Neurophysiol 78:1108–1119

36

THE USE OF COARSE AND FINE PERIPHERAL INFORMATION DURING THE FINAL PART OF FIXATIONS IN SCENE PERCEPTION

Martien Wampers and Paul M. J. van Diepen

University of Leuven, Belgium

1. INTRODUCTION

A large body of evidence exists, showing that visual stimuli are simultaneously analyzed by a number of quasi-independent channels (Campbell and Robson, 1968; Blakemore and Campbell, 1969; Blakemore and Sutton, 1969), each sensitive to a limited range of spatial frequencies. These channels seem to differ with respect to temporal characteristics: Low spatial frequencies appear to be processed faster than high spatial frequencies (Breitmeyer, 1975).

The spatial content of visual stimuli can be determined by Fourier analysis. This mathematical technique furthermore allows isolation of a predefined frequency range. Selective removal of low spatial frequencies generates an image that preserves coarse, global information like luminance. Maintaining the high spatial frequencies of an image preserves fine details like contours and edges at the expense of the contrast over broad spatial regions. When visual information processing is indeed biased towards a coarse-to-fine analysis, coarse (low frequency) image information will be available more rapidly than detailed (high frequency) image information. Hence coarse information will exert more influence on the initial stages of visual processing.

Experimental data support the hypothesis that visual information integration proceeds in a coarse-to-fine order. Parker et al. (1992) showed that the order in which sequences of spatially filtered images are presented, greatly influences the perceived quality of the compound picture. They presented their subjects sequences consisting of three images. The sequences either ran from low to high or from high to low spatial frequencies. A sequence took 120 ms, each constituent image being available for 40 ms. Subjects judged the quality of the combined picture on a four-point rating scale. Their was a significant effect of order of spatial frequency presentation: the perceived quality of the composed image was rated significantly higher when frequency information was presented according to a coarse-to-fine analysis than when frequency information was displayed in the reversed order.

Current Oculomotor Research, edited by Becker *et al.*
Plenum Press, New York, 1999.

Schyns and Oliva (1994) also provided evidence for the faster integration of low spatial frequencies as compared to high spatial frequencies. Subjects performed a matching to sample task. Hybrid stimuli consisting of the high spatial frequencies of one scene and the low spatial frequencies of another scene were presented for 30 or 150 ms, followed by the 40 ms presentation of a mask. Subsequently, an unfiltered comparison stimulus was displayed. Subjects indicated whether or not hybrid and comparison stimulus represented the same scene. With an exposure duration of 30 ms, hybrids and comparison stimuli were matched when they shared the low spatial frequencies. When the exposure duration was 150 ms, hybrid and comparison stimulus were regarded as representing the same scene when they had the high spatial frequencies in common. From these results, it was concluded that the early stages of visual processing are dominated by the coarse, low frequency content of an image whereas high spatial frequencies govern later processing phases.

The preference for a coarse-to-fine order in information acquisition does not imply that high frequency information is not utilized during the initial stages of visual processing. In a minority of the trials with an exposure duration of 30 ms, subjects declared that hybrid and comparison stimulus depicted the same scene even though these two stimuli only shared high frequency information. Hence, high frequency information can be used from the onset of visual processing. This was also illustrated by means of a priming paradigm. Schyns and Oliva (1996) tested whether the two components of a hybrid stimulus could prime the recognition of two normal pictures, namely the full frequency images associated with the low and high frequency elements of the hybrid. A hybrid stimulus was presented for 30 ms followed by a 40 ms mask presentation. Then a full frequency image was shown that had to be categorized as fast as possible. It was observed that images containing either the low or the high spatial frequencies of the hybrid were primed equally effective. The priming rates were comparable to those obtained when the prime consisted of only one spatial scale (high or low spatial frequencies), indicating that in the case of a hybrid prime, the effect of the high frequency component is not attenuated by the presence of low frequency information or vice versa. High and low frequency information are apparently both available at the start of visual processing.

High spatial frequency information may even be more effective in directing the visual analysis, such as was shown by Parker et al. (1996). Subjects performed a same-different comparison task. A full frequency image of a face (the target stimulus) was displayed for 500 ms. The presentation of a comparison stimulus followed after an interval of 1 s. The comparison stimulus either showed a full frequency image for the whole 500 ms or contained a sequence of two images: high or low frequency information during the first 100 ms and a full frequency image for the remaining 400 ms. The full frequency picture was compatibel with the preceding frequency information in half of the trials. Subjects then judged whether or not target and comparison stimulus represented the same face. When the frequency information available during the first 100 ms was compatibel with the undegraded information shown during the following 400 ms, high and low frequencies primed the identification equally effective. Clearly, the result of this experiment provides no evidence for a coarse-to-fine analysis but suggests that high and low frequency information are equally useful during early visual processing. However, if the initially presented frequency information was irrelevant, high frequencies proved to be significantly more disruptive than low frequencies, indicating an initial dominance of high spatial frequency information.

It should be noted that stimulus presentation times are relatively short in all cited experiments. Therefore, results can't be extrapolated unequivocally to natural viewing situation. To create an ecologically more valid situation, we allowed subjects to explore stimuli up to 30 s. When subjects thought they had sufficiently inspected the stimulus to perform the experimental task, they self-terminated the stimulus presentation. Only in a minority of trials subjects actually used the full 30 s, indicating that they had ample time to visually process the presented stimuli.

Furthermore, in all studies mentioned above, fovea and periphery were always manipulated simultaneously. Taking into account the limitations of the human eye, one can however expect a differential use of spatial frequency information as a function of retinal eccentricity. We focused on the use of spatial frequencies in peripheral vision. The spatial frequency content of the peripheral image was manipulated, while foveal information remained undegraded. When peripheral information is degraded throughout fixations by spatial frequency filtering, high frequency information results in a better performance than low frequency information (Wampers and van Diepen, 1998). By varying the moment during fixations at which peripheral information is degraded, we tested the hypothesis that visual scenes are processed according to a coarse-to-fine strategy. If visual scenes are processed according to a coarse-to-fine strategy, we can expect that low frequency information dominates performance during the initial part of fixations. This was experimentally investigated (van Diepen and Wampers, 1996) by manipulating the frequency information (high, low, or medium spatial frequencies) available during the first 150 ms of each fixation when subjects explored computer designed full-colour drawings of scenes in the context of a search task. No significant differences were observed between filter conditions. The filter conditions also did not differ from a control condition that showed a blanked periphery and hence did not contain any useful peripheral information. It was concluded that initially, peripheral information is of minor importance and is mainly needed during the later part of fixations (e.g. for the selection of a new saccade target). This hypothesis is supported by the finding of Van Diepen et al. (1995) revealing that the first 45–75 ms of fixations are sufficient to extract the foveal information necessary for object identification. Possibly, little peripheral information is obtained during that period.

The present study examined the role of spatial frequencies during the final part of fixations, by degrading the peripheral information a preset delay after the beginning of each fixation.

2. EXPERIMENT 1

In the first experiment, we tried to determine if peripheral information is needed during the final part of fixations and which spatial frequencies are primarily used during that period. This was done by showing normal, unmanipulated peripheral information during the first 100 ms of each fixation. After that interval, the periphery was degraded by maintaining only high, low or medium spatial frequencies or by blanking the periphery with the average scene colour. Performance was evaluated by means of five dependent variables: scene inspection time, number of fixations, fixation duration, saccadic amplitude and number of errors. When peripheral information is processed according to a coarse-to-fine sequence, we can expect that high frequency information guides visual processing during the final part of fixations. Hence, the presence of high frequency information in peripheral vision was predicted to yield the best performance.

2.1. Method

2.1.1. Stimuli. Stimuli were created from the laboratory's collection of 3D-models consisting of 12 scene backgrounds, 112 objects and 40 non-existing objects (non-objects). Non-objects are meaningless, closed volumes with a size and shape similar to that of real objects.

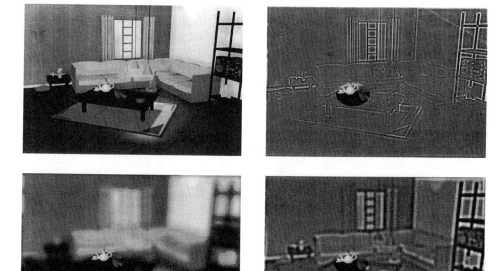

Figure 1. The normal (upper left), high-frequency (upper right), low-frequency (down left) and medium-frequency (down right) versions of a filler scene containing three non-objects. A window is placed at a possible fixation location. Within the window, the normal image is visible. In the experiments, images appeared in colour.

The backgrounds were furnished with a number of probable objects, all in likely positions, and rendered in full colour from a standard view point. A second version of these scenes was obtained by reorganising the present objects and adding one non-object to each scene. Besides these 24 targets, 24 filler scenes were created using a different point of view. Additionally, two or three non-objects were added to each filler scene and the constituent objects of the targets were as far as possible replaced by other ones. Two filler versions of each scene were created.

By means of Fourier filtering, we created a low- (LF), medium- (MF) and a high-frequency (HF) version of each of the resulting scenes. The LF-versions only maintained the spatial frequencies below one cycle/degree of visual angle which produced images that only contained coarse, global information at the expense of detailed information. The HF-versions of the scenes preserved the spatial frequencies above three cycles/degree of visual angle. This created images that contained fine details like edges but lost e.g. colour information. Spatial frequencies between one and three cycles/degree were kept in the MF-version. The resulting MF-pictures contained more colour and luminance information but less detail than the HF-versions.

2.1.2. Subjects. Eight subjects participated in the experiment. All had normal or corrected to normal vision. Some of them had experience with eye movement research in unrelated experiments.

2.1.3. Procedure and Design. Subjects were told that they would participate in an experiment on the nature of image processing and were instructed to explore images of realistic scenes for the presence of a variable number of non-objects. They were asked to localise the non-existing objects as fast as possible while maintaining a high level of accuracy. As soon as subjects had determined the number of non-objects present, they self-terminated the scene presentation by pressing a button thus allowing the registration of global scene inspection time. When there was no response within 30 s, the trial ended automatically. Subjects could then indicate their answer and got feedback about the correctness of their answer . After the instructions, the subjects were seated at 125 cm from the display with their head steadied by a bite-bar and a head-rest. Subjects were told that their eye movements would be measured to change information around the area where they were looking.

The eye tracker was then calibrated. After a succesful calibration a practice block consisting of five trials was initiated. Each trial included the following events: First, a fixation dot was presented in the middle of the display. A 300 ms fixation on that point triggered the scene presentation. During the scene exploration, eye movements were measured to position an elliptic window (3.5 x 2.6 visual degrees) at the fixation point. Inside the window, the undegraded image was presented troughout the fixation. Outside the window (peripherally), the unmanipulated image was shown during the first 100 ms of each fixation. After that period, the peripheral information (outside the window) was replaced by one of the filtered scene versions (HF-, LF-, and MF-condition) or blanked with the average scene colour (Uniform condition) for the rest of the fixation. When subjects were of the opinion that they located all non-objects, they pressed the right of two response bottons which initiated the presentation of a response display. When the maximally permitted period for scene examination (30 s) had expired, the response screen was shown automatically. The response display consisted of two rows of five boxes containing the numbers 0–9. Subjects had to fixate the digit that equaled the number of non-objects they had detected. The fixated number lit up and could be passed as an answer by pressing the left of the two response buttons. Subsequently, feedback on the exactness of the response was provided.

Each subject saw four blocks of 24 trials. Stimuli were randomly assigned to those four blocks with the restrictions that each block contained 12 targets and 12 fillers and that each number of non-objects appeared 6 times within a block. Consequently, one half of the target scenes contained no non-objects, the other half one non-object. The same was true for the filler scenes, six fillers appeared with 2 non-objects, the other six with three non-objects. Across blocks, each scene appeared twice in each version. Only one version of each target and filles scene appeared within a block.

Conditions were counterbalanced across blocks and randomly assigned to the scenes with the following restrictions: each condition had to appear six times within each block, three times coupled with a target, three times with a filler. Each target had to be combined with each condition in one of the four blocks. For every subject, each condition had to be combined with six targets containing no non-objects, and six targets containing one non-object. Over a set of four subjects, each condition had to be combined twice with each target in the no non-object version, and twice with each target in the one non-object version. This resulted in four counterbalanced series of condition assignments for four subjects receiving the normal trial order. The other four subjects received the same scene-condition combinations but in reversed trial order. Between blocks, subjects was given a short break. The whole experiment took about 90 minutes.

2.1.4. Apparatus. Eye movements were recorded with a Generation-V dual-Purkinje-image eye tracker (Crane and Steele, 1985). The system has an accuracy of 1 min of arc at a 1000 Hz sampling rate. It was interfaced to a 486 PC that stored every sample of the eye's position. For each sample, the computer made an on-line decision about the eye state: fixation , saccade, blink or signal loss. Eye state and position were fed into a second 486 PC, controling the stimulus presentation (Van Rensbergen and De Troy, 1993). This second PC contained two Truevision ATVista Videographics Adapter boards (henceforth called 'Vista 1' and 'Vista 2') and was linked with a third 486 PC, also containing an ATVista board. The three vistas were synchronized and connected to a video switcher that enabled Vista 1 to select between the Vista 2 and Vista 3 image on a pixel-by-pixel basis (van Diepen, 1997). Vista 3 contained the normal scene version whereas Vista 2 contained the manipulated scene version that had to be presented outside the window. The Vista 1 video output functioned as a key-signal for the video switcher to select Vista 3 pixels inside the oval window, and Vista 2 pixels outside the window. The Vista 1 key signal could be repositioned very quickly to move the window to the desired screen position (van Diepen et al., 1994). The detection of a new fixation initiated the timing of the window's disappearance. Whenever the eye moved less than 5 min of arc over a 5 ms period, it was regarded as the start of a new fixation. At that time, the stimulus computer determined during which video frame the normal scene should be replaced by the undegraded scene plus window, in order to approximate the requested delay of 100 ms as closely as possible. The timing algorithm ensured that on average, half of the changed stimulus had appeared on the display after 100 ms. Stimuli appeared in 60 Hz interlaced NTSC mode on a barco 6351 CRT with a 756 x 486 resolution, and subtended approximately 16 x 12 degrees of visual angle.

2.2. Results

All subsequent analyses pertain to the data of the 12 target scenes only. Total scene inspection time, mean fixation duration, number of fixations, mean saccadic amplitude, and number of errors were computed for each scene presentation. Total scene inspection time was defined as the time that elapsed between the onset of the stimulus and the occurrence of a right button press or the scene offset. Scene inspection time ranged from 1.3 s to 27 s. Mean scene inspection time was 6.2 s. The distribution of scene inspection time was normalized by means of a logarithmic transformation. The number of errors was defined as the absolute difference between the counted number of non-objects and the actual number of non-objects present in the scene. All saccades and fixations that were preceded or followed by signal loss or blinks, were excluded from the analyses as well as fixations on or near non-objects. The remaining saccades and fixations on average accounted for 78% of the total scene inspection time.

All data were entered in a repeated-measures subject (8) x condition (4) analysis of variance. The Huynh-Feldt sphericity estimator was used to correct for circularity assumption violations. Following a significant main effect of condition, all pairwise contrast were tested with the Tukey procedure using contrast specific error terms. An alpha level of .05 was adopted for all statistical tests. Unexpectedly, none of the analyzed contrasts reached significance. The mean condition values and the main effect statistics are shown in table 1.

2.3. Discussion

Availability of filtered stimulus information in peripheral vision during the later part of fixations did not improve performance compared to the control condition, where peripheral information was completely removed. Together with the van Diepen and Wampers (1996) findings with respect to peripheral stimulus degradation during the early part of

Table 1. Results of experiment 1

	M								
	LF	MF	HF	Uniform	CI	MSE	$F(3,21)$	$\Theta_{H\text{-}F}$	p
Inspection time*	0.734	0.731	0.704	0.713	±0.027	0.00138	1.06	0.99	.39
	(5.42)	(5.38)	(5.06)	(5.16)					
Number of fixations	14.2	14.6	13.6	14.1	±1.41	3.666	0.36	0.59	.68
Fixation duration (ms)	286	281	279	293	±8.4	131.96	2.45	0.91	.099
Saccadic amplitude (deg)	3.36	3.28	3.35	3.19	±0.164	0.0497	1.02	0.72	.39
Number of errors	0.125	0.188	0.146	0.271	±0.128	0.0303	0.96	0.42	.38

Note. CI = within-subject confidence interval, using the pooled error term (Loftus and Masson 1994, formula 2). $\Theta_{H\text{-}F}$ = Huynh and Feldt's estimator of nonsphericity. The reported p Values for the main effects of periphery type are obtained by multiplying the degrees of freedom of the F distribution by $\Theta_{H\text{-}F}$, whenever this estimator was smaller than one. Since none of the main effecrs was significant at the α = .05 level, no Tukey test was performed. *Inspection times were log-transformed. Corresponding antilog values (the geometrical means, in seconds) appear enclosed in parentheses.

fixations, the present findings could be interpreted as evidence that peripheral information is hardly used at all. Wampers and van Diepen (1998) however showed that degradation of peripheral information throughout fixations decreased performance. Possibly, no critical period for the acquisition of peripheral image information exists. Alternatively, the present experiment failed to interfere with peripheral stimulus utilisation during the later part of fixations, due to the fact that spatial frequency information was removed from the image but not masked. Possibly, a sufficiently useful iconic stimulus representation remained available that compensated for the distal stimulus degradation. The latter possibility is tested in Experiment 2.

3. EXPERIMENT 2

To prevent that removed spatial frequency information could still influence performance, we used the same paradigm as in experiment 1 but masked the spatial frequencies that were removed from the image by replacing them by the corresponding spatial frequencies from a pattern mask. In this way, we hoped to prevent temporal integration of information and to determine which spatial frequencies are preferentially used during the final part of fixations.

3.1. Method

3.1.1. Stimuli. The same stimuli as in experiment 1 were used. Additionally, 12 masks were created by means of a 3D modelling program. From each mask, three frequency versions were constructed by removing one specific spatial frequency range (either high, low or medium spatial frequencies), producing images that preserved high and low, high and medium or low and medium spatial frequencies respectively. The resulting versions were randomly merged with the filtered stimulus versions so that the combined image enclosed the complete frequency spectrum. For example, the HF-version of a farm scene was combined with a randomly chosen mask version containing low and medium spatial frequencies.

The undegraded stimulus version was shown inside as well as outside the window during the first 100 ms of each fixation. During the following part of fixations, the unmanipulated periphery was replaced by a stimulus+mask combination that maintained high, low or medium frequency information of the stimulus and replaced the other stimulus frequencies by the corresponding spatial frequencies of the mask.

3.1.2. Subjects. Sixteen subjects, with normal or corrected to normal vision, participated in the experiment. None of the subjects had participated in experiment 1, but some subjects had experience with eye movement research in unrelated experiments.

3.1.3. Procedure and Design. The same procedure and design were used as in experiment 1.

3.1.4. Apparatus. The same experimental setup as in experiment 1 was used.

3.2. Results

All subsequent analyses pertain to the data of the 12 target scenes only. Total scene inspection time, mean fixation duration, number of fixations, mean saccadic amplitude, and number of errors were computed for each scene presentation. Scene inspection time ranged from 0.4 s to 28.5 s with a mean of 6.4 s. The distribution of scene inspection time was normalized by means of a logarithmic transformation. The number of errors was defined as the absolute difference between the counted number of non-objects and the actual number of non-objects present in the scene. All saccades and fixations that were preceded or followed by signal loss or blinks, were excluded from the analyses as well as fixations on or near non-objects. The remaining saccades and fixations accounted for on average 92% of the total scene inspection time.

All data were entered in a repeated-measures subject (16) x condition (4) analysis of variance. The Huynh-Feldt sphericity estimator was used to correct for circularity assumption violations. The mean condition values and the main effect statistics are shown in table 2.

The main effect of the frequency manipulation on saccadic amplitude and global scene inspection time failed to reach significance. A significant main effect of the experimental manipulation was present for fixation duration. However, none of the pairwise comparisons between fixation duration means reached significance. The other dependent variables were not affected by the experimental manipulation.

3.3. Discussion

When the availability of useful peripheral frequency information is limited to one spatial frequency range by means of masking, we find that fixation durations are influenced by the frequency manipulation. The results show a tendency for high frequency peripheral information to be most benificial for task performance, mean fixation durations being 11 ms shorter in the HF-condition compared to the LF- and MF-conditions. The same pattern of results was observed for global scene inspection time: Global scene inspection times in the HF-condition were on average 0.5 s shorter than in the LF- and MF-condition, albeit not significantly. Hughes et al. (1984) found evidence showing that lower spatial frequencies mask a given frequency more effectively than higher spatial frequencies. Hence, the present experiment potentially underestimates the HF-advantage. These

Table 2. Results of experiment 2

	M				CI	MSE	F(3,45)	$\Theta_{H\text{-}F}$	p
	LF	MF	HF	Uniform					
Inspection time*	0.826	0.821	0.789	0.785	± 0.025	0.002	2.76	0.87	.06
	(6.70)	(6.62)	(6.15)	(6.10)					
Number of fixations	21.3	21.5	20.4	20.5	± 1.067	4.492	0.94	1.06	.43
Fixation duration (ms)	298.02	298.31	287.14	288.12	± 6.514	168.007	3.54	1.01	.02
Saccadic amplitude (deg)	3.09	3.07	3.06	2.93	± 0.088	0.031	2.66	1.09	.07
Number of errors	0.22	0.15	0.24	0.20	± 0.079	0.024	1.04	0.91	.39

Note. CI = within-subject confidence interval, using the pooled error term (Loftus and Masson 1994, formula 2). $\Theta_{H\text{-}F}$ = Huynh and Feldt's estimator of nonsphericity. The reported p Values for the main effects of periphery type are obtained by multiplying the degrees of freedom of the F distribution by $\Theta_{H\text{-}F}$, whenever this estimator was smaller than one. Since none of the main effecrs was significant at the a = .05 level, no Tukey test was performed. *Inspection times were log-transformed. Corresponding antilog values (the geometrical means, in seconds) appear enclosed in parentheses.

findings suggest that high frequency information is prefered in peripheral vision during the final part of fixations. Hence, the use of a coarse-to-fine strategy in the processing of peripheral information can not be ruled out. This interpretation is not contradicted by the observation that the results in the HF- and Uniform-condition are indistinguishable. Blanking the periphery does not mask iconic memory. Consequently, some information remains available for visual processing. The comparable results in the HF- and Uniform-condition suggest that high frequency information is preferentially used from iconic memory.

There are a number of possible reasons why peripheral degradation during the later part of fixations hardly affected scene exploration compared with the uniform condition. First, the two spatial frequency ranges that are removed from the periphery after 100 ms, are replaced by the corresponding frequencies of one mask, producing a very strong percept of the mask. This can reduce the impact of the peripheral spatial frequencies that are stimulus relevant, when, at higher levels of visual processing, the information, supplied by the different spatial frequency channels, has to be integrated. At that point, interference can occur between the information of the different frequency channels. The influence of the scene-relevant peripheral information on the final interpretation of the stimulus will be reduced since more weight will probably be given to the frequency information available from the mask because two groups of channels contain compatibel mask information whereas only one group of channels contains stimulus information. In summary, the dominant presence of mask information can disturb the perception of relevant peripheral information. In future research we therefore plan to replace every frequency range that is removed from the periphery by the corresponding frequencies of different masks. Second, the large display changes produced by the experimental manipulations can severely disrupt the ongoing scene perception, reducing possible effects. Presumably, the display changes not only influenced peripheral information extraction but also strongly disrupted the normal eye guidance processes. Saccades in the filter conditions possibly were attracted automatically by parts of the suddenly appearing and highly perceptible mask structure whereas in the Uniform-condition saccade targets needed to be chosen on the basis of information available in iconic memory. This could explain why saccadic amplitudes tended to be slightly (though not significantly) longer in the filter conditions than in the Uniform-condition. Further research will therefore apply more gradual stimulus transitions.

4. GENERAL DISCUSSION AND CONCLUSION

Two experiments were conducted to study which kind of peripheral information is preferentially used during the final part of fixations. In Experiment 1, no significant effect of the different kinds of peripheral information was observed. It was assumed that this was due to the possibility to combine the undegraded information available during the first part of fixations with information obtainable from iconic memory. As information was simply removed from peripheral vision by the experimental manipulation, information in iconic memory was not masked and remained available for further processing. This hypotheses was tested in Experiment 2 where information was not only removed from the periphery but also masked. The results of experiment 2 suggested that high frequency information was more useful during the later part of fixations than low and medium frequency information. This is compatibel with a coarse-to-fine strategy of information processing. Decisive evidence for the occurence of a coarse-to-fine analysis requires gradual changes in the peripherally available frequency information throughout fixations. Therefore, in future research the peripheral available information will be changed in gradual stages, starting with limited frequency information and adding spatial frequencies until the full-frequency image is displayed at the end of the fixation. Varying the order in which the frequency information is supplied should allow to pass judgement upon the preference for a coarse-to-fine or a fine-to-coarse analysis.

REFERENCES

Blakemore C, Campbell FW (1969) On the existence of neurons in the human visual system selectively sensitive to the orientation and size of retinal images. J Physiol (Lond.) 203: 237–260.

Blakemore C, Sutton P (1969) Size adaptation: A new aftereffect. Science 166: 245–247.

Breitmeyer BG (1975). Simple reaction times as a measure of the response properties of transient and sustained channels. Vision Res 15: 1411–1412.

Campbell FW, Robson JG (1968) Application of Fourier analysis to the visibility of gratings. J Physiol (Lond.) 197: 83–298.

Crane HD, Steele CM (1985) Generation-V dual-Purkinje-image eyetracker. Applied Optics 24: 527–537.

Hughes HC, Layton WM, Baird JC, Lester LS (1984) Global precedence in visual pattern recognition. Percept Psychophys 35: 361–371.

Loftus GR, Masson MEJ (1994) Using confidence intervals in within subject designs. Psychon Bull Rev 1: 476–490.

Parker DM, Lishman JR, Hughes J (1992) Temporal integration of spatially filtered visual images. Perception 21: 147–160.

Parker DM, Lishman JR, Hughes J (1996) Role of coarse and fine spatial information in face and object processing. J Exp Psychol Hum Percept Perf 22: 1448–1466.

Schyns PG, Oliva A (1994) From blobs to boundary edges: Evidence for time- and spatial-scale-dependent scene recognition. Psychol Sci 5: 195–200.

Schyns PG, Oliva A (1996, September) Flexible taskdependent scale encodings of complex visual stimuli. Paper presented at the workshop on spatial scale interactions, Durham, UK.

van Diepen PMJ (1997) A Pixel-resolution video switcher for eye contingent display changes. Spat Vis 10: 335–344.

van Diepen PMJ, De Graef P, d'Ydewalle G (1995) Chronometry of foveal information extraction during scene perception. In J.M Findlay, R.W.Kentridge, & R. Walker (Eds.) Eye movement research: Mechanisms, processes and applications. Elsevier, Amsterdam, pp 349–362.

van Diepen PMJ, De Graef P, Van Rensbergen J (1994) On-line control of moving masks and windows on a complex background using the ATVista Videographics adapter. Behav Res Meth Instr Comp 26: 454–460.

van Diepen PMJ, Wampers M (1996) Scene exploration with Fourier filtered peripheral information. Manuscript submitted for publication.

Van Rensbergen J, De Troy A (1993) A reference guide for the Leuven dual-PC controlled Purkinje eyetracking system (Psych. Rep. No. 145). Laboratory of Experimental Psychology, University of Leuven, Belgium.

Wampers M, van Diepen PMJ, d'Ydewalle G (1998) The use of coarse and fine peripheral information during scene perception. Manuscript in preparation.

37

EYE MOVEMENTS DURING FREE SEARCH ON A HOMOGENOUS BACKGROUND

Ulrich Nies, Dieter Heller, Ralph Radach, and Birgit Bedenk

Technical University of Aachen
Institute of Psychology
Jaegerstr. 17-19, D-52056 Aachen.

1. INTRODUCTION

Searching for small targets within a large homogenous area is common to many quality control tasks, where inspectors have to detect irregularities in industrial products (Bloomfield 1975; Megaw and Richardson 1979). For example in CRT manufacturing, inspectors have to search for a large variety of flaws, e.g. bubbles and stones, differing in contrast, size and appearance. The minimal diameter for irregularities that have to be identified is 0.4 mm. The inspector's task is difficult because of low target visibility, homogeneity of the glass surface and the short time allowed for inspection. The aim of the present research was to identify visuomotor and perceptual determinants of search performance as a base to design training programs for improvement.

A major determinant of detection rate in visual search tasks is the visual processing of parafoveal and peripheral information (see e.g. Findlay and Gilchrist 1998, for a discussion). Extrafoveal visual performance is often described in terms of the "useful field of view" (Bouma 1978), the area around the point of fixation, within which a certain type of visual information can be acquired. The useful field of view (UFV) has been quantified for a variety of tasks, e.g. for recognition of small objects in complex scenes (Nelson and Loftus 1980) and for detecting small peripheral targets while driving (Miura 1987). In reality, the useful field of view will not be marked by a sharp boundary but rather constitute a spatial gradient of decreasing visual performance.

The spatial distribution of fixations across the search field should have substantial impact on performance. Ideally, fixations should be distributed such that the whole search field is covered by adjacent UFV's. A systematic scanning pattern with interfixation distances of about the diameter of the UFV should lead to an optimal result. In practice, even extensively trained quality control inspectors will not exhibit this ideal eye movement pattern. However, a question of interest is up to which degree inspectors do indeed search systematically.

The case of searching very small targets within a homogenous area is unique in that it represents the lower end of complexity in visual search. The analysis of eye movements

Current Oculomotor Research, edited by Becker *et al.*
Plenum Press, New York, 1999.

269

in this context may therefore reveal general principles of search processes especially with respect to the role of the useful field of view and to search strategies. In the present chapter we report results of two recent experiments that address these issues using a computer simulation of CRT screen quality control.

2. EYE MOVEMENTS DURING FREE SEARCH

2.1. Method

In the course of extensive pre-experiments, involving a large variety of targets and a total of 30 inspectors, we created a realistic laboratory simulation of the search task. The external validity of the simulation was tested by comparing search performance with actual work performance of the same inspectors. A correlation of $r = .78$ between these two measures indicates that the demands posed by the simulation program are comparable to those in real quality control.

Targets were presented on an 21" EIZO Flexscan 6500 monochrome monitor at a viewing distance of 50 cm on a homogenous grey background (19 candela/m²). The search field subtended 27.7 x 23.1 cm (31 x 26 deg.). Two different targets were used in the main experiment, for which detection rates of 50 percent and 70 percent had been established in the pre-experiments. Target 1 simulated a bubble and was created by two light pixels (1 pixel 0.3 mm wide) surrounded by 6 darker ones. Luminance of the light centre was 39.1 candela/m² and luminance of the darker periphery 5.4 candela/m². Target 2 resembled a stone and consisted of 4 relatively dark pixels of 12 candela/m², arranged in a square. Both targets were presented 40 times. 20 target free trials (flawless screens) were included. Targets were distributed equally across the search field.

Subjects started a search trial by clicking a large button in the centre of the screen. Button and mouse cursor disappeared and after one second an acoustic signal indicated the beginning of the search. At the same time, the target was displayed on positive trials. Subjects were instructed to finish the trial with a mouse click as soon as they detected a target. After the search period, the target was removed, a two alternative choice displayed and subjects were asked whether there had been a target on the screen. On positive answers, subjects had to locate the target with the mouse cursor. When requested, subjects received a mouse manipulation training. All subjects took part in 20-trial search training with performance feedback on every trial.

The experiment was run in two series. In the first series, six inexperienced students (2 female, 4 male; mean age 26.9 years) participated. Since the search area was smaller in the eye movement study as compared to the pre-experiments, we reduced the display time from 12 seconds (equivalent to the real task) to 8.3 seconds. However, when running nine quality control inspectors (all male, mean age 33.9 years) in a second series, it turned out that they felt rushed and unable to perform their usual search routine. Therefore we set search time back to 12 seconds for these participants. Each subject performed 100 trials plus 20 training trials. All participants had normal or corrected to normal visual acuity.

Eye movements were recorded from the left eye using an infrared pupil reflection AMTech 3 eye tracker sampling at 200 Hz. A bite board and a forehead rest were used to minimise head movements. A calibration routine was run at the beginning of the experiment and after each block of 25 trials. To encourage subjects to search properly, individual detection rates were presented after the experimental session.

2.2. Results

Mean detection rate reached 82.9 percent, while false alarms were negligible (1.6 percent). Individual performance varied between 100 percent (two experts) and 65 percent. Novices detected 76 percent and experts 87 percent of the targets, which was probably in part due to the different search times allowed (see above). Detection rate for target 1 was significantly lower than for target 2 (79 vs. 87 percent; $t_{(14)} = 2.81$; $p < .05$). There was no significant correlation between foveal visual acuity as determined using a Titmus vision tester and search performance ($r = .06$; $n = 15$).

Subjects fixated on average 3 times per second. Mean fixation duration was 285 ms, mean saccadic amplitude 7.5 deg. There were substantial differences between subjects in these parameters (fixation duration range: 215 - 415 ms; saccade amplitude range: 4.2 - 10.7 deg.) but no significant differences between experts and novices. Both parameters did not significantly correlate with search performance (fixation duration $r = -.28$; saccade amplitude $r = .21$).

2.2.1. Useful Field of View. To estimate the extent of the useful field of view, fixations were determined that had resulted in target detection. Fixations were defined as "successful" when they were immediately followed by a saccade to the target. Fixations preceding the successful fixation were classified as "unsuccessful". To estimate detection performance as a function of retinal eccentricity, for every trial the distance between target location and the position of the selected fixations was determined. Performance was then computed as the proportion of successful fixations relative to all selected fixations (sum of successful and unsuccessful fixations) for a given target-fixation distance (in 1 deg. steps).

Within a range of 1 deg. almost all fixations were successful. Performance declined gradually up to an eccentricity of 3 deg., where the drop-off became somewhat steeper. Targets farther away than 6 deg. were nearly undetectable (see figure 4, where this function is compared to the one obtained in experiment 2). Figure 1 shows 4 individual examples for the spatial distribution of "successful" vs. "unsuccessful" fixations within an 8 x 6 deg. area centred around the search target. To illustrate the large interindividual variation in size and shape of the useful field of view, ellipses were fitted to the 50 percent and 70 percent performance level. The useful field of view as defined by the 70 percent performance level extended on average 3.3 deg. horizontally and 2.7 deg. vertically (note that the overall detection probability inside the field is much higher than 70 percent since this criterion is reached only at its outer limits). The individual 70 percent thresholds were between two and four deg. and showed a significant correlation with search performance ($r = .73$; $p < .01$).

An analysis of the relation between fixation duration, eccentricity and detection probability indicated that there is a continuous improvement of performance with increasing fixation duration up to about 200 milliseconds (see figure 2). Although subjects made many fixations that were of longer duration, this did not significantly contribute to detection probability.

2.2.2. Distribution of Fixation Locations. To analyse the spatial distribution of fixation locations, the search field was divided into eight areas of equal size (along the major axes together with a division into an edge and a centre region). An analysis of variance with the number of fixations (completed target free trials only) as the dependent variable revealed significant differences for the factors height ($F(1;14) = 6.57$; $p < .05$) and edge vs. centre ($F(1;14) = 12,33$; $p < .05$). It is noteworthy that despite the statistical signifi-

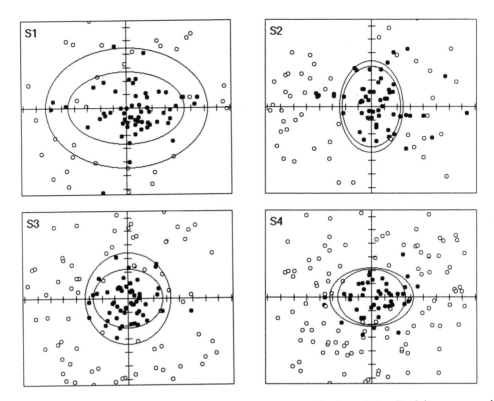

Figure 1. "Successful" (solid circles) vs. "unsuccessful" (open circles) fixations within a 8 x 6 deg. area around the search target. Ellipses are fitted corresponding to 70 percent (inner ellipses) and 50 percent (outer ellipses) detection performance. Subjects 1 and 4 were the participants with the largest and smallest extent of the UFV. The atypical shape of the UFV in Subject 2 may be related to his vertical "column" by "column" search strategy.

cance the difference in fixation density is rather small. The highest difference (edge 55% vs. centre 45%) means that 11 out of 20 fixations were placed in the edge region.

   2.2.3. Individual Search Strategies. Theoretically, an optimal search would require to keep track of all fixation positions within a scanpath in order to leave no parts of the search field uncontrolled and not to control other parts more than once. The associated

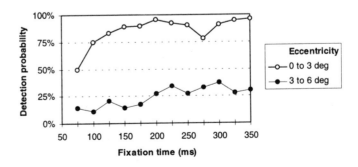

Figure 2. Detection probability as a function of fixation duration for targets near and far from the fixation point.

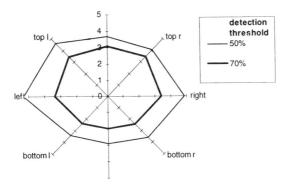

Figure 3. Estimated useful field of view in experiment 2. Depicted are the 50 and 70 percent iso-detection lines for the 8 target orientations.

memory load can be minimised by using a search strategy, i.e. a prespecified scanpath for each screen (Arani et al. 1984). Thus, it could be hypothesised that the similarity of the scanpaths of one subject is positively correlated with performance. However, the similarity of scanpaths can not be easily quantified, considering the usual variability in eye movement parameters.

Our first approach to assess scanpath similarity was a qualitative rating by human observers. Twenty scanpaths per subject (target free trials) were visualised on a computer screen. Three independent raters compared the scanpaths of each participant, searched for recurring patterns and rated their consistency. For ten subjects, similarities between trials could be seen. Each of these ten participants had an idiosyncratic way to search the screen, for example a reading-like scanning pattern or a clockwise search along the borders with a following scan through the centre. Based on the ratings, these participants could be subdivided into two groups. Five participants had nearly the same pattern in all trials. The other five showed comparable patterns but used different ones in some trials or lost their way over time on trial. In the paths of the remaining five subjects, no similarities between trials could be seen, so each screen was searched in a unique way. Contrary to the hypothesis, the non-consistent group performed better (97.3 percent, mean corrected for display time) than the other two (88 percent and 85.3 percent, mean corrected for display time).

For a quantitative assessment, we selected the most characteristic fixations of each scanpath on the basis of two criteria: distance to the preceding fixation (> 10 deg.) and change of direction (> 45 deg.). Out of approximately 35 fixations per scanpath, between

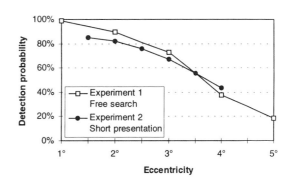

Figure 4. Comparison of detection probability as a function of target eccentricity for experiment 1 and 2.

five and fifteen fixations remained, marking the "cornerstones" of the path. To assess the similarity of two paths, we calculated the mean difference in spatial direction orientation between the connections of these characteristic fixations. On this measure, 0 deg. would indicate a maximum and 90 deg. a minimum of similarity.

The mean similarity value was 55° for all subjects. Individual values ranged between 13 and 88°. These similarity values were in good correspondence with the classification described above. The five participants with high ratings for consistency had a mean value of 27 deg., the intermediate group 49 deg. The group without consistent scanpaths reached a value of 84 deg. which is near the value expected with random paths (90°). Differences between experts and novices were rather small (experts 53.6 deg.; novices 57.4 deg.). The correlation of similarity values and search performance indicated a tendency against the hypothesis ($r = .22$; n.s.).

3. PSYCHOPHYSICAL DETERMINATION OF THE USEFUL FIELD OF VIEW

In experiment 1, the useful field of view proved to be a major determinant of search performance. However, its extent was estimated only indirectly. The difference between this procedure and a direct psychophysical determination of detection performance can bee seen in analogy to the distinction of perceptual span and visual span in reading. While visual span is based on the performance level in tachistoscopic extrafoveal letter identification tasks, perceptual span refers to the actual reading performance under the conditions of a complex, dynamic task (O'Regan et al. 1983, O'Regan 1990). A similar distinction has been proposed by Shioiri and Ikeda (1989) for the case of picture perception.

We were interested in the question to what extent the indirect UFV estimation from our eye movement study would correspond to a direct psychophysical test including a systematic manipulation of target direction and eccentricity. At first hand, a brief presentation of the target somewhere in the periphery appears to be the adequate experimental set-up for this purpose. However, the sudden appearance of the target leads to an almost perfect detection even at high eccentricities due to transient stimulation. It is quite difficult to counter this effect by masking the area beforehand with a large random dot pattern. Therefore, the method described below was developed which uses a concurrent transient stimulation of a simultaneously appearing saccade goal to mask the appearance of the detection target (Herzberg 1996).

3.1. Method

Subjects fixated on a central fixation cross and started the trial by a mouse click. After 400 ms the fixation cross disappeared and a second fixation cross appeared either to the left or right at an eccentricity of 8 deg. Subjects were instructed to make a saccade as fast as possible to the new fixation cross. In the vicinity of the second cross the target was simultaneously displayed. After a total presentation time of 500 ms, the whole area was masked by a large circular random dot pattern. Subjects were then asked to locate the position of the target with the mouse cursor or press a button to indicate that they did not detect a target. Viewing distance was set to 50 cm. The same hardware as in experiment 1 was used.

In a pre-experiment, eye movements were recorded (AMTech ET 3, see experiment 1) to ensure that subjects were indeed able to perform the task in the intended way, i.e. presentation time was neither too short nor too long to allow for one primary saccade and appropriate detection. Latency of the saccade was 180 ms on average and fixation duration on the second fixation cross before masking 176 ms. 77 percent of the critical fixations were located within 2 deg. around the second fixation cross. These data indicate that the presentation time used in the experiment was suitable for the intended task.

In the main experiment, three different targets were used, two of which were identical to those in experiment 1 (the third target was introduced for reasons not related to the current discussion). They were placed at six different eccentricities (1.5 to 4 deg. in 0.5 deg. steps). Target direction was varied in steps of 45 deg. around the fixation point. Each combination of the four independent variables (saccade direction, type of target, target direction, target eccentricity) was presented four times in random order. 248 target free trials were included, making up to a total of 1400 trials per subject. 20 naive students participated as subjects.

3.2. Results

Detection performance was tested with a four factor within subjects ANOVA using an arcsin transformation of percent correct. Due to violations of variance homogeneity degrees of freedom had to be corrected using the Huyhn-Feldt (hf) or Greenhouse-Geisser (gg) method.

The direction of the primary saccade did not show any significant differences ($F(19;1) = 0.22$), therefore results for left and right presentation were pooled in subsequent analyses. Detection rate of the three targets proved to be significantly different ($F(1.95; 37) = 43.55; p < .001;$ hf corrected). The order of the detection rate for the different targets was equivalent to that in the visual search experiments.

The distance between second fixation cross and target had a strong effect on detection rate ($F(1.5; 28.7) = 203.18; p < .001;$ gg corrected). A post hoc analysis of linearity revealed a significant linear decrease of detection rate with increasing distance ($F(1;19) = 249.7; p < .001$). At a distance of 1.5 deg., detection rate was 85 percent, whereas at 4 deg. it had dropped to 43 percent. Finally, direction of the target had a significant effect on detection rate ($F(7;133) = 10.27; p < .001$) with targets on the horizontal meridian yielding best performance.

The form of the useful field of view was determined using iso-detection lines computed for 50 and 70 percent performance thresholds. In figure 3, the elliptical form of the resulting UFV can be clearly seen. Target detection was worst in locations below the fixation cross. As in experiment 1, there were large differences in UFV size between subjects. The best participant had more then 70 percent detection frequency at 4 deg. eccentricity, indicating that her UFV extends beyond the range used in the experiment. On the contrary, the participant with the smallest UFV did not reach 70 percent at 1.5 deg.

Figure 4. presents a comparison of experiment 1 and experiment 2 with respect to the relation between detection and target distance. The apparent similarity indicates that in the specific search task used in our study, there is very little difference between a psychophysical visual span and a perceptual span as determined indirectly from eye movement data.

4. DISCUSSION

Our analysis of eye movements during free search of small targets on a homogenous background showed that there is no simple relation between general eye movement parameters and search performance.

A very powerful determinant of performance proved to be the extent of the useful field of view as assessed by determining the fixation that led to target detection. There were remarkable differences between subjects in the size and shape of the useful field of view. Whether the extent of the UFV is a stable individual factor or whether it is dependent from state variables like motivation and attention cannot be resolved within the scope of this study.

The striking similarity between detection performance as a function of target distance between experiment 1 and 2 has methodological implications. It shows that performance in a dynamic visual search task can be predicted accurately by a psychophysical determination of the useful field of view. This is interesting also from a theoretical point of view. In a complex visual search field or within a natural scene, object identification performance will in most cases be lower, as compared to a tachistoscopic one-object presentation. Several factors can be made responsible for this difference: The presence of similar extrafoveal objects ("lateral masking", see e.g. Huckauf et al., in press), a narrowing of the useful field of view due to foveal processing load (Ikeda and Takeuchi 1975), demands of saccade programming on visual processing resources, and increasing load on spatial working memory while keeping track of the scanpath. In our task, no other objects are present, masking and response competition are impossible and "foveal" processing load reduced to a minimum. Therefore, we can interpret the similarity of the results of our two experiments as indicating that the two remaining factors, saccade programming and spatial memory do not interfere with processing of fine detail within the useful field of view. At least under conditions of a homogenous visual field with clearly defined spatial co-ordinates, the programming of saccades to distant positions appears to be carried out either with minimal resources or in parallel with local visual processing.

In our analysis of eye movements during free search, no advantage of a "regular" search strategy could be established. This may seem surprising, but it has been shown before that search behaviour of experts can be closer to a random walk model as compared to an ideal observer model (Kundel et al. 1987). Our results are in line with Gale and Worthington's (1983) findings on scanpaths in radiology. While they showed that it is possible to train specific visual strategies (i.e. advised scanning patterns) when searching for small coin lesions in X-ray images, it turned out that this type of training did not lead to improvements in detection performance.

As the results of our analysis show, the placement of fixations relative to search targets turned out to be a critical factor for search performance. We therefore assumed, that it would be useful to induce a systematic and exhaustive scanpath with every fixation having the same chance to be placed near to a target. This was accomplished in a subsequent series of experiments (Bedenk, in preparation) by segmenting the search area into rectangular quadrants which were to be fixated one by one. We are currently running a study using the same simulated quality control task as in experiment 1. The search field is divided into 25 segments and subjects are instructed to fixate once in the centre of each segment. Preliminary results indicate that search performance does indeed increase by about 7 percent for easy targets and 12 percent for more difficult targets and that especially participants with low or medium performance in free search profit from this technique.

REFERENCES

Arani T, Karwan MH & Drury CG (1984) A variable-memory model of visual search. Human Factors 26: 631–639

Bedenk B (in preparation) Visuelle Inspektion homogener Flächen. Leistungsverbesserung durch die Segmentierung der Suchfläche (Visual inspection of homogenous areas. Performance improvement by segmenting the search field). Doctoral dissertation, Technical University of Aachen

Bloomfield JR (1975) Theoretical approaches to visual search. In: Drury CG, Fox JG (eds) Human Reliability in Quality Control. Taylor & Francis, London, pp 19–29

Bouma H (1978) Visual search and reading: eye movements and functional visual field. In: Requin J. (ed) Attention and Performance VII. Erlbaum, Hillsdale, N.J. pp. 115–147

Findlay JM, Gilchrist ID (1998) Eye movements and visual search. In: Underwood G (ed) Eye guidance in reading and scene perception. Elsevier, Amsterdam, pp 297–314

Gale AG, Worthington BS (1983) The utility of scanning strategies in radiology. In: Groner R, Menz RC, Fisher DF, Monty RA (eds) Eye movements and psychological functions: International Views. Erlbaum, Hillsdale, N. J., pp 43–52

Herzberg F (1996) Bestimmung der optimalen Größe des Suchraumes bei visueller Produktendkontrolle (Determination of the optimal size of the search field in visual product inspection). Unpublished Master Thesis, Technical University of Aachen

Huckauf A, Heller D, Nazir T (in press) Lateral masking: limitations of the feature interaction account. Perception & Psychophysics

Ikeda M, Takeuchi R (1975) Influence of foveal load on the functional visual field. Perception & Psychophysics 18: 255–260

Kundel HL, Nodine CF, Thickman MD, Toto L (1987) Searching for lung nodules. A comparison of human performance with random and systematic scanning models. Investigative Radiology 22: 417–422.

Megaw ED, Richardson J (1979) Eye movements and industrial inspection. Applied Ergonomics 10: 145–154

Miura T (1987) Behaviour oriented vision: functional field of view and processing resources. In: O'Regan JK, Levy-Schoen A (eds) Eye Movements: From Physiology to Cognition. Elsevier, Amsterdam, pp 487–498

Nelson WW, Loftus GR (1980) The functional visual field during picture viewing. J Exp Psy: Human Learning and Memory 6: 391–399

O'Regan JK (1990) Eye movements and reading. In: Kowler E (ed) Reviews of oculomotor research: Vol.4. Eye Movements and Their Role in Visual and Cognitive Processes. Elsevier, Amsterdam, pp 395–453

O'Regan JK, Levy-Schoen A, Jacobs AM (1983) The effect of visibility on eye-movement parameters in reading. Perception & Psychophysics 34, 457–464

Shioiri S, Ikeda M (1989) Useful resolution for picture perception as a function of eccentricity. Perception 18: 347–361

38

IS THERE ANY NEED FOR EYE-MOVEMENT RECORDINGS DURING REASONING?

W. Schroyens, W. Schaeken, W. Fias, and G. d'Ydewalle

Laboratory of Experimental Psychology
University of Leuven
Tiensestraat 102, B-3000 Leuven, Belgium.

1. INTRODUCTION

In experimental research on the psychology of reasoning one mostly uses the nature and frequency of conclusions to reasoning problems as a measure of the cognitive processes involved in reasoning. Less often, researchers use problem solving latencies as an additional measure. We aimed to add more fine-grained measures to the field of reasoning research: namely those obtained by registering eye-movements. At the same time we ventured that those measures might also be obtained without the use of eye-movement registration equipment. By displaying the constituent clauses of reasoning problems contingent upon the movements of a mouse-cursor, we expected to obtain results equally sensitive to the difficulty of making particular inferences. In order to tackle these questions we conducted some studies in which the negations paradigm was applied to the conditional inferences task. Jargon being what it is, we will first explicate what conditional reasoning is about, how conditional reasoning can be investigated with the conditional inferences task and how the negations paradigm is applied to the conditional inferences task. Only then are we in the position to elaborate the hypothesized difficulties in drawing inferences about conditionals with negative constituent clauses; difficulties which were expected to be reflected in eye-movement measures if these are to provide a sensible measures to reasoning processes.

1.1. Conditional Reasoning and the Conditional Inferences Task

Conditional reasoning, that is, reasoning about sentences containing a propositional connective like 'if_then_', is a widely investigated aspects of the psychology of reasoning (see Evans, Newstead, & Byrne, 1993). Conditional reasoning is often investigated with the conditional inference task. In this task, reasoners are given conditional inference problems based on two premises. Four basic conditional inference problems are set by a categorical premise that either affirms or denies either the antecedent (p) or consequent (q) of

Current Oculomotor Research, edited by Becker *et al.*
Plenum Press, New York, 1999.

Table 1. The conditional inference problems set up by an affirmation or denial of a negative or affirmative antecedent or a negative or affirmative consequent in the conditional

Conditional	Problem type			
	MP	AC	DA	MT
If p, then q				
Categorical Premise	p	q	not p	not q
Conditional	q	p	*not q*	*not p*
Conclusion				
If p, then not q				
Categorical Premise	p	not q	not p	q
Conditional	not q	p	**q**	*not p*
Conclusion				
If not p, then q				
Categorical Premise	not p	q	p	not q
Conditional	q	*not p*	*not q*	**p**
Conclusion				
If not p, then not q				
Categorical Premise	not p	not q	p	q
Conditional	not q	*not p*	**q**	**p**
Conclusion				

Note: 'AA' = affirmation of the antecedent; 'AC' = affirmation of the consequent, DA = denial of the antecedent, 'DC' = denial of the consequent. Conclusions typed in bold require eliminating a double negation to infer the conditional conclusion and negative conclusions are underscored.

a conditional (if p then q). In the first section of Table 1 we give a formal representation of these conditional inference problems, along with the conclusion which is classically being called the conditional inference. Affirming the consequent (q) as the inference to the *affirmation of the antecedent problems* (AA: if p then q; p) is a logically valid conclusion, and corresponds to the Modus Ponendo Ponens argument in propositional logic. Affirming the antecedent (p) as a conclusion to the *affirmation of the consequent problems* (AC: if p then q; q) is not invalid. Affirming the antecedent when the consequent is affirmed is valid only in case of a bi-conditional (If and only if p, then q). As for the AC problems, the conditional inference to the *denial of the antecedent problems* (DA: if p, then q; not p), that is, denying the consequent (not q) is not a logically valid conclusion. Finally, the conditional inference to the *denial of the consequent problems* (DC: if p then q, not q) is that of denying the antecedent (not p). This conditional inference is logically valid and in formal propositional calculus the argument is known as the Modus Tollendo Tollens argument. Since reasoners are invited to make an inference about the consequent in the case of the AA and DA problems, we refer to the consequent of these problems as the *'inferential clause'*. Analogously, the inferential clause of the AC and DC problems is the antecedent because reasoners are invited to make an inferences about it.

1.2. Conditional Reasoning with Negations

In investigating the impact of negations on the conclusions that people draw from conditional inferences problems, mostly the negations paradigm is applied to the conditional inference task. In the negations paradigm one systematically permutes the presence of a negation in the antecedent or consequent of the conditionals used to set up conditional inference problems. In Table 1 we show the sixteen conditional inferences problems with their conditional conclusion, as they can be constructed by applying the negations paradigm. Two hypotheses have been proposed to explain or predict the effects of introducing negation in the inferential clause of a conditional: (I) negative conclusion bias and (ii) double negation elimination.

In reviewing the literature on conditional reasoning with negatives, Evans (1993) discussed a *negative conclusion bias*: Reasoners would prefer negative conclusions over affirmative conclusions. That is, people would be more likely to draw the conditional inference when the inferential clause in the affirmation problems is negative and when the inferential clause in the denial problems is affirmative. To explain the mechanism of the bias, he says that affirmative conclusions are maybe filtered out, due to some caution principle (see, Pollard & Evans, 1980). Being cautious under uncertainty might work in favor of negative conclusions because the likelihood of a falsifying instance for a negative conclusion is smaller than the likelihood of observing a falsifying instance for an affirmative conclusion.

Evans et al. (1995) conducted a series of experiments in order to test for negative conclusion bias. Overall, they found no reliable evidence for negative conclusions being preferred over affirmative conclusions to the AC or AA problems. That is, higher proportions of conditional inferences were only made on the denial problems with an affirmative inferential clause. As such, Evans et al. (1995) suggested an alternative hypothesis to negative conclusion bias. This hypothesis can be labeled '*double negation elimination*'. If reasoners have to negate a negation, less conditional inferences will be made, because they have to eliminate this double negation (see e.g., Evans, 1972). The heart of the problem with double negation seems to lie in the inference 'not [not-p], therefore [p]'. Since people do not need to deny the inferential clause to solve the affirmation problems, a negative inferential clause will have no effect on the affirmation problems (AA and AC), but will influence the two denial problems: DC inferences will be harder with a negative antecedent and DA inferences will be harder with a negative consequent.

2. A COMPARISON OF EYE MOVEMENT AND MOUSE MOVEMENTS

2.1. Introduction

In the following we present the results we obtained in conducting two studies on conditional reasoning with negations (See Schroyens et al. 1998). In the first experiment we used the eye-movement registration technique. For the second experiment we developed a novel procedure based on mouse cursor movements. In both experiments we presented the participants with 64 conditional inferences problems: Four instances of each of the 16 conditional inference problems with negations (see Table 2). The participants in the eye-movement experiment (N = 31) were first confronted with the problem presented on a computer screen. They could take as long as they wanted to derive their solution to a problem and had to press a button when they had found their solution, after which they could select their conclusion among a set of four answer-alternatives. From the eye-movement data, we abstracted three measures which were expected to extent standard problems solving latencies. That is, we abstracted the reading times on the three clauses which constitute the conditional inference problems: The antecedent, the consequent and the categorical premise.

Table 2. Differences (negative minus affirmative antecedent or consequent) on the percentages of conditional inferences (%), the reading times on the antecedent (A), consequent (C) and the categorical premise (CP)

| | Antecedent Polarity | | | | Consequent Polarity | | | |
| | | Reading times | | | | | Reading times | |
	%	A	C	CP	%	A	C	CP
Affirmation of the antecedent (AA)								
Eye Movements	-5.0	0.51	0.39	0.20	-2.6	0.21	0.43	0.21
Mouse movements	3.6	1.11*	0.44	0.68*	-4.2	0.12	0.62*	0.46
Affirmation of the Consequent (AC)								
Eye movements	*±16.0**	*1.10**	*0.45*	*0.13*	-14.4*	0.39	0.64	0.46
Mouse movements	*±16.8**	*1.60**	*0.43*	*0.55*	-8.2	0.10	0.87	0.63
Denial of the antecedent (DA)								
Eye movements	+8.7	0.56	0.39	0.20	***-33.2****	***0.78****	***0.68****	***0.22***
Mouse movements	+10.4	1.25	0.58	0.28	***-31.8****	***0.50***	***1.16****	***0.04***
Denial of the Consequent (DC)								
Eye movements	***-37.0****	***1.48****	***1.58****	***0.20***	+5.0	0.03	0.17	0.22
Mouse movements	***-36.1****	***3.15****	***1.63****	***0.26***	-7.5	0.17	0.40	0.56

Note: Marked differences are significant (α = .01), differences typed in bold require the elimination of a double negation when the inferential clause is negative, and underscored differences involve a negative conclusion.

In the second experiment we registered the mouse-cursor movements. Participants (N = 35) had to point a mouse cursor within soft-ware defined boundaries around the antecedent, consequent and categorical premise before they could see the content of these clauses. They were initially presented with incomplete antecedent 'if ...', an incomplete consequent 'then ...' and an incomplete categorical premise 'There is ...'. When moving the mouse cursor across the antecedent region it would become completely visible and when moving to mouse cursor within the region defined around the consequent, the antecedent would become masked again, and the consequent would become completely visible. Participants could look to the constituent problem clauses as long and a many times as they wanted. As in the eye-movement study, the antecedent reading times were calculated as the total time the mouse cursor (alternatively the eyes) pointed within the soft-ware defined boundaries around the antecedent and the same for the reading times of the consequent and the categorical premise.

3. RESULTS AND DISCUSSION

Table 2 gives the difference scores (negative versus affirmative antecedent or consequent) for the percentages of conditional inferences, the reading times on the antecedent, consequent and categorical premise. In both the eye-movement and mouse-movement study, the results were analyzed by means of analyses of variance. In the following we will discuss the results as a function of the different questions that gave rise to these experiments.

3.1. Double Negation and/or Negative Conclusion Bias?

Obviously, given that the same problems were used in the respective studies, response patterns would not differ between the two studies. Indeed, its a prerequisite to compare the eye-movement and mouse-movement data. First, as can be seen in Table 2 and as expected, a negation in the inferential clause resulted in a reliable decrease of the percentages of conditional inferences for both denial problems (DA and DC). Participants less frequently made the denial inferences when they had to deny a negative inferential clause. Second, we can not reject the null-hypothesis that a negative inferential clause in AC problems does not affect the ease of making the AC inferences (pace, Evans et al., 1995). The participants in both studies preferred negative conclusions above affirmative conclusions. In the literature, negative conclusion bias and double negation elimination are mostly pitted against each other in terms of either the one or the other. Since it falls beyond the scope of the present article we will not elaborate and suffice with noting that there are both theoretical and empirical grounds for abandoning the presumption that negative conclusion bias and double negation elimination are mutually exclusive processes (see Schroyens et al., 1998, submitted).

3.2. Do Eye-Movements Reflect Difficulties in Reasoning?

As can be seen in Table 2, the pattern of effects observed on the constituent reading times look very promising concerning the use of eye-movement measures. When the presence of a negation reliably affected the percentages of conditional inferences on particular problems, the reading times on the constituent problems clauses were also reliable affected. And, most importantly, the increased reading times were most particularly observed on those constituent problem clauses which affected the percentages of conditional inferences when it was negative.

However, the eye-movements also exhibited *spill-over effects* which indicate that the link between manifest eye-movement patterns and latent processes such as the difficulty of double negation elimination is not as stringent as one might have hoped for. The decrease in the percentages of denial inferences with a negative inferential clause were not only associated with increased reading times of the inferential clause itself. The other clause was also reliably effected by the polarity of the inferential clause. These spill-over effects, however, are not unprecedented and have been reported in literature on word processing and reading. Though certainly revoking the idea of eye-movements providing a 'mirror to the soul', these findings have not impinged the usefulness of eye-movement measures.

3.3. Eye Movements versus Mouse Movements

The global pattern of effects observed in the mouse-movement study indicates that our procedure of presenting constituent problem clauses contingent upon movements of a mouse cursor is also sensitive to the difficulties of reasoning about negations. The reading times on the constituent clauses of the problems which were reliably effected by the presence of a negation in the inferential clause reveal essentially the same pattern of effects as the one observed in the eye-movement study.

However, in comparison with the eye-movement measures, the mouse-movement experiment showed effects which suggest that their use is not as advantageous as those of eye-movement data. As can be seen in Table 2, the antecedent and consequent reading times of the AA problems increased significantly when this clause contained a negation, despite the fact that the AA inferences were not affected. In addition, the reading times of the inferential clause of the AC, DA, and DC problems all showed a reliable interaction between the polarity of the antecedent and the consequent. Specifically, in the case of an asymmetrical conditional, that is a conditional in which either the antecedent or the consequent was negative ([if not p, then q] and [if p, then not q]) the presence of a negation increased the reading times of both the antecedent and the consequent as compared to the reading times of the respective clause in the symmetrically affirmative conditional [if p, then q]. In the case of a symmetrically negative conditional [if not p, then not q], the reading times on both the antecedent and the consequent were generally longer than those on the symmetrically affirmative conditional [if p, then q] but generally shorter than either one of the asymmetrical conditionals.

We suspect that the interactions between the polarity of the antecedent and consequent, are induced by the characteristics of the task. First, moving a mouse cursor is not an activity engaged in as spontaneously and automatically as moving ones eyes to a particular region of interest. Second, representing asymmetrical conditionals in working memory would be more difficult than representing a symmetrical conditionals. One must not only represent whether a negation is present or not, but also has to keep count of whether the negation is present in the antecedent or consequent. As such, as compared to symmetrically negative conditionals, the participants would more frequently move the mouse cursor over both the antecedent and consequent of asymmetrical conditionals. Obviously, the simple main effects we reported could only have come about when the relative increase on the reading times of the antecedent and consequent differs as a function of whether or not these clause serve as the inferential clause of a particular type of problem.

4. GENERAL CONCLUSIONS

The present study focussed on three questions. First, do people exhibit negative conclusion bias or difficulties in eliminating a double negation, or both? Our results suggest that both negative conclusion bias and double negation elimination are part of the cognitive mechanism invoked in reasoning about negative conditionals. Second, can we use eye-movement measures to constrain and test hypotheses about human reasoning? Our results indicate that eye-movement measure can be used to obtain more fine-grained measure than global problem solving latencies. Reading times of the inferential clause and generally not the reading times on other constituent problem clauses, reflected the supposed difficulties of coping with a negation in that inferential clause. Hence, eye movement measures at least provide evidence converging upon the difficulty of reasoning with negative conditionals. And, more general, eye-movement measures might provide additional constraints to the cognitive mechanisms invoked to account for reasoning about other types of problems. Third, can a procedure more readily applicable than the eye-movement registration technique provide equally sensitive measures? Our procedure of mouse-movement registrations seems to do so. So it would seem that there is no need for eye-movement registration in reasoning about negative conditionals. However, our procedure also set specific task demands which result in effects occluding the hypothesized reasoning mechanisms. Hence, from a theoretical point of view, we must prefer eye-movement registrations.

REFERENCES

Evans, J. St. B. T. (1972). Interpretation and 'matching' bias in a reasoning task. *Quarterly Journal of Experimental Psychology, 24*: 193–199.

Evans, J. St. B. T. (1993). The mental model theory of conditional reasoning: Critical appraisal and revision. *Cognition, 48*:1–20.

Evans, J. St. B. T., Clibbens, J., & Rood, B. (1995). Bias in conditional inference: Implications for mental models and mental logic. *Quarterly Journal of Experimental Psychology*, 48A: 644–670.

Evans, J. St. B. T., Newstead, S. E., & Byrne, R. M. J. (1993). *Human reasoning: The psychology of deduction.* Hillsdale, NJ: Erlbaum.

Pollard, P., & Evans, J. St. B. T. (1980). The influence of logic on conditional reasoning performance. *The Quarterly Journal of Experimental Psychology, 32*: 605–624.

Schroyens, W., Schaeken, W., Fias, W., & d'Ydewalle, G. (1998). *Bias in propositional reasoning with negative conditionals.* Psychological reports (N° 230), Laboratory of Experimental Psychology, University of Leuven, Belgium.

Schroyens, W., Schaeken, W., Fias, W., & d'Ydewalle, G. (submitted). *Bias in propositional reasoning with negative conditionals.* Paper submitted for publication.

39

A NEW WAY OF LOOKING AT AUDITORY LINGUISTIC COMPREHENSION

Brooke Hallowell

Ohio University School of Hearing and Speech Sciences
208 Lindley Hall
Athens, Ohio

1. INTRODUCTION

Methods currently being developed for the use of eye movements in the assessment of linguistic comprehension have important clinical and research applications. These methods may be particularly useful for the assessment of severely neurologically impaired patients whose motoric response capabilities are limited to the degree that-regardless of linguistic involvement-they would demonstrate poor or even no responses on traditional tests of linguistic comprehension. Recent methodological developments have been focused on stimulus design, testing protocols, dependent measures, and instrumentation.

2. WHY USE ALTERNATE INDICES OF COMPREHENSION?

The recognition of competence versus performance issues in the process of differential diagnosis of communication disorders is especially important in neurologically impaired patients. Most items in traditional tests of language comprehension used with neurologically impaired patients require some overt response on the part of the patient. A failure to respond (or to respond correctly) does not necessarily indicate a failure to comprehend, especially in patients with severe motoric difficulties (Rosenbeck et al 1984). It is important that we consider alternate nonverbal means of comprehension assessment in order to make our inferences some patients' comprehension abilities more valid (Hallowell 1991).

3. WHY USE SPONTANEOUS EYE MOVEMENT MEASURES TO STUDY COMPREHENSION?

Advantages of using eye movements to index auditory comprehension include: provision of information about intact comprehension ability (currently unavailable for severely inexpressive patients); allowance for stimulus adaptations to control for perceptual,

Current Oculomotor Research, edited by Becker *et al.*
Plenum Press, New York, 1999.

attentional, and oculomotor deficits; reduced reliance on patients' understanding of verbal instructions regarding testing; allowance for real-time measurement of comprehension; and allowance for testing of a broad range of verbal stimulus types. Additionally, eye movements are often preserved even in cases of severe motoric and cognitive deficits (Leigh and Zee, 1983).

For the present purposes, spontaneous eye fixations are studied as subjects view scenes or pictures in verbal and nonverbal conditions. Not requiring conscious planning and execution, spontaneous fixations are differentiated from volitional and intentionally directed eye fixations, as used with some augmentative communication systems. This is an important distinction, given the potential for apraxic deficits that may affect oculomotor programming of intentional eye movements in some patients.

4. METHODOLOGICAL ISSUES IN THE USE OF EYE MOVEMENT MEASURES FOR THE STUDY OF COMPREHENSION

The design of visual and verbal stimuli and of the testing protocol must be done very carefully in order to increase our confidence that where a subject looks yields information about what linguistic and graphic information the subject is processing. Some of the issues requiring particular attention are:

- means of controlling for possible effects of peripheral vision
- means of controlling for possible differences between foveal and attentional fixation
- means of controlling for physical stimulus properties of visual stimuli (e.g., color, luminance, size, and complexity of individual objects) on scanning patterns
- means of controlling for the redundancy or predictability of visual and verbal stimuli
- determination of optimal numbers of nontarget foils within visual stimuli
- determination of optimal semantic relationships between visual "target " stimuli and visual foils, and between visual and verbal stimuli
- means of controlling for contextual constraints on information processing
- rationale for the use of various possible units of eye movement analysis in the quantification of differences between scan patterns
- rationale for the use of various possible statistical methods in eye movement analysis
- design of verbal stimuli which vary in length and complexity as well as the types of responses they require from subjects

5. THE STATE OF THE ART

Methodological developments in the use of eye movement measures to assess linguistic comprehension have thus far involved experimentation using language-normal subjects. It is important to assess the eye movement testing protocols using subjects who clearly understand a verbal stimulus pertaining to a visual stimulus in order to and validate testing protocols which are under development.

Experimental testing protocols using a variety of verbal and visual stimulus types have been designed to evoke significant differences in fixation patterns in verbal as compared to nonverbal (free-scanning) conditions. In a free-scanning condition no questions or instructions are presented to subjects. Subjects look at the same visual arrays which are later shown in the verbal condition. In a verbal condition a question or instruction is presented to subjects and is immediately followed by the presentation of a test picture. Because a verbal stimulus ideally leads a comprehending subject to orient to a specific target or sequence of targets of the visual array, and because a prior orientation assumed for a given picture is likely to be recalled on subsequent exposures to that picture (Stark and Ellis 1981), the free-scanning condition is presented first.

Data from one study in which 20 language-normal subjects viewed pictures in both verbal and nonverbal conditions yielded a contrast between conditions according to one dependent measure, the proportion of total fixation time subjects spent looking at a "target" picture within a matrix of pictures. A brief description of this study is presented below.

6. EXPERIMENTAL PROTOCOL FOR EXAMINING DIFFERENCES IN SCANS BETWEEN VERBAL AND NONVERBAL CONDITIONS

Following a series of pilot experiments designed to examine numerous methodological issues, an experiment was performed to assess the effectiveness of one protocol to evoke differential scanning patterns under verbal compared to nonverbal conditions, to study the relationship among several possible dependent measures used in scan analysis, and to examine the effects of various visual and verbal item types on scan patterns.

6.1. Method

6.1.1. Subjects. Twenty subjects with a mean age of about 23 years participated.

6.1.2. Materials. Visual stimuli for the free-scanning and verbal conditions were photographic slides of 22 black-and-white four-picture matrices. All matrices were presented on a rear-projection screen 200 cm from the subjects. Eighty-eight verbal stimuli exhibiting a broad range of grammatical complexity and length typical of test items used in traditional language comprehension tests were designed for the verbal condition. The number of picture foils subjects need to look at before responding accurately, and the type of verbal response required of a subject-if any-were also varied. Prior to experimentation, each subject was randomly assigned to one of four subject groups to allow for counterbalancing of pictures designated as targets within matrices across trials.

6.1.3. Instrumentation. Electro-oculographic (EOG) techniques (system bandwidth 0 to 35 Hz, with resolution better than 0.5 degrees) were used to record horizontal and vertical eye positions.

6.1.4. Procedure. The order of trials for each condition was randomized. For the free-scanning condition subjects fixated on a center reference point (for calibration purposes), then scanned each of the 22 test matrices for 10 seconds. For each verbal trial, subjects fixated on a center reference point for calibration purposes and were presented a pre-recorded digitized speech stimulus. Again, eye position was recorded during 10 seconds of scanning of the picture matrices.

Table 1. Means and standard deviations for
difference between verbal and free-scanning
conditions in terms of proportions of durations
per scan spent looking at targets

Subject group[a]	Difference between conditions (verbal - free-scanning)	
	Mean	SD
Group A	.293	.220
Group B	.209	.272
Group C	.314	.238
Group D	.262	.247
Total	.270	.244

[a] n = 90 per group

6.2. Results and Discussion

An analysis of variance on differences between conditions in terms of the proportion of total duration subjects spent fixating a "target" was implemented on four between-groups levels of subject group. Although the free-scanning condition itself does not involve the definition of target versus nontarget pictures, "targets" corresponding to verbal condition targets are designated for scans in the nonverbal condition for purposes of comparison. Means and standard deviations of differences in proportions of fixation duration allotted to targets for each subject group may be found in Table 1.

There was no significant effect for subject groupings [F (3,350) = 2.992; p = .031]. Data were therefore collapsed across subject groups for an examination of overall differences between the verbal and free-scanning conditions.

Data pertaining to the proportion of the total duration of fixations in a scan that subjects spent looking at a target yielded a significant main effect for condition [t (353) = 20.6, $p < .0001$]. During verbal trials subjects spent greater proportions of fixation durations on targets than they did during free-scanning trials. There were no significant differences among nonverbal condition trials in terms of the proportions of fixation durations spent on targets, ensuring no biasing effects of target picture position on the results.

Language-normal subjects fixated significantly longer on targets of visual stimulus matrices after a verbal stimulus than they did with no prior stimulus. The contrast between conditions assures us that testing for linguistic comprehension using eye movement responses with this testing protocol is feasible.

7. NEW DIRECTIONS

Continued development of eye movement applications for assessing linguistic comprehension involves further research. Some of the most critical issues currently being addressed are:

- optimal stimulus adaptations for neurologically impaired patients, including adaptations for patients with visual field deficits and visual neglect;
- controlled manipulation of semantic relationships among visual target and foil stimuli and verbal stimuli;

- testing of methodological validity and reliability, using patients with known linguistic processing deficits and normal subjects;
- establishment of assessment protocols with a remote pupil-center/corneal reflection system to allow for less subject constraint and set-up time; and
- application of testing protocols to other areas of information.

REFERENCES

Hallowell, B (1991) *Using eye movement responses as an index of linguistic comprehension.* The University of Iowa.

Leigh JR, Zee D (1983) *The neurology of eye movements.* FA Davis, Philadelphia

Rosenbeck JC, Kent RD, LaPointe LL (1984) Apraxia of speech: An overview and some perspectives. In: Rosenbeck JC, McNeil MR, Aronson AE (eds), *Apraxia of speech.* College Hill Press, San Diego, pp 1–72

Stark L, Ellis SR (1981) Scanpaths revisited: Cognitive models direct active looking. In: Fisher DF, Monty RA, Senders JW (eds), *Eye movements: Cognition and visual perception.* Erlbaum, New Jersey, pp 193–226.

40

EYE MOVEMENT-BASED MEMORY ASSESSMENT

Robert Althoff, Neal J. Cohen, George McConkie, Stanley Wasserman,
Michael Maciukenas, Razia Azen, and Lorene Romine

Beckman Institute
University of Illinois at Urbana-Champaign

1. ABSTRACT

We introduce here a new indirect (implicit) measure of memory based on eye move-ment monitoring. Eye movement data collected while participants were viewing images of faces showed that viewers process repeated items differently than novel items. Participants viewed repeated items with fewer eye fixations to fewer regions and more randomness (i.e. less *constraint*) in their eye movement patterns. We term this effect the "eye move-ment-based memory effect". Thus far, it appears that the effects of experience on eye movements generalize across different eyetrackers, types of visual stimuli, and types of prior exposure to the stimuli. Moreover, we show that the effects occur separately from explicit remembering by testing amnesic patients -- i.e. patients with a profound impair-ment in learning and remembering of new declarative memory. Even in these patients who showed impairment learning the faces presented to them, there was evidence of prior proc-essing in the eye movement data in the same direction as normal controls. With this in mind, we argue that certain of these eye movement measures can provide a useful index of procedural memory and that the use of eye movement measures as an indirect (implicit) measure of memory provides direct evidence that previous experience does indeed change the *nature* of perceptual processing.

2. INTRODUCTION

The nature of the eye movements elicited in viewing scenes has been the subject of research aimed at understanding aspects of perceptual processing. Although the movement of the eyes is not necessary to process a scene, eye movements are involved in the proc-essing of that scene (Antes and Penland 1981; Parker 1978). The manner in which the eyes move has been shown to be related to physical aspects of a scene such as luminance or texture of the objects (Antes 1974; Buswell 1935; Mackworth and Morandi 1967) as well as to certain semantic attributes of the scene, such as the suitability or plausibility of

Current Oculomotor Research, edited by Becker *et al.*
Plenum Press, New York, 1999.

particular objects or object features in that scene (Parker 1978; Loftus and Mackworth 1978; Biederman et al. 1974). For example, Loftus and Mackworth (1978) showed that viewers fixate more frequently, earlier, and with longer durations on objects that are out of place in a scene (e.g., an octopus in a farm scene). The influence of such semantic factors on eye movements indicates the importance of the prior knowledge that viewers bring to the viewing situation, and suggests the utility of eye movement monitoring in revealing memory effects on perceptual processing.

In the work presented here we show that previous exposure exerts significant effects on eye movements to visual stimuli. Different patterns of eye movements are elicited during viewing of previously presented materials than during viewing of novel materials. This change in eye movement patterns, involving differences in the number of regions within a stimulus sampled during viewing, the number of fixations made, and the amount of constraint or predictability of transitions among successively sampled regions, is termed the *eye movement-based memory effect.* It provides the basis for a new indirect (implicit) measure of memory. The eye movement-based memory effect permits us to extend previous work on indirect measures of memory, providing evidence that the nature of perceptual processing is changed by previous exposure

This paper describes the methods we have used to assess eye movement patters, characterizes the nature of the generalizability of the eye movement-based memory effect, and considers its implications for our understanding and measurement of memory. In a series of studies we show that the effects of prior exposure on eye movements are robust across different classes of stimulus materials, different types of prior exposure, and different task situations. In addition, we show that the eye movement-based memory effect scales with the number of prior exposures and does *not* depend upon explicit remembering of the stimuli.

3. METHODS

A major focus of our work has been to integrate the recent advances in eye tracking technology and the quantification of eye movement data into a method that can be used for the investigation of memory function. The methods described below represent the latest installment of this work, much of which has been integrated into a comprehensive analysis tool, EMTool.

3.1. Apparatus

These experiments were performed with two different eyetrackers. The Forward Technologies Dual Purkinje Image - Generation V eyetracker had high spatial accuracy (error less than 1/4 degree of visual angle) and high temporal accuracy, sampling eye position at 1000 Hz. The Applied Science Laboratories (ASL) R4000 remote eyetracker used floor-mounted optics with a near-infrared light source and calculated eye position using a video-based pupil-corneal reflection technique, sampling at 60 Hz. With signal filtering and averaging, the spatial accuracy of this eyetracker was between 1/2 and 1 degree of visual angle, without the necessity of fixing the head of the participant.

In an initial calibration phase and then in all experiments, eye (gaze) position in X and Y position on the screen were sent to the computer, which also collected information about when the stimuli are being presented, and what behavioral responses were produced. Data analyses were then performed in a series of stages that permit determination of fixation location and the eye movements made between them, description of the data in terms of a set of structural variables, and finally, the exploration of differences in eye movement behavior elicited by familiar versus unfamiliar materials.

3.2. Mapping X,Y Data onto Stimulus Locations

The first stage of data analysis entailed reducing the continuous data (X,Y coordinates sampled every 1 or 16.7 msec), segmenting it into a series of eye fixations separated by saccadic eye movements, and producing a fixation-based data matrix having one row for each saccade-fixation pair. The data obtained during the calibration task were used to map the average of the eye position values obtained during each eye fixation to a location in the photograph that had been examined, thus indicating direction of gaze (in terms of stimulus coordinates) during that fixation (McConkie 1981). Multiple dependent variables were then derived from the reduced data matrices for each photograph viewed by each person. These consisted of the number of eye fixations made during the viewing period for that photograph (NF), the number of regions sampled (NR), and entropy measures that indicate the degree of predictability or constraint in the sequence of fixations during viewing of that picture. These entropy measures will be described below.

3.3. Defining Regions of Interest

Eye position was usually tied to stimulus features that were of particular salience to the viewer. One can then describe how the viewer moves his or her eyes by defining regions and looking at the transitions made between these regions. One could define regions on a face as "eyes," "nose," "mouth," and "other" as done by Walker-Smith et al. (1977). As reasonable as this is for faces, however, it is somewhat problematic for stimuli other than faces where the set of features of the picture is not as well defined across stimuli. Instead of taking this *a priori* approach, we defined "regions of interest" that are repeatedly sampled by viewers, defined for each viewer for each stimulus individually. Indeed, the distribution of X,Y positions of a viewer's eyes for a particular scene was typically clustered in particular salient regions. Thus, we defined the regions with an automated clustering routine based on proximity among neighboring fixation locations. A nearest neighbor rule was used such that any two fixation locations within a criterion distance were assigned to the same region. Any fixation not within the criterion distance from any other fixation was considered its own region.

3.4. Calculation of Measure of Constraint

After clustering the eye movements, analyses were performed to determine the pattern of transitions between the regions of interest. To conduct these analyses, the data for each image viewed by each participant were transformed into (Markov) transition matrices, indicating the transitions between successive fixations. These transition matrices permitted specification of the extent to which fixations to particular regions were constrained by the location of prior fixations. First-order matrices indicated 1-step transitions among regions for immediately successive fixation locations. Second-order matrices indicated 2-step transitions, embodied in 3-dimensional transition tables.

These transition matrices permitted examination of the extent of constraint produced, or the amount of predictive information provided by, the immediately preceding fixation location (in first-order transition matrices) and by the two immediately preceding fixation locations (in second-order transition matrices). This was determined by calculating the *entropy* (or randomness) contained in the individual cells of the first-order or second-order Markov matrix, embodying the transitions among the regions, above and beyond what would be expected on the basis of the row and column totals. If the movement of the eyes to various regions were completely unconstrained by the location of previous fixations, then fixations would be distributed across the cells of the transition matrix in accordance only with the probability of totals fixations landing in a given location. In this situation, there would be much entropy or randomness in the viewing pattern -- i.e. all transitions in the matrix cells could be predicted by the proportions in the row and column totals (what Stark and Ellis (1981) refer to as "stratified-random" viewing). By contrast, to the extent that the fixations were distributed in a fashion where the probability of making some transitions was other than what would be predicted by chance alone (what Stark and Ellis (1981) refer to as "deterministic" viewing), there would be evidence that eye movements are constrained in moving to particular locations dependent on the previous fixation location.

We quantified the amount of constraint in these Markov matrices by looking at the amount of entropy in the row and column totals and the amount of entropy in each individual cell. Using I to represent entropy in a given cell, a quantification of entropy within all of the cells of the matrix can be computed as Icell = $Sum[P(i)*log_2(1/P(i))]$, where P(i) is the relative probability of the event in the cell of the matrix. Similarly, the entropy contained in the expected matrix can be computed on the basis of the row and column total cells as Icolumn totals Irow totals. In this manner, one can compute a measure of first-order constraint (or, conversely, a measure of entropy reduction), S1 = [Icolumn totals + Irow totals - Icell]/ Icolumn totals. In this measure, if the pattern of eye movements is close to being random, Icell will be very nearly equal to the summation of the column and row entropy. On the other hand, if there is very little randomness in the signal, i.e. if the eye movement patterns are highly constrained, then Icell will be smaller than the expected values from the row and column totals and this measure will be near 1. Similar analyses of the second-order matrices yield a measure of second-order constraint, S2.

3.5. Interpretation of Constraint Measures

A high level of constraint (i.e. an S1 or S2 with a value near 1) indicates a pattern of eye movements that follow some specific, probabilistic manner of movement, different from the pattern expected by chance. For example, eye movement patterns to a particular face in which viewing of the right eye invariably leads to a transition to viewing of the left eye exhibit a high level of constraint. When these values are closer to 0, all of the transition probabilities in the body of the matrix can be explained by the row and column totals, which means that there is completely stratified-random viewing. In this case, the transitions between regions of the picture are explained more by relative, overall probabilities of fixating a region and not by specific point-to-point transition.

A striking example of the ability of these constraint measures to pick up on underlying patterns in a series of eye movements comes from an experiment by Althoff and Cohen (1998a). In this experiment, 18 undergraduates from the University of Illinois were run in two sessions of a face processing experiment. In each session viewers saw 96 faces, 48 of which were famous and 48 of which were not famous. In the first session, participants were asked to make a famous/not famous judgment to each face, responding with a button press. No constraints were placed on their eye movement patterns by our instructions. In the second session, two weeks later, the participants viewed the same 96 faces, but were asked to perform one of two intentional scanning strategies to the faces, in which

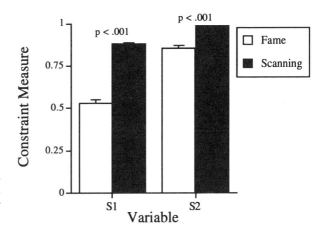

Figure 1. First and second order constraint measures (S1 and S2, respectively) show higher constraint for patterned scanning.

we imposed very specific constraints on their eye movement patterns. In these conditions, viewers were asked to look at the items either as if they were reading (i.e., "look from left to right from the top to bottom of the face") or to look at the features of the face in a particular order (e.g., "look to the top of the head, left eye, right eye, nose, and mouth in that order"). The different instructions for these two sessions produced very different amounts of constraint in their eye movements, as revealed by our measures of constraint. As shown in Figure 1, eye movements produced under intentional scanning instructions were more constrained on both first-order and second-order measures of constraint, confirming that nonrandom patterns of eye movements exhibit higher levels of constraint on these information measures.

4. CHARACTERISTICS OF THE EYE MOVEMENT-BASED MEMORY EFFECT

Having described the methods for assessing patterns of eye movements and how these measures can detect constrained viewing, we can now document and characterize four basic features of the eye movement-based memory effect.

4.1. The Eye Movement-Based Memory Effect Distinguishes between Repeated and Novel Stimuli

The basic phenomenon is reported in two experiments in Cohen et al. (1998). In one experiment, 17 viewers saw images of famous (pre-experimentally familiar) and non-famous (pre-experimentally novel) faces. In the other experiment, 20 participants saw images of previously seen and of novel buildings (buildings from the University of Illinois campus of from a different campus unfamiliar to these viewers). In both experiments, participants exhibited fewer fixations to fewer regions with less constraint in viewing previously seen materials while the pattern of viewing for novel materials was more constrained, and had more fixations to more regions (Figure 2).

The differences in the design of the two experiments permitted us to document that the eye movement-based memory effect extends across materials, to both faces and buildings, and across types of prior exposure. The prior exposure to famous faces was undoubt-

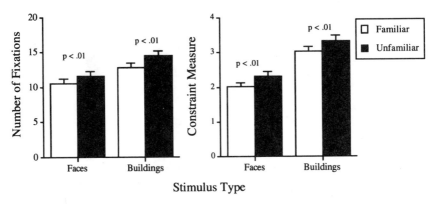

Figure 2. Previously seen items are viewed with fewer fixations and less constraint across class of stimuli and type of prior exposure.

edly through images like the ones the subjects viewer in the experiment; it is unlikely that subjects had ever seen the famous people depicted in the images. By contrast, subjects had real-world exposure to the campus buildings -- i.e. their experience was with the objects depicted in the images

In processing an item, viewers move their eyes around the display, sampling and encoding the salient information. It appears that in processing novel items the eyes follow a stereotypic but idiosyncratic path. This was suggested by the work of Walker-Smith, Gale and Findlay (1977) in a face processing task. They found that across viewers there were differences in the amount of time spent on different features of a face but that within a single viewer the amount of time spent fixating certain regions of a face was relatively constant, even across tasks with different requirements. Parker (1978) observed that when asked to perform a task involving the detection of changes in a scene, viewers exhibited stereotypic fixation patterns that could be disrupted when changes were detected in peripheral vision.

The early eye movement work by Noton and Stark (1971), Stark and Ellis (1981), and Walker-Smith et al. (1977), suggested that viewers might exhibit a more stereotypic (but idiosyncratic) pattern of eye movement sampling for novel items compared to previously studied ones. Having a stereotypic processing pattern that would permit efficient extraction of information from new materials makes good sense; such a stereotypic pattern would *not* be needed when viewing already familiar materials, at least once recognition occurs. The findings from our work, reported above, confirm this idea. Eye movements to novel items are indeed more constrained than to previously seen items. Together with our finding of more fixations to more regions in viewing novel items, it seems that sampling behavior for novel materials, whether faces or buildings, is optimized for extracting information in a stereotypic way.

4.2. The Eye Movement-Based Memory Effect Generalizes across Different Task Constraints

In the experiments discussed thus far, eye movements were collected while the subject was making familiarity judgments about the stimuli. Although the eye movements were incidental to the behavioral response, it seems important to demonstrate that the ef-

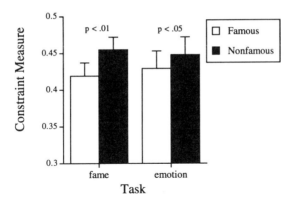

Figure 3. Higher constraint for nonfamous faces even when task is unrelated to fame.

fects of prior processing on our eye movement measures can be obtained regardless of the task being performed; i.e., that the eye movement-based memory effect indexes the effects of prior processing even when viewers are performing tasks that have nothing to do with judgment of prior occurrence.

This was addressed in Experiment 1 of Althoff and Cohen (1998a), in which 18 participants were tested on two occasions separated by two weeks. In one session, they made happy/not happy decisions to 96 faces (48 of which were famous and 48 of which were nonfamous); in the other session they made famous/not famous judgments to the same faces. As can be seen in Figure 3, the eye movement-based memory effect, as indexed here by differences in S1 between repeated and novel items, emerged regardless of the task being performed.

4.3. The Eye Movement-Based Memory Effect Increases with Increasing Amounts of Prior Exposure

In Althoff and Cohen (1998b), we explored the sensitivity of the eye movement-based memory effect to varying amounts of prior exposure. The number of prior exposures to items was manipulated within the experiment, permitting us to assess the patterns of eye movements to items as they go from novel to increasingly familiar. For each of our eye movement variables, we looked for the emergence of an eye movement-based memory effect as repetitions increased. As shown in Figure 4, there was an increasing separation of the values on several variables (number of fixations, number of regions, and the constraint measures S1 and S2) for repeated versus novel items, as a function of the number of repetitions -- i.e. the eye movement-based memory effect scaled with the number of prior exposures.

In documenting the relationship between amount of prior exposure and the size of the eye movement-based memory effect, this experiment also confirmed that the differences in eye movement patterns between previously seen versus novel items can occur *within* items. In previous experiments, previously seen items and novel items were physically different stimuli -- famous versus nonfamous faces and on-campus versus other-campus buildings. Thus, despite careful matching of the stimuli across repeated versus novel categories, it remained possible that we were picking up stimulus item effects rather than repetition effects. The Althoff and Cohen (1998b) study ruled out this possibility by show-

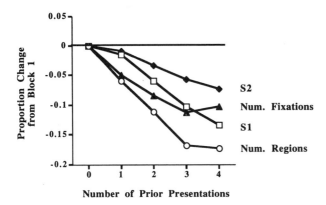

Figure 4. Increasing amounts of exposure leads to incrementally fewer fixations to fewer regions with less constraint.

ing that the eye movement-based memory effect emerged as items were repeated within the experiment.

4.4. The Eye Movement-Based Memory Effect Is Separate from Explicit Remembering of Items

To what extent are the effects of prior exposure on eye movement patterns driven by the explicit remembering of the items? We have been referring to the eye movement effects as an indirect measure of memory because they are seen even in the absence of the instructions to the subjects to explicitly remember the stimuli. But, given that viewers in these experiments can recognize many items, what is the relationship between that recognition and the eye movement-based memory effect? We explored this question by conducting eye movement studies with amnesic patients with severe declarative memory deficits who are impaired in their explicit remembering of the items being shown.

Althoff et al. (1993) tested one well-characterized, severely amnesic patient on a set of 96 faces, 48 of which were famous and 48 nonfamous. This patient, A.S., was able to recognize only 7 of the 48 famous faces on standard behavioral testing, and yet her eye movement patterns still discriminated between famous and nonfamous faces. Following this work, Althoff and Cohen (1998b) tested a set of 7 memory-impaired individuals in a multiple repetitions experiment like that described above. We showed that even when recognition performance for items was significantly impaired compared to college-aged controls (indeed, after 5 exposures to a face the amnesic patients were still very near chance recognition performance), the eye movement-based memory effect persisted -- as shown in Figure 5 using S1 as a measure.

5. CONCLUSIONS

We have shown here that eye movement patterns differ for previously seen versus novel items; that previous exposure to visual stimuli changes the way in which they are subsequently viewed. The effects of experience on eye movements -- what we have termed the eye movement-based memory effect -- was shown to generalize across different eyetrackers, classes of visual stimuli, types of prior exposure to the stimuli, and type

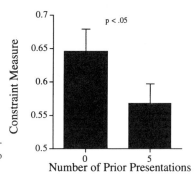

Figure 5. Despite being impaired at recognition of the items, amnesic patients show a normal eye movement-based memory effect to repeated items.

of task being performed. The methods we have developed for detecting and for characterizing the eye movement-based memory effect were outlined.

The effects of prior exposure on eye movement patterns were shown to occur even in the absence of explicit remembering of the stimuli, in amnesic patients with severe deficits of declarative memory, and to be sensitive to (indeed, scale with) increasing numbers of prior exposure to the stimuli.

Eye movement monitoring provides a new methodology for the study of multiple memory systems in the brain and of the way in which we are shaped by our experience. We have long argued that some effects of prior experience arise from the on-line tuning and modification of specific cortical and subcortical networks (and of the specific processing operations they support) engaged during the original processing task, causing changes in subsequent processing (Cohen and Eichenbaum 1993). The changes in eye movement patterns observed here for previously seen materials provide the best evidence yet that previous exposure to the to-be-tested materials alters the nature of the perceptual processing those items will subsequently receive. Such a conclusion could previously only be inferred from increases in speed and accuracy of responding in priming and skill learning tasks.

Future work will help to clarify which specific measures, and in which combinations, are the most effective in distinguishing between repeated and novel items, and we are in the process of testing powerful multivariate classification procedures which may allow us to reliably distinguish among viewers with different viewing histories.

REFERENCES

Althoff RR, Cohen NJ (1998a) Eye movement-based memory effect: A re-processing effect in face perception. Submitted for publication.

Althoff RR, Cohen NJ (1998b) The emergence of the eye movement-based memory effect. Manuscript in preparation.

Althoff RR, Maciukenas M, Cohen NJ (1993) Indirect assessment of memory using eye movement monitoring. Soc Neurosci Abstr 19: 439.

Antes JR (1974) The time course of picture viewing. J Exp Psychol 103(1): 62–70.

Antes JR, Penland JG (1981) Picture context effects on eye movement patterns. In:Fisher DF, Monty RA, Senders JW (eds), Eye movements: cognition and visual perception. Lawrence Erlbaum Associations, Hillsdale, NJ, pp 157–170.

Bachevalier J, Brickson M, Hagger C (1993) Limbic-dependent recognition memory in monkeys develops early in infancy. Neuroreport 4(1): 77–80.

Biederman I, Rabinowitz JC, Glass AL, Stacy EW (1974) On the information extracted from a glance at a scene. J Exp Psychol 103(3): 597–600.

Buswell GT (1935) How people look at pictures. University of Chicago Press, Chicago.

Cohen NJ, Althoff RR, Webb JM, McConkie GW, Holden JA, Noll EL (1998) Eye movement monitoring as an indirect measure of memory. Submitted for publication.

Cohen NJ, Eichenbaum HE (1993) Memory, amnesia, and the hippocampal system. MIT Press, Cambridge, MA.

Graf P, Schacter DL (1985) Implicit and explicit memory for new associations in normal and amnesic subjects. J Exp Psychol Learn Mem Cogn 11(3): 501–518.

Goldman-Rakic PS (1988) Topography of cognition: Parallel distributed networks in primate association cortex. Annu Rev Neurosci 11: 137–156.

Loftus G, Mackworth NH (1978) Cognitive determinants of fixation location during picture viewing. J Exp Psychol Hum Percept Perform 4(4): 565–572.

Mackworth NH, Morandi AJ (1967). The gaze selects informative details within a picture. Percept Psychophys 2: 547–552.

McConkie GW (1981) Evaluating and reporting data quality in eye movement research. Behav Res Methods Instrum 13(2): 97–106.

Noton D, Stark L (1971). Scanpaths in saccadic eye movements while viewing and recognizing patterns. Vision Res 11: 929–942.

Parker RE (1978) Picture processing during recognition. J Exp Psychol Hum Percept Perform 4(2): 284–293.

Stark L, Ellis SR (1981) Scanpaths revisited. In:Fisher DF, Monty RA, Senders JW (eds), Eye movements: cognition and visual perception. Lawrence Erlbaum Associations, Hillsdale, NJ, pp 157–170

Tulving E, Schacter, DL (1990) Priming and human memory systems. Science 247: 301–306.

Walker-Smith GJ, Gale AG, Findlay JM (1977) Eye movement strategies involved in face perception. Perception 6: 313–326.

Whitlow SD, Althoff RR, Cohen NJ (1995) Deficit in relational (declarative) memory in amnesia. Soc Neurosci Abstr 754.

41

VISUAL AND VERBAL FOCUS PATTERNS WHEN DESCRIBING PICTURES

J. Holšánová, B. Hedberg, and N. Nilsson

Lund University Cognitive Science

Are there similarities between the way in which we perceive pictures visually and the way we describe them verbally? How can units in eye movement data be compared to units in spoken language data? One of the most important hypotheses is that there are similar principles for processing visual and verbal information (Just and Carpenter, 1976; Chafe, 1994).

Ever since Yarbus' classic observations (1967), eye movements have been thought to reflect cognitive processes. Buswell (1935) suggests that in a visual experience, the centre of fixation is the centre of attention at a given time, and Just and Carpenter (1976) advocates a strong eye-mind relation: What is being fixated equals what is being processed. Underwood and Everatt (1992), on the other hand, argue that one current fixation can measure past, present and future information acquisition. In our setting we suggest that, what is being focused visually and described verbally, is also attended to mentally.

Four subjects studied a picture, taken from a children's book. Their eye-movements were registered with the help of an eye tracker (50 Hz pupil and corneal reflex system). The picture was then covered, the subjects were asked to describe the picture from memory and their eye movements were, once again recorded. The visual patterns from these two phases were compared and the spoken descriptions, varying from 55 to 135 seconds, were transcribed and segmented into intonation units and centres of interest (Chafe, 1994).

The picture was overlaid with maps of the verbal focuses, based on the intonation units, and the visual and verbal focus patterns were compared (see Fig. 1). Intonation units, referring to specific picture elements, are either summarising, localising, epistemic, or substantive, whereas other intonation units are oriented towards interaction (Holšánová, 1997:28).

To summarise the results of our study; we can clearly identify two general patterns, in the eye movement data: An initial general survey followed by examination phase, consisting of several detailed examinations (also found by Buswell, 1935:142). Similar patterns can also be identified in the spoken language descriptions, but are differently distributed.

Current Oculomotor Research, edited by Becker *et al.*
Plenum Press, New York, 1999.

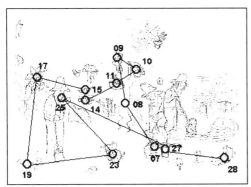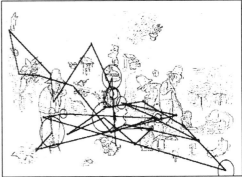

Figure 1. Left: Focus movements in the spoken description, based on intonation units. Right: Eye movement patterns during verbal description.

Another similarity between the visual and verbal data concerns re-examination of picture elements. As an extension to Yarbus' (1967) claims about observers repeated returns to certain picture elements, we can distinguish patterns of comparing activity. Our subjects create classes of similar objects, relations and traits and the objects are compared within this class.

Furthermore, we have found that, both in the eye movement data and the verbal data, unusual parts of the picture attract the viewer's attention. Although this does not happen in the initial observation phase, it happens later on in the session as the viewer becomes more acquainted with the picture.

When describing the picture from memory, the subjects direct their gaze at certain locations on the white board in front of them. These locations correspond very well to the actual locations of the picture elements, as if the subjects were looking for them. We have found striking similarities between the eye movement patterns and the patterns of the verbal focuses.

REFERENCES

Buswell, GT (1935) *How people look at pictures.* A study of the psychology of perception in art. Chicago: The University of Chicago Press.

Chafe, W (1994) *Discourse, Consciousness, and Time, The Flow and Displacement of Conscious Experience in Speaking and Writing.* The University of Chicago Press: Chicago, London.

Holšánová, J (1997) Bildbeskrivning ur ett kommunikativt och kognitivt perspektiv. (Picture description from a communicative and cognitive perspective). *LUCS Minor 6.* Lund University.

Just, MA, Carpenter, PA, (1976) Eye fixations and cognitive processes, *Cognitive Psychology* 8:441–480.

Underwood, G, Everatt, J (1992) The Role of Eye Movements in Reading: some limitations of the eye-mind assumption. In: E Chekaluk and KR Llewellyn (Eds.), *The Role of Eye Movements in Perceptual Processes*, Elsevier Science Publishers B. V., Advances in Psychology, Amsterdam, vol. 88:111–169.

Yarbus, AL (1967) *Eye Movements and Vision* (1st Russian edition, 1965). New York: Plenum Press.

42

VISUAL ATTENTION TOWARDS GESTURES IN CONVERSATION

Kenneth Holmqvist and Marianne Gullberg

Department of Cognitive Science
Lund University
S-222 22 Lund, Sweden
Department of Linguistics
Lund University
S-223 62 Lund, Sweden

1. INTRODUCTION

Interactional studies of gaze behaviour have established that listeners will typically focus on a speaker's face (Fehr and Exline 1987, Yarbus 1967). Gesture research, on the other hand, has shown that listeners actually attend to gestural information (Berger and Popelka 1971; Cassell, McNeill and McCullough, in press; Rogers 1978). However, little is known about how gestural information is attended to visually–foveally or peripherally.

We performed a pilot study using modern eye tracking techniques (the SMI iView headset). We measured the visual focus and the eye movements of two subjects listening to a story told by other subjects in their direct visual field. The two speakers, one a native Swede, the other a native French woman, told their story in Swedish to a native Swedish listener and in French to a native French listener. This combination allowed for control of the speaker's language proficiency level and the possible effect thereof on the listener's perception of the speaker's gestures. Non-native speakers often use gestures to elicit correct words, and native listeners could therefore be expected to focus on the gestures of a non-native speaker as part of their co-operative behaviour.

The ecological validity of the design–and the minimal disturbance of the eye tracker on the interaction–was supported by the fact that the number of gestures and feedback signals in these data did not deviate from those produced in an identical design where no eye tracker was used (Gullberg 1998).

The gesture data were analysed into four different gestures categories: iconic, metaphoric, and deictic or pointing gestures, and beats (McNeill 1992).

Current Oculomotor Research, edited by Becker *et al.*
Plenum Press, New York, 1999.

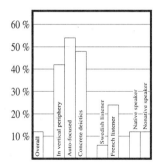

Figure 1. Frequencies of gestures focused by the listener.

2. RESULTS

The results from our study are summarised in Figure 1.

Listeners visually focused on 29 out of 245 speaker gestures (11.8 %). A gesture counts as focused if it is fixated by the listener for a minimum of 160 ms. Three factors were identified in the data which made listeners significantly more likely than average to focus on speaker gestures.

1: Vertical periphery. The vertical periphery is defined as the space below the speaker's elbows when the arms are hanging loosley at the sides. 42.8% of the gestures performed in this area were focused, as opposed to only 8.6% in the horizontal periphery. This tendency to focus on gestures produced in the vertical periphery can be assumed to be a function of the physiology of the human visual field which is wider than it is high.

2: Concrete pointing. 47.0 % of the concrete deictic gestures were focused. Pointing has the function to direct listener gaze to the target. Often, the target is within reach and will converge with the gesture, making the listener focus on both. No other gesture type was focused significantly more often than the average.

3: Auto-focus. 53.8 % of the gestures auto-focused by the speaker were also focused by the listener, as exemplified in Figure 2. Streeck (1993) claims that auto-focus is a means for the speaker to indicate by visual deixis that the gesture is relevant. An alternative explanation to the auto-focus effect instead considers discourse structure. When the speaker in the data looks at her own hand, she is acting as a character in the narrative, a sales person at a pharmacy, who is looking at a medical prescription. By doing this, the speaker mimetically moves to a different discourse level and space, viz. the pharmacy in the story. Since the speaker has moved to the pharmacy, the listener finds him- or herself in the same discourse space, i.e. the pharmacy. The listener therefore acts as an observer would in the pharmacy, looking at the same medical prescription as the speaker. The collective move to a different discourse level and space thus results in the alignment of interlocutors' focus.

The linguistic proficiency level of the speaker did not appear to influence listeners' fixation behaviour, neither with respect to the amount of fixations, nor to gesture type.

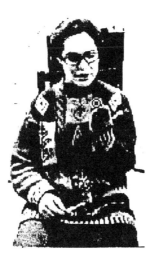

Figure 2. Gesture focused by both speaker (auto-focus) and listener.

There are important individual differences in gaze behaviour concerning the duration and frequency of fixations (4.8% for the Swedish vs. 27.3% for the French listener). However, the three factors conditioning whether a gesture is focused or not appear to be valid across speakers.

REFERENCES

Berger KW, Popelka GR (1971) Extra-facial gestures in relation to speech reading. Journal of Communication Disorders 3: 302–308.

Cassell J, McNeill D, McCullough KE (in press) Speech-gesture mismatches: Evidence for one underlying representation of linguistic and nonlinguistic information. Pragmatics & Cognition.

Fehr BJ, Exline RV (1987) Social visual interaction: A conceptual and literature review. In: Siegman AW, Feldstein S (eds) Nonverbal behavior and communication. Erlbaum, Hillsdale, pp 225–326.

Gullberg M (1998) Gesture as a communication strategy in second language discourse. Lund University Press, Lund.

McNeill D (1992) Hand and mind. What the hands reveal about thought. Chicago University Press, Chicago.

Rogers WT (1978) The contribution of kinesic illustrators toward the comprehension of verbal behavior within utterances. Human Communication Research 5:54–62.

Streeck J (1993) Gesture as communication I: Its coordination with gaze and speech. Communication Monographs 60:275–299.

Yarbus A (1967) Eye movements and vision. Plenum Press, New York.

43

MODELLING EXPERIENTIAL AND TASK EFFECTS ON ATTENTIONAL PROCESSES IN SYMMETRY DETECTION

C. Latimer, W. Joung, R. van der Zwan, and H. Beh

University of Sydney

1. INTRODUCTION

The effects of attention and scanning strategies on symmetry detection have been discussed by several investigators, Locher et al. (1993) and Wenderoth (1994) being good examples. Wenderoth showed that the salience of vertical and horizontal symmetry can be manipulated by varying the range of stimuli presented, and attributes this to effects on the scanning or attentional strategies adopted by subjects. Locher et al demonstrated that scanning patterns on symmetrical displays could be manipulated by instructions and task requirements. In this paper, we look at the effects of task requirements and experience on the distribution of eye movements and fixations on symmetrical dot patterns. It is possible to link eye movements and fixations to attention by creating tunnel vision stimulus conditions, using fixation contingent displays or simply by using large stimulus patterns. In our studies, we are using large patterns together with control conditions in which the same patterns are presented at a size small enough not to require eye movements. The underlying assumption is that if we can reproduce the same order of reaction times and errors in both contexts, then the overt eye movements and fixations on the large patterns may be valid indices of small, covert attentional shifts that occur naturally on the small versions of the patterns, but which cannot otherwise be observed. We report data from one participant with five years experience viewing, constructing and manipulating symmetrical patterns and one participant without such experience. Future work will compare the eye movements and fixations of architects, and designers and those of inexperienced controls.

2. METHOD

2.1. Stimulus Materials

Patterns were constructed within 20 x 20 matrices with probability of a cell being filled set at 0.3. Large patterns subtended 30 degrees of visual angle and were viewed on a

Current Oculomotor Research, edited by Becker *et al.*
Plenum Press, New York, 1999.

17-inch Monitor from 40 cms. Small patterns subtended 3 degrees of visual angle and were viewed for 200 msec from 38 cms.

2.2. Procedure

In one condition, while eye movements and fixations were recorded, participants judged symmetry/asymmetry in a random sequence of 20 asymmetric and 20 symmetric patterns (5 from each axis of symmetry: vertical, horizontal, positive oblique and negative oblique). In another condition, participants judged axis of symmetry in a random sequence of 40 patterns (10 patterns from each axis of symmetry). These two conditions were repeated with small patterns and without eye-movement recording. Patterns were presented by a Power Macintosh and SuperLab software. Detection times were recorded by key press with millisecond resolution, and eye movements and fixations were recorded by an Ober2 infrared sensing system.

3. NEURAL NETWORK SIMULATIONS

Is there any basis for predicting how experimental subjects will scan patterns for symmetry? Artificial neural networks can be used to assess the information content and location of differentiating regions within a set of patterns. We have trained back-propagation networks with 20 x 20 input units, 24 hidden units and 4 output units (1 output unit for each axis of symmetry) on the patterns presented to experimental participants. After training with 20,000 patterns (5,000 each axis of symmetry) networks display 95% accuracy when classifying 2,000 unseen patterns. By analysing the hidden units of such networks and observing where and how weight is assigned to regions of the input array, it is possible to determine objectively the most and least differentiating regions of the pattern set (Latimer and Stevens 1994; Latimer et al. 1994). It was predicted that experienced participants, with their more efficient scanning strategies for detecting symmetry, would concentrate more attention on these more differentiating regions of the pattern set than inexperienced participants.

4. RESULTS

Figure 1(C) is a three-dimensional representation of the pattern of weight placement on the regions of the 20 x 20 binary patterns. The matrix of input units has been reduced to 5 x 5. Viewpoint is from the bottom-left corner of the patterns and input matrix. Column height indicates magnitude of weight with white topped columns signifying positive and black-topped columns signifying negative weight. It can be seen from Figure 1 (A), where column height indicates fixation time, that the experienced participant has distributed her attention in a manner similar to the distribution of weights in the network with more fixations on the centre and diagonal regions. By contrast, the pattern of fixations of the inexperienced participant depicted in Figure 1(B) is less structured and unlike the distribution of weight in the network.

Turning now to the detection times for the small control patterns not requiring overt eye movements, it is clear from Figure 2 that the patterns of mean detection times for the large and small patterns across axes are quite similar, particularly in the case of the experienced participant. This suggests that the overt eye movements produced by the large pat-

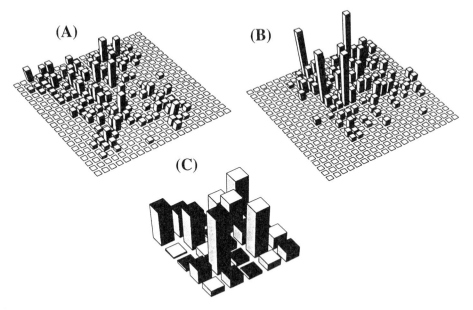

Figure 1. A comparison of the cumulative fixation times on regions of the stimulus patterns by the experienced and inexperienced participants and the weights assigned to regions by the neural network. Views are from the bottom-left corner of the patterns and screen. (A) Cumulative fixation time for the experienced participant. (B) Cumulative fixation time for the inexperienced participant. (C) Connection strength between array of input units and hidden units in the neural network. Black-topped and white-topped columns signify negative and positive weights respectively.

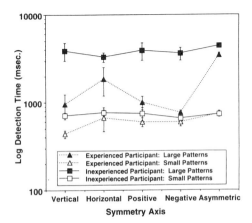

Figure 2. Participants' detection times for large and small patterns as a function of symmetry axis.

terns may be valid indices of the normal, covert attentional shifts produced by the small patterns and that the distributions of fixation time in Figure 1 (A) and (B) are not mere artefacts of the adopted experimental methods.

5. CONCLUSIONS

Experience produces marked effects on attentional processes in symmetry detection. In general, our experienced participant demonstrated a more structured and efficient distribution of attention than our inexperienced subject. Objective assessment of the information and differentiation in sets of symmetrical patterns by way of artificial neural networks may provide a basis for prediction of the attentional strategies of experienced subjects.

REFERENCES

Latimer C, Joung W, Stevens C (1994) Modelling symmetry detection with back-propagation networks. Spatial Vision 8: 415–431
Latimer C, Stevens C (1994) Eye movement measures and connectionist models of form perception. In Ballesteros S (ed) Cognitive approaches to human perception. Erlbaum, Hillsdale NJ, pp 91–121
Locher P, Cavegn D, Groner M, Muller P, d'Ydewalle G, & Groner R (1993) The effects of stimulus symmetry and task requirements on scanning patterns. In: d'Ydewalle G. Van Rensbergen J, (eds.) Perception and cognition: Advances in eye movement research. North Holland, Amsterdam, pp 59–69
Wenderoth P (1994) The salience of vertical symmetry. Perception 23: 221–236

44

EYE MOVEMENTS WHILE VIEWING A FOREIGN MOVIE WITH SUBTITLES

Mariko Takeda

Department of Psychology
Faculty of Education, Wakayama University
930 Sakaedani, Wakayama 640-8510, Japan

1. INTRODUCTION

It is very popular that foreign movies are presented with Japanese subtitles in Japan. In the case it is necessary to gain both verbal and pictorial information through the visual channel. As for how information on subtitled television or movie was processed, d'Ydewalle, Praet, Verfaillie & van Rensbergen (1991) and Kogo & Kishi (1996) analyzed eye movements. d'Ydewalle & Gielen (1992) discussed on many aspects of viewing subtitles. However, it is yet unclear whether skilled viewers process subtitles effectively or not. The purpose of this study was to examine the following two questions: (1) Are there any differences of visual behavior between those who are accustomed to foreign movies with subtitles and those who have little experience in viewing such movies, and (2) Are there any differences between when subjects are instructed to pay their attention to verbal information in the subtitles and when to pictorial information?

2. METHOD

2.1. Subjects

Twelve undergraduates served as subjects. Half of them belonged to the group with much experience (H group), those who liked to view movies and were accustomed to foreign movies with subtitles, and the other half belonged to the group with little experience (L group), those who had less interests in movies, scarcely viewed them, and were not accustomed to movies with subtitles. Both were selected from sixty undergraduates by a questionnaire which consisted of thirty items.

Current Oculomotor Research, edited by Becker *et al.*
Plenum Press, New York, 1999.

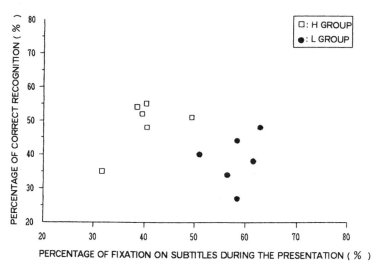

Figure 1

2.2. Procedure

Eye movements of each subject were recorded by Nac Eye-mark recorder (type V) while viewing an American movie with Japanese subtitles that no subjects had viewed. Three instrusction conditions (within-subjects variable) were given: (1) the control condition in which they were just instructed to view the movie, (2) the subtitle condition in which the subjects were instructed to focus their attention on the subtitles to understand the contents of the movie, and (3) the picture condition in which they were instructed to look at details to understand the contents of the movie. The order of (2) and (3) was counterbalanced among the subjects. Three one-minute scenes from the movie were presented, counterbalanced within each condition. Presentation of the subtitles occupied 77.7?t. A recognition-and-comprehension test was administered after each condition. The test consisted of thirty items, ten for the subtitles, ten for the contents, ten for details of the picture.

3. RESULTS AND DISCUSSION

Cumulative fixation-duration on the subtitles was caliculated. Under all the instruction conditions the H group spent less time to view the subtitles than the L group, as Table 1 shows.

Table 1. Mean cumulative fixation-duration
on the subtitles in seconds

	Condition		
	Control	Subtitle	Picture
H group	19.0 (3.37)	20.3 (5.64)	17.5 (2.38)
L group	27.1 (2.76)	28.9 (5.06)	26.2 (4.37)

Standard deviation in parentheses

Table 2. Mean score of the recognition-and-comprehension test

Items	Condition		
	Control	Subtitle	Picture
H group			
Subtitles	4.75 (1.30)	6.33 (1.41)	5.88 (2.09)
Contents	5.13 (1.36)	6.13 (1.36)	5.88 (1.36)
Details	4.50 (1.58)	5.50 (0.50)	3.88 (1.69)
Total	14.38 (3.04)	18.25 (2.28)	15.63 (3.57)
L group			
Subtitles	4.13 (1.54)	5.25 (1.92)	5.75 (2.33)
Contents	4.00 (2.06)	4.75 (1.09)	4.25 (1.09)
Details	3.13 (1.17)	4.25 (1.09)	3.63 (0.99)
Total	11.25 (3.03)	14.25 (3.38)	13.63 (2.34)

Standard deviation in parentheses

The 2 (experience: H, L) X 3 (instruction: control, subtitle, picture) ANOVA yielded significant main effect for experience ($F (1,10)=38.56$, $p<.001$). However, for the score of the recognition-and-comprehension test, even for the recognition of the subtitles, the H group was more superior to the L group, as Table 2 shows. The ANOVA yielded significant main effects for experience, $F(1,14)=6.874$, $p<.05$; and for instruction, $F(2,28)=6.624$, $p<.01$. d'Ydewalle & Gielen (1992) pointed out that the distribution of attention between different channels of information while watching television is developed in childhood. This fact suggests that effective viewing behavior in processing both pictorial and verbal information was brought about by experience in viewing movies with subtitles. The recognition-and-comprehension score in the subtitle condition was significantly higher than that in the control condition. It is true that the attention to the subtitles, verbal information, could take an important role on the recognition. However it should be noted that not the amount of fixations on the subtitles but the effective viewing behavior is related to the comprehension, as Figure 1 also shows.

ACKNOWLEDGMENT

This study is a co-work with Miss Asami Sakamoto, graduated from Wakayama University in 1996.

REFERENCES

Kogo C, Kishi M (1996) Analysis of eye movement during the viewing of subtitled movies. Jpn J Educ Technol 20:161–166 (In Japanese)

d'Ydewalle G, Gielen I (1992) Attention allocation with overlapping sound, image, and text. In Rayner K (Ed.), Eye Movements and Visual Cognition. pp.415–427 New York: Springer Verlag.

d'Ydewalle G, Praet C, Verfaillie K, van Rensbergen J (1991) Watching subtitled television: Automatic reading behavior. Communic Res 18:650–666

45

DIFFERENCE OF SHAPE CONSTANCY IN UPPER AND LOWER VISUAL FIELDS

Takahiro Yamanoi,[*] Kazuya Kubo, and Hiroshi Takayanagi

Department of Electronics and Information Engineering
Faculty of Engineering, Hokkai Gakuen University
South 26 Jo, West 11 Chome, Central Ward
064-0926 Sapporo, Japan

1. ABSTRACT

Functions of human vision have been developed to adapt to ecological restrictions. Especially, the position in early vision is neurophysiologically different between objects in the upper visual field (UVF) and in the lower visual field (LVF). In recent years, we have studied the relationship between shape constancy and eye movement. In this study, we investigate differences of shape constancy in the UVF and in the LVF.

We performed psychophysical experiments using three types of boards (circle, square and lozenge: square turned 45 deg.) as comparison stimuli and graphic patterns on a CRT as standard stimuli. The perspective shape was displayed on the CRT as if it was inclined at angles of 10, 25, 35, 45, 55, 65 and 80 deg, respectively. Subjects were asked to actually make the shape equal to the pattern on the CRT.

The results of the test determined by the difference between two mean values show a difference at a significance level of 2.5% between the UVF and the LVF. Subjects exhibited the tendency to look at the upper end of the stimulus in case of the UVF but not in the case of the LVF.

2. INTRODUCTION

When we observe objects inclined toward us, we see them not as shapes indicated by the laws of perspective but as the shapes these objects 'really' possess. This charac-

---
[*] E-mail:yamanoi@eli.hokkai-s-u.ac.jp

Current Oculomotor Research, edited by Becker *et al.*
Plenum Press, New York, 1999.

teristic of perception is called 'shape constancy.' In recent years, we have studied the relationship between shape constancy and eye movement. Previc studied functional specialization in the upper visual field (UVF) and in lower visual field (LVF) in the human (F. H. Previc 1990). According to his study, the position in the early vision is neurophysiologically different with an object in the UVF and in the LVF. In the present study, we have investigated differences of shape constancy and eye movements related to objects in the UVF and the LVF.

3. APPARATUS

We used three reference objects: circle, square and square turned 45 deg. Each object was made of white acrylic board and suspended by a thin pole embedded in the central horizontal axis of the frontal plane. Objects are divided into upper and lower halves so as to be displayed in the UVF and the LVF, respectively. Acrylic boards can spin around the pole. For the standard objects, we made corresponding perspective shapes of the inclined objects by computer graphics on the CRT of a microcomputer. Vertical length of each object would vary as if it were inclined forward or backward in relation to the subjects.

4. METHODS

Psychophysical experiments were done using acrylic boards of three shapes (circle, square and lozenge: square turned 45 deg.) ; real objects and graphic patterns on CRT.

The perspectives of the shape, as displayed on the CRT as a standard stimulus was manipulated so as to appear to be inclined at angles in 10, 25, 35, 45, 55, 65, and 80 deg., respectively. Shapes composed of acrylic board and used as a comparison stimulus were inclined forward toward the subjects or backward away from subjects. Number of subjects is nine and each of them was mounted an eye mark camera. Eye movements of the subjects were also registered by an eye mark recorder.

5. ANALYSIS

We revised the Thouless index (R. H. Thouless 1931) as a degree of shape constancy. Revised Thouless index is defined by $Z = (\log S - \log P) / (\log W - \log P)$, where W is the length of the standard object from the center of rotational axis to the apex perpendicular to the axis, P is the length of the orthogonal projection of W to the frontal plane, and S is the length of the comparative object corresponding to W. By a statistical test, we analyzed the difference in shape constancy between the UVF and LVF and between for-

Table 1. Difference in shape constancy
between directions of inclination of objects

Visual Field	Directions of Inclination: Forward vs. Backward
UVF	Statistically significant difference
LVF	No statistically significant difference

Table 2. Difference in shape constancy
between the UVF and the LVF

Direction of Inclination	Visual Field: UVF vs. LVF
Forward	UVF < LVF
Backward	No statistically significant difference

ward and backward inclinations. Test of paired-difference by t-distribution were applied to the data. Eye movements of the subjects were also analyzed.

6. RESULTS

First, we examined the difference between orientations of inclination in the UVF and in the LVF. With the UVF, the tendency of shape constancy was greater in forward inclinations than in backward inclinations, with a difference at significance level of 2.5%. With the LVF, no statistical difference was observed between backward and forward inclination (Table 1).

Secondly, we examined the difference between visual fields in each orientation of inclination. In the case of forward inclination, no statistically significant difference was observed between the UVF and the LVF. In the case of backward inclination, neither was a statistical difference observed, however, the degree of shape constancy was larger in the LVF than in the UVF (Table 2).

Most of fixation points of eye movement in the UVF were coincident with the upper apexes of the boards and the graphic patterns. On the contrary no tendency was found in distributions of the fixation points.

7. CONCLUSION

In the present study, we found partial differences in shape constancy between the UVF and the LVF. This suggests the possibility of the functional specialization in the UVF and the LVF as well as the positional specialization. By the results of analysis of eye movement, it might be noted that a linear process in the UVF and a nonlinear process in the LVF are used.

REFERENCES

Holmes G (1945) The organization of visual cortex in man. Proc Royal Soc B132: 348–361
Previc FH (1990) Functional specialization in the lower and upper visual fields in humans: Its ecological origins and neurophysiological implications. Behav Brain Res 13: 519–575
Thouless Rh (1931) Phenomenal regression to the real object I. Brit J Psychol 21: 339–359

46

OCCURRENCE AND FUNCTION OF VERY SHORT FIXATION DURATIONS IN READING

Ralph Radach,[1] Dieter Heller,[1] and Albrecht Inhoff[2]

[1]Technical University of Aachen
Institute of Psychology
Jaegerstr. 17, D-52064 Aachen
[2]State University of New York at Binghamton
University Center
Binghamton, NY 13902-6000

1. BACKGROUND: READING FIXATIONS AND EYE MOVEMENT CONTROL

Fixation durations during reading range from less than 50 ms to more than 1 second with means in the order of 220 ms to 250 ms and standard deviations of approximately 80 ms to 100 ms. An interesting property of frequency distributions of fixation duration is the gradual increase in the relative frequencies up to approximately 140 ms followed by a much steeper increase for longer fixation durations until the modal fixation duration interval is reached. According to McConkie et al. (1994), this change in the slope of frequency distributions is of functional significance: The duration of fixations of 140 ms or less is determined by information obtained during the pior fixation, the duration of longer fixations is controlled 'on line', by properties of fixated text so that departing saccades can be "directly controlled".

There is good evidence in favour of such a functional distinction. For example, McConkie et al. (1985) replaced words in a contemporary novel with orthographically irregular letter strings and compared initial fixations on these strings to fixations on normal words. The comparison indicated that relative fixation duration frequencies were very similar in the two text conditions for durations up to 140 ms. The two distributions differed, however, when longer-duration fixations were considered, suggesting that at least 140 ms (including afferent and efferent transmission time, central processing and movement preparation) are necessary for the orthographic manipulation to have an effect on fixation durations. Experiments involving the masking of text at some delay after the beginning of a fixation provide converging evidence. On the basis of fixation duration distributions under different masking conditions, Morrison (1984) concluded that fixations

Current Oculomotor Research, edited by Becker *et al.*
Plenum Press, New York, 1999.

shorter than about 150 ms reflect instances of saccade programming that are not based on the processing of visual information from the current fixation.

The present chapter extends this work in several directions. First, we distinguish two types of short duration fixations during reading and use this distinction to examine the generality of very short fixation durations over subjects. Second, we delineate conditions that are conducive to the occurrence of very short fixations and, third, examine the success with which two models of eye movement control can explain their occurrence in normal reading.

2. CORRECTIVE SACCADES AND SHORT FIXATIONS IN READING

A large portion of short fixations in reading can be accounted for by corrective movements. The 'classic case' are corrections following the large return sweep saccades that bring the eyes form the end of a line to the beginning of the next line (e.g. Dearborn 1906, Heller 1982). When reading lines of about 22 deg. (corresponding to about 81 letters) from a computer monitor, as many as 68 percent of all return sweeps are followed by a further leftward saccade. These saccades, obviously aimed to correct return sweep undershoots, move the eyes on average 6 letters toward the beginning of the line (Hofmeister at al., this volume). Fixations between return sweep and the subsequent corrective saccade to the left are of short duration, usually forming a narrow distribution with a peak of about 140 ms to 160 ms.

It has long been known from basic oculomotor research that the latency of corrective saccades is a function of the saccadic error. For errors of 1 deg. or less, correction latencies are similar to latencies of normal goal directed saccades. For errors exceeding 2–4 deg., latency approaches an asymptotic minimum and variability is substantially reduced (Becker 1989). Assuming letter position 3 or 4 to be the target location for return sweeps (Heller and Radach, 1992), and given the large return sweep undershoots reported by Hofmeister et al. (this volume), most correction latencies are likely to fall into the latency minimum. Therefore, we assume return sweep correction latencies to provide a good estimation of the individual minimum duration of directly controlled fixations in reading.

There are two possible objections against this assumption. It could be argued that return sweeps and corrections are programmed in a grouped fashion, as one 'package', being part of a general scanning routine. This argument can be rejected on the basis of Hofmeister et al's finding that return sweep latencies and landing positions as well as corrective saccades are identical for left justified and unjustified text. Clearly, return sweep corrections are aimed relative to the current line beginning and hence programmed on the basis of local visual information rather then global scanning routines.

Another objection could be that correction latencies overestimate the minimum duration of directly controlled fixations as text information will be acquired during these fixations and their duration will vary as a function of cognitive (i.e. lexical) processing. Hofmeister (1997) tested this hypothesis by comparing return sweep correction latencies for normal reading vs. scanning of 'z'-strings arranged in a text-like spatial layout (Inhoff et al. 1993). Frequencies of corrective saccades differed only by 2 percent and latencies were 4 ms longer for 'z'-strings. These results should not be taken to indicate that no text information can be acquired during correction latencies. They do show, however, that the presence of meaningful text is not the determining factor for the occurence and duration of these fixations.

3. PARTITIONING FIXATION DURATION DISTRIBUTIONS

3.1. An Individual Example

Is there a distinct population of fixations whose duration is shorter than the duration of fixations that precede corrective saccades? To examine this possibility, we attempted to partition the general fixation duration distribution into several sub-distributions (see also Hogaboam, 1983). Specifically, we discriminate fixations depending on whether they are preceded and followed by a progressive (right-directed), a regressive (left-directed) or a return sweep movement. Of special importance is the distinction between sequences that end with an outgoing progressive vs. regressive saccade.

We selected two subjects from a standard reading experiment to demonstrate the logic of this approach. In the experiment, an interesting popular science text was presented in pages of 6 to 7 lines of text, each containing up to 72 letters. Each letter subtended 1/3 deg of visual angle on a CRT screen. Apparatus and method were as described in Hofmeister et al. (this volume).

We start with the two fixation duration distributions shown in figure 1 (top panel), including 8202 fixations for subject 1 and 7762 fixations for subject 2. As can be seen, the two distributions are quite similar, with mean fixation durations being 210 ms for subject 1 and 189 ms for subject 2. Obviously subject 1 made far less fixations shorter then 120 ms as compared to subject 2, but there is no hint of any qualitative difference between the two distributions.

The center panel of Figure 1 shows distributions for two types of fixations: fixations that follow the return sweeps and precede a subsequent corrective saccade toward the left and fixations that precede regressions during sentence reading. The distributions are nearly identical for both subjects with durations of fixations prior to regressions showing much more variation and a large tail toward longer fixation durations. The fact that peaks for regressions and return sweep corrections are very similar and the respective distributions largely overlap points to the possibility that in normal reading many regressive saccades are of corrective nature.

The bottom panel of Figure 1 presents the result of subtracting the cases included in the center panel from the overall distributions shown in the top panel. Also excluded are all fixations peceding or following return sweeps. In subject 1, the segment of short fixations is effectively removed from the distribution. In subject 2, however, a bimodal distribution with a distinct population of very short fixations emerges. The striking bimodality is also present when plotting the fixation duration distributions for the patterns progression-progression, regression-progression separately, which is not done here because of space limitations. The overall proportion of very short fixations in subject 2 (individual range from 80 to 120 ms) amounts to 14 percent, which is an unusually high rate. We have identified another three subjects, from a total of 14 readers who participated in two passage reading experiments, who show bimodal distributions of fixations prior to progressive saccades with total proportions of very short fixations of 9 to 12 percent. Individual boundaries of the brief fixation range were between 80 ms and 130 ms in these subjects.

If the fixation duration preceding a corrective saccade defines the minimum latency of saccades that are programmed on-line, then saccades departing from fixations of even shorter durations must be controlled on a functionally different basis, i.e. by computations that precede the onset of the fixation. We assume that a population of such functionally distinctive brief fixations is present when an individual fixation duration distribution prior to progressive saccades (as in the bottom panel of figure 1) shows a separate peak some-

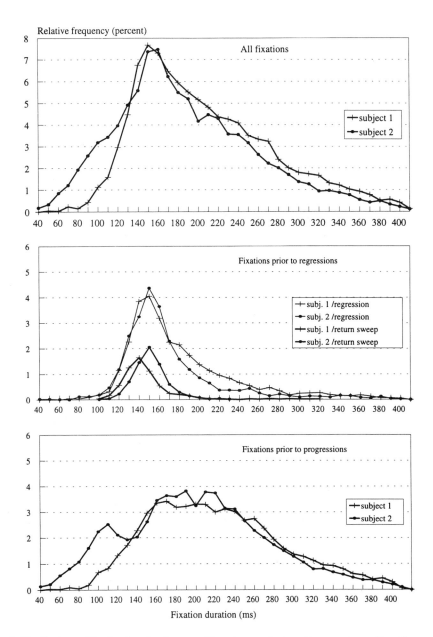

Figure 1. Distributions of fixation duration for two subjects in a standard reading experiment. Top: General distributions including all fixations made. Center: Distributions including fixations prior to regressions extending less then 20 letters (n=2225 and n=1951 for subjects 1 and 2) as well as fixations following return sweeps and prior to regressions (n=595 and n=543). Bottom: Distributions of fixations before progressions including the fixation patterns progression-progression (n=2706 and n=3435) and regression-progression (n=1845 and n=1651).

where between 80 ms and 130 ms with the modal value of the peak being at least 20 ms below the individual mean corrective saccade latency (see center panel of figure 1). When these conditions are met, we refer to the respective brief fixations as "fast fixations".

3.2. How Frequent Are Very Short Fixations in Reading?

Up to now we have applied the technique of partitioning fixation duration distributions to a total of 54 subjects from a variety of reading experiments. Looking at individual distributions of fixations prior to progressive saccades, a distinct population of fast fixations can be found in 20 to 25 percent of these readers, depending on how many observations are required for the definition of a "distinct population".

We will now give an overview on the frequency of very short fixations among 24 participants of a recent sentence reading experiment. For this purpose we follow Inhoff et al. 1993 in defining a range between 80 ms and 130 ms as "very short fixations". In table 1 subjects are ordered according to their rates of very short fixation frequencies. The sample includes cases where the criteria for a separation of "fast fixations" are met as well as cases with unimodal fixation duration distributions and readers with almost no fixations in the critical range.

As table 1 shows, there is considerable variation among normal readers in the proportion of very short fixations. Values range from 12 to below 0.5 percent for fixations with incoming and outgoing progressions and from 18 to 0 percent for fixations after regressions and prior to progressions. Most important is the fact that in nearly all participants the proportion of very short fixations is substantially smaller when a regressive saccade follows.

It should be noted that the data presented in table 1 are from a sentence reading experiment where participants were instructed to read carefully in order to detect pragmatic inconsistencies. It is our impression that under the less constraint situation of reading pages of prose text for comprehension, the number of very short fixations (and also the proportion of "fast fixations") is somewhat higher. This hypothesis cannot be tested on the basis of the available data, as large enough groups of subjects having read continuos text vs. single sentences under otherwise identical conditions are not yet available. When statistically significant, this difference would provide a further interesting example of how eye movement control can vary as a function of reading intention (Heller and Radach, this volume).

4. THE PROGRAMMING OF FAST FIXATIONS

The literature offers two theoretical accounts for the occurrence of fast fixation durations in reading. One account is related to the concept of "express saccades". These saccades, with latencies in the order of about 100 ms are frequently found in the gap paradigm, where a fixation point is removed prior to the onset of a peripheral target. Fischer (1992) interprets express saccades as generated by a visuomotor reflex that is normally under the control of cortical activity. The occurence of express saccades in the gap paradigm is attributed to the early triggering of a state of "disengaged attention" as induced by the offset of the fixation point. Express saccades in reading may occur when the attentional system stays in the disengaged stage for longer than normal periods of time, i.e. the reader has difficulties in switching to the engaged state. The resulting oculomotor

Table 1. Means and standard deviations of fixation durations as well as
proportions of very short fixations for three fixation patterns
(progression – progression, regression – progression and progression – regression).
N is the number of observations per subject.

	Fixation duration (ms)		Proportion of fast fixations (percent)			
	Mean	SD	prog – prog	regr – prog	prog – regr	N
1	207	(81)	12.14	16.55	4.72	2002
2	199	(75)	11.48	9.01	2.83	2125
3	207	(80)	8.64	12.81	4.34	2711
4	212	(81)	9.10	9.19	3.92	2374
5	224	(81)	8.58	12.27	3.08	2490
6	208	(78)	5.61	15.43	5.61	1814
7	215	(75)	2.94	19.01	2.49	1910
8	224	(76)	5.10	18.35	3.54	1970
9	227	(78)	5.25	10.42	1.39	2513
10	229	(84)	4.19	8.91	2.30	1915
11	231	(83)	3.83	5.11	1.89	2541
12	235	(83)	1.24	13.93	6.38	1720
13	243	(84)	3.22	4.84	2.16	2874
14	251	(83)	2.38	2.65	1.26	2367
15	247	(86)	2.02	2.64	1.40	2156
16	239	(82)	1.66	6.37	1.26	2040
17	242	(77)	2.34	3.85	0.00	1819
18	228	(77)	2.44	5.05	4.55	1594
19	242	(81)	1.42	3.85	2.12	2647
20	232	(71)	1.16	17.74	1.37	1679
21	255	(84)	0.36	6.19	1.63	1405
22	248	(74)	0.61	2.13	1.06	1552
23	236	(78)	0.14	0.00	0.00	1156
24	234	(76)	0.54	0.00	0.00	1462
Mean	230	(79.5)	4.02	8.60	2.47	2035

problems are assumed to include a rather unstable fixation with a tendency to execute more saccades. Most importantly, saccades will have shorter reaction times and there will be an increased amount of express saccades.

When comparing dyslexic and non-dyslexic readers in the gap task, Biscaldi and Fischer (1994) and Biscaldi et al. (1994) found an increased proportion of express saccades in dyslexics. They also identified subjects who made many express saccades in the standard overlap task (with no offset of the fixation point prior to the target onset). On the basis of a rather strict criterion of 40 percent express saccades and less than 150 ms mean latency in the overlap task, 23 percent of their dyslexic readers and 6 percent of their normal readers were classified as "express makers". Using a more relaxed definition, the proportion of subjects with express latencies in the normal population will be closer to the proportion of subjects with fast fixations during reading. Very short fixations during reading functionally could be equivalent to express saccades in the gap paradigm, i.e., they could be controlled by a low level visuomotor reflex system. In the following , this possibility will be referred to as the "express latency hypothesis".

Alternatively, fast fixations could occur when there is temporal overlap in the programming of successive saccades, as indicated by double-step experiments (Becker and Jürgens 1979, see also Deubel 1984, Findlay and Harris 1984). Morrison (1984) interpreted the results of his masking experiments in terms of a partially parallel saccade programming mechanism that has become one of the core ingredients of "attention-based" models of eye movement control in reading (but note the recent modifications e.g. in Rayner, Reichle and Pollatsek 1998). In Morrison's theory, a saccade to a new word is always preceded by a shift of attention occuring after a certain amount of lexical processing on the current word has been completed. When the parafoveal word is easy to process, it is possible that a second shift of attention takes place before the outgoing saccade has been committed to action. Depending on how quickly the second attention shift occurs, several scenarios are suggested, including skipping the first parafoveal word (N+1), landing half-way between word N+1 and word N+2 (similar to an amplitude transition function in the double-step literature) or making a very short fixation on N+1 before going to N+2. This latter scenario is interesting in the current context, because it suggests a functional explanation for fast fixations during reading. In the following, this specific account will be referred to as the "sequential attention shift model".

The tight coupling between shifts of attention (thought of in terms of a lexical processing beam) and saccade programming suggested by Morrison (1984) has recently been questioned (see e.g. Underwood & Radach, 1998, for a discussion). However, the objections raised against details of attention-based models of eye guidance are not necessarily critical for a parallel processing account of fast fixations, as lexically driven attention shifts need not to be the triggering events for parallel saccade programming. The general hypothesis that temporal overlap in the programming of subsequent saccades is the functional base for fast fixation in reading will be referred to as the "parallel programming hypothesis".

4.1. Fast Fixations and Incoming vs. Outgoing Saccades

According to the parallel programming hypothesis, saccades prior to fast fixations should be of relatively small amplitude. In the terminology of the sequential attention shift model (Morrison 1984; Rayner & Pollatsek 1989) this would be described as follows: When two attention shifts are made in rapid succession, the first is likely to go to an adjacent target (e.g. a short word that is easy to process), hence its amplitude should be relatively small. Similarly, saccades departing from a fast fixation should be of relatively small amplitude, if they are directed towards the goal of the second attention shift, presumably consisting of the next or second next word in the text. It is important to note that these predictions are also valid for a more general account that is not tied to lexical/attentional processing as a saccade trigger. The occurence of fast fixations in reading can be compared to the case of two-step responses in the double-step paradigm. The critical constraint is that the shorter of two possible saccades (e.g. a saccade to the next word as opposed to skipping it) is assumed to be the default, at least in the majority of cases. This can bee seen in analogy to an uncrossed double step situation where the first and second saccade of a two step response will both be shorter then the amplitude of a single step response.

The express latency hypothesis does not allow a prediction for incoming saccades, as in the gap and overlap paradigms only latencies and subsequent saccades are studied. For outgoing saccades, however, a prediction can be derived from Fischer and Weber (1993). They conducted a gap experiment with target distances ranging from 0.5 deg to 10 deg and plotted saccade latency against saccade amplitude. The number of express latencies was substantially reduced for amplitudes smaller then 4 deg. and there were almost no

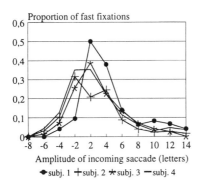
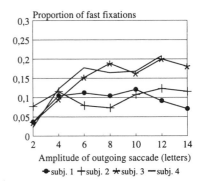

Figure 2. Left panel: Proportion of fast fixations as a function of incoming saccade amplitude. Negative numbers on the abscissa refer to regressive (right to left) incoming saccades. Included are observations with outgoing progressive saccades of up to 20 letters. Right panel: Proportion of fast fixations as a function of outgoing saccade amplitude. Every data point represents at least 50 observations.

express latencies prior to saccades below 2 deg, hence saccades following very short fixations should not be of atypically short amplitude.

Figure 2 examines these predictions by looking at the relation between fixation duration and the amplitude of saccades directed toward (incoming saccade) vs. away from the fixation (outgoing saccade). The proportion of fast fixations is plotted as a function of the amplitude of incoming (left panel) vs. outgoing (right panel) saccade size for four subjects from a standard reading experiment. All four subjects showed a distinctive peak of fast fixations in their distributions of fixation durations before progressive saccades which is the base for the proportions depicted in figure 2. As the figure indicates, there is indeed an increase in the proportion of fast fixations for smaller incoming saccades. This is in accordance to the prediction based on the sequential attention shift model (Morrison 1984). However, larger outgoing saccades are clearly associated with a larger proportion of fast fixations. This is contrary to the prediction of the attention shift model but corresponds to the latency-amplitude relation reported by Fischer and Weber (1993) for express saccades.

4.2. Fast Fixations and Subsequent Regressions

One oculomotor phenomenon that can provide different predictions for both hypotheses are regressive saccades made after fast fixations. Reasons for making regressions in reading can be summed into three classes: higher level comprehension problems, word processing difficulties and misplacements of the eyes (Vitu and McConkie, 1998). If fast fixations in reading are reflexive, as suggested by the express latency hypothesis, they should constitute an unexpected event. If not disrupting the normal flow of visual information processing, the reduction of the available fixation duration by about 100 ms should at least lead to serious word recognition problems causing a massive increase in regressions back to the location where the fast fixation occured. On the contrary, the parallel programming hypothesis assumes that fast fixations occur because the saccade to the critical location has become unnecessary, hence processing is not hampered and no excessive increase in regression frequency is predicted. Figure 3 shows the proportion of regressive saccades made when the prior fixation duration had been in the fast fixation range. First, the figure replicates the common finding that more regressions are made following longer progressive saccades (e.g. Vitu and McConkie 1998). It also shows that the frequency of regres-

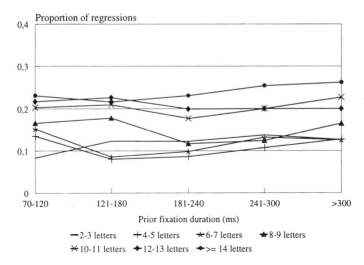

Figure 3. Proportion of outgoing regressive saccades as a function of prior fixation duration for different incoming saccades amplitudes (2–3 to >13 letters). Pooled data from four subjects (n=12129). Every data point represents more then 50 observations.

sions subsequent to fast fixations is only marginally increased, as should be expected from short fixations in general. There is no evidence of any disruption in the flow of continous reading caused by fast fixations.

5. GENERAL DISCUSSION

Our examination of local fixation patterns revealed a distinct population of very short fixations in a subgroup of adult normal readers. Fast fixations emerged when the distribution of corrective saccade latencies was subtracted from the general frequency distributions of fixation durations. In the distributions of all readers showing this phenomenon, the modal value of the fast fixation peak is at least 20 ms shorter then the modal value of corrective saccade latencies (after return sweeps). We see this as indicating that these very short fixations do not reflect corrections of misplaced fixation positions and that they are not controlled by visual input acquired during the brief fixation.

The fact that relatively few very short fixations are found before outgoing regressive saccades is in agreement with recent findings by Radach and McConkie (1998). They claim that progressive interword saccades as well as progressive and regressive refixation saccades are all part of a predominant low level-based mode of eye movement control. Regressive interword saccades appear to be controlled on a different base, presumably related to an interruption of the usual routine mode by programming one goal-directed regression saccade. Based on these considerations, we propose that fast fixations are also part of the normal, fairly automatic control mode. Our preliminary observation of more very short fixations in casual prose reading as compared to careful sentence reading is in line with this idea.

So far there has been only one study looking explicitly for the conditions under which very short fixations in reading can be found. Inhoff et al. (1993) manipulated attentional demands by asking subjects to read a passage of text several times and, in a second experiment, replaced the text by strings of 'z' arranged in a word-like fashion. These manipulation did neither lead to an increase in the number of very short fixations nor did fast fixations show up as a separate population in the normal reading conditions. We assume that two reasons can be made responsible for the apparent difference to the results of the present study. First, in the Inhoff et al. (1993) study, each participant contributed only a few hundred observations to each condition. Therefore, individual sub-distributions could not be analysed and fast fixations made by some participants can well have been buried in group variance. Also, Inhoff et al. (1993) partitioned their distributions in a different way, looking exclusively at cases with progressive incoming saccades. This may have produced a mixture of fixation patterns with and without fast fixations, further reducing the chance of finding distinct fast fixation populations.

Our finding of an increased number of fast fixations following short incoming saccades is compatible with the sequential attention shift model (Morrison 1984), whereas the reduced number of fast fixations before short outgoing saccades is not. In order to accomodate this result, a more relaxed version of the parallel processing hypothesis is required that would allow for a modification of the "second" movement amplitude prior to or during the fast fixation. The reduction of fast fixation prior to small saccades is similar to the finding by Fischer and Weber (1993) of a sharp reduction in the number of express latencies for shorter target eccentricities. A problem with this analogy is that the phenomenon is not exclusive to the occurence of express latencies, but applies to saccade latencies in general (see O'Regan, 1990, for a discussion of the saccadic "dead zone" and its relevance for fixations in reading). Quite compelling is the absence of a massive increase in regression frequency after making fast fixations. On the basis of this result we tend to believe that the parallel programming hypothesis is the better candidate to explain fast fixations in reading. At present this conclusion must be considered tentative, however. A more stringent test would be to select groups of subjects on the basis of their reading data and ask them to perform the original tasks in the gap overlap and double step paradigms. These experiments are currently being done.

ACKNOWLEDGMENTS

We wish to thank R. Kresser and M. Schroeder for their help in preparing this chapter.

REFERENCES

Becker W (1989) Metrics. In: Wurtz RH, Goldberg ME (eds.) The Neurobiology of Saccadic Eye Movements. Elsevier, Amsterdam, pp 13–61

Becker W Jürgens R (1979) An analysis of the saccadic system by means of double step stimuli. Vision Res 19: 967–983

Biscaldi M, Fischer B (1994) Saccadic eye movements of dyslectics in non-cognitive tasks. In: Ygge J Lennerstrand G (eds) Eye Movements in Reading. Pergamon, Oxford, pp 245 - 259

Biscaldi M, Fischer B, Aiple F (1994) Saccadic eye movements of dyslexic and normal reading children. Perception 23: 45–64

Dearborn W F (1906) The psychology of reading. Archives of Philosophy, Psychology, and Scientific Methods

Deubel H (1984) The evaluation of the oculomotor error signal. In: Gale A., Johnson G. (eds) Theoretical and Applied Aspects of Eye Movement Research. Elsevier, Amsterdam, pp 55–62

Findlay, J Harris, R (1984) Small Saccades to Double-Stepped Targets Moving in two Dimensions. In: Gale A, Johnson G (eds) Theoretical and Applied Aspects of Eye Movement Research. Elsevier, Amsterdam, pp 71–78

Fischer, B (1992) Saccadic reaction time: implications for reading, dyslexia and visual cognition. In Rayner K (ed) Eye movements and visual cognition. Scene perception and reading. Springer, New York, pp 31–45

Fischer B, Weber H (1993) Express Saccades and Visual Attention. Behavioral and Brain Sciences 16: 553–610

Heller D (1982) Eye movements in reading. In: Groner R, Fraisse P (eds) Cognition and Eye Movements. Deutscher Verlag der Wissenschaften, Berlin, pp 139–154

Heller D, Radach R (1992) Returning to an unanswered question: On the role of corrective saccades in text reading (Abstract). International Journal of Pychology 27: 55

Hofmeister J (1997) Über Korrektursakkaden beim Lesen von Texten und bei leseähnlichen Aufgaben. (On corrective saccades in reading and reading-like tasks.) Unpublished doctoral dissertation, Rheinisch-Westfälische Technische Hochschule, Aachen

Hogaboam (1983) Reading patterns in eye movement data. In: Rayner K (ed) Eye Movements in Reading. Perceptual and Language Processes. Academic Press, New York, pp 309–332

Inhoff A Topolski R Vitu F, O'Regan K (1993) Attention demands during reading and the occurrence of brief (express) fixations. Perception & Psychophysics 54: 814 - 823

McConkie GW, Kerr PW, Dyre BP (1994) What are 'normal' eye movements during reading: Toward a mathematical description. In: Ygge J, Lennerstrand G (eds), Eye movements in reading. Pergamon, Oxford, pp 315–328

McConkie GW, Underwood NR, Zola, D, Wolverton, GS (1985) Some temporal characteristics of processing during reading. Journal of Experimental Psychology: Human Perception and Performance 11: 168–186

Morrison RE (1984) Manipulation of stimulus onset delay in reading: Evidence for parallel programming of saccades. Journal of Experimental Psychology: Human Perception and Performance 10: 667–682

O'Regan JK (1990) Eye movements and reading. In: Kowler E (ed) Reviews of oculomotor research: Vol.4. Eye Movements and Their Role in Visual and Cognitive Processes. Elsevier, Amsterdam, pp 395–453

Radach R, McConkie G (1998) Determinants of fixation positions in reading. In: Underwood G (ed) Eye guidance in reading and scene perception. Elsevier, Oxford, pp 77–100

Rayner K, Reichle E D, Pollatsek A (1998) Eye movement control in reading: An overview and a model. In Underwood G (ed) Eye guidance in reading and scene perception. Elsevier, Oxford, pp 243–268

Vitu F, McConkie G (1998) On regressive saccades in reading. In: Underwood G (ed) Eye guidance in reading and scene perception. Elsevier, Oxford, pp 101–124

47

THE PLANNING OF SUCCESSIVE SACCADES IN LETTER STRINGS

Cécile Beauvillain, Tania Dukic, and Dorine Vergilino

Laboratoire de Psychologie Expérimentale, URA 316 CNRS
Université René Descartes
28, rue Serpente, Paris 75006, France

1. INTRODUCTION

Reading is the most remarkable ordered scanning performance that people can acquire. This behavior relies on saccadic eye movements which direct the gaze to a new location in the text. Such orienting movements are produced with highly automated routines, in an environment of complex structures which offer a variety of potential targets for the eye. For the selection of one target position among many alternatives recognition processes are necessary. We will focus here on one aspect of this behavior that is concerned with the planning of successive movements within words. During reading, subjects frequently direct their gaze to two successive positions in a word, hence bringing the fovea to different parts of the words. In recent years, the conditions under which refixations take place have been investigated. It has been shown that the probability of refixation depends on the word length and the position of the initial fixation on a word (O'Regan et al. 1984 ; McConkie et al. 1988). In addition, the probability of refixation was found to be influenced by lexical factors such as word frequency (McConkie et al, 1988; Vitu, 1991) and lexical information integrated during the first fixation (Beauvillain, 1996; Pynte, 1996).

The aim of this chapter is to explore one aspect of this behavior that involves the programming of refixation saccades within words. The fixation-saccade-refixation sequence requires the selection of successive target position within word. There are various dynamic mechanisms that can account programming of the first and refixation saccades. Possibility one is that only the next intended movement is programmed. Accordingly, the first movement is computed before the first saccade, and the second movement prior the second refixation saccade during the initial fixation. Possibility two is that the coordinates of both saccades are mapped before the first movement. We present two experiments out of a series of studies performed in the lab which investigate how the visual information given before the primary and refixation saccade influences the calculation of the refixation saccade amplitude in reading-like situation. In the first experiment, we used a step paradigm in which the target letter string that elicited the primary saccade was shifted during

Current Oculomotor Research, edited by Becker *et al.*
Plenum Press, New York, 1999.

333

this saccade. The motor response data obtained show that, for the majority of responses, the refixation saccade does not correct the artificially induced fixation error. Rather, the amplitude of the refixation saccade has a relatively constant value that is mainly a function of the letter string length. The second experiment investigated the effect of length information given before and after the primary saccade on the refixation saccade amplitude. Evidence is provided for a preprogramming of the refixation saccade based on visual information integrated before the execution of the primary saccade. The amplitude of the refixation saccade is modified on the basis of new visual length information displayed during first fixation only for responses triggered 130 msec after the length shift.

2. THE PROGRAMMING OF REFIXATION SACCADE

The double step paradigm was implemented to study goal directed saccades in which the displacement of a target leads to consecutive correction saccades (Becker and Jürgens, 1979 ; Deubel et al. 1982). The investigations developed with this technique have shown that the displacement is not perceived by the subject but is taken into account by the oculomotor system that programs and executes a correction saccade to reach the target. Results of our first experiment indicates that saccades elicited by the letter string position shift are not typical «correction saccades», that is saccades that correct fixation errors induced by the shift. Clearly, basic characteristics of saccade programming in reading fundamentally differ from the ones revealed by studies using single dots as targets. Our experiment focused on small target steps within the range of typical first fixation positions observed in reading. Three different lengths of stimuli were used : 7-, 9- and 11-letter strings. To control for the linguistic properties of the different length stimuli, nonsense letter strings were constructed sharing the same initial letters. These letter strings could be read easily as they were composed of letter sequences that were orthographically and phonologically regular in French. First, subjects were instructed to fixate a cross displayed on a screen. After a delay, a target letter string was displayed at a visual angle of 2°30 from the initial fixation point which was remove simultaneously. This was the signal for the primary saccade. During this saccade, the whole target letter string was displaced by one or two character-spaces, in the same or opposite direction to the direction of the primary saccade. Subjects were required to read the letter string as quickly as possible, and then to fixate a cross displayed at three character-spaces after the ending of the letter strings. Eight subjects participated in 3 blocks of 300 hundred trials.

Eye position was registered with a Bouis oculometer system and sampled at 500Hz. Absolute resolution of the eye tracker was 6 min of arc, whereas a character-space equaled 30' of visual angle. Vision was binocular and head movements were restricted by a biteboard and a forehead rest. Stimuli were displayed on a CRT screen (Hewlett Packard 1310A; P15 phosphor) that was interfaced by a fast graphics system.

Figure 1 (a-b) shows the distributions of landing positions as well as the of the refixation saccade amplitudes for the different steps of 11-letter sequences. Similarity between refixation amplitude distributions for each step is illustrated in Fig. 1b. Obviously, appropriate oculomotor response to a target displacement in a reading task is a refixation saccade reaching the second part of the letter string as observed in no displacement control condition. This saccadic behavior strongly differs from saccadic responses observed in double step experiments with a single target where a consecutive correction saccade is triggered, bringing the foveal line of sight to the target position. Our data reveal that refixation saccade amplitude is constant and is not affected by the displacement conditions. The same pattern is observed for 7- and 9-letter strings. Experimental results presented in

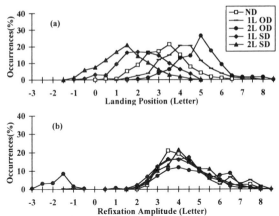

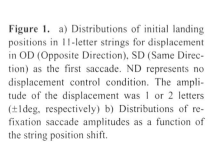

Figure 1. a) Distributions of initial landing positions in 11-letter strings for displacement in OD (Opposite Direction), SD (Same Direction) as the first saccade. ND represents no displacement control condition. The amplitude of the displacement was 1 or 2 letters (±1deg, respectively) b) Distributions of refixation saccade amplitudes as a function of the string position shift.

Figure 2 indicate that refixation saccade amplitude is not calculated on the basis of the distance that separates the position of the first fixation from the string ending boundary. mainly determined by the string length. For fixation positions located at 7 or 8 characterspaces from the letter string ending boundary, refixation amplitude depends on the string length. This means that the effective refixation saccade is not computed during the first fixation on the basis of the distance that separates the position of the first fixation from the end of the letter string. Such a mechanism should have predicted a similar refixation saccade amplitude for letter sequences of various lengths when the distance between the first fixation position and the ending boundary was similar. Rather, refixation amplitude still depends on the string letters when the distance from the first fixation position to the string ending boundary is similar for the different string lengths.

Note that the observed correction saccades only occurred for opposite direction conditions. In this case, different types of saccadic reactions are observed. First, one-fixation data in which secondary saccades left the letter string. Figure 3 shows low mean frequency of refixations for opposite direction displacements. Such responses are a consequence of initial fixations very near the center of the letter string. This corresponds with the well known observation that the refixation frequency in reading is lower when first fixation is located near the word center. Second, regressive saccades which correct the error artificially induced by the target step. These regressive corrective saccades represent

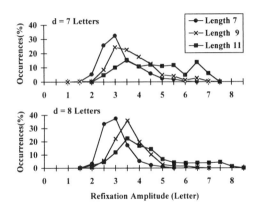

Figure 2. Distributions of amplitude of refixation saccades on 7-, 9- and 11-letters strings as a function of the distance between the first fixation position and the string ending boundary.

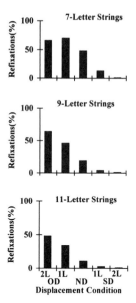

Figure 3. Occurrences of single fixations on 7-, 9-and 11-letter strings as a function of the string position shift condition.

25%, 16%, and 13% of the responses for respectively 7-,9- and 11-letter strings. Regressions are observed for initial fixations located beyond the center of the letter string. The higher frequency of these corrective responses for 7-letter strings may be due to the position of initial fixations that is more likely to overshoot the letter string center. Indeed, the first saccade usually landed at a position that will be increasingly closer to the geometric string center as the strings gets shorter. The remaining saccadic reactions were progressive refixation saccades whose amplitude does not consider the opposite direction step.

Except these saccadic responses obtained when the eye overshoot the string center, our results do not support a mechanism selecting a precise target position as the goal for the refixation saccade. Clearly, there is no evidence in our data of either shortening nor lengthening of refixation saccade amplitude as a function of the first fixation position. This suggest that refixation amplitude saccade is coded in a movement of a constant amplitude.

3. THE PLANNING OF SUCCESSIVE SACCADES

The previous experiment showed that the refixation saccade amplitude is mainly computed on the basis of string length information. However, it should be of interest to determine whether such this information is integrated by the saccadic computation system to determine the refixation saccade amplitude. Possibility one is that both primary and refixation saccades are planned and computed before the primary saccade, based on target length integrated before the execution of the first movement. Possibility two is that the calculation of the amplitude of refixation saccade only begins during the first fixation. In order to examine the ability of the saccadic system to calculate the amplitude of the refixation as a function of the visual information given before and after the primary saccade, the following experiment was designed to test the effects of length shift on the amplitude of the refixation saccade. The primary saccade triggered by the first target letter string dis-

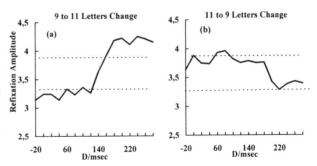

Figure 4. Amplitude of the refixation saccade as function of the Delay (interval between the length shift and the second saccade) in the (a) 9 to 11 Letters shift (b) 11 to 9 Letters shift. Negative values correspond to refixation saccades triggered before the length shift while positive values correspond to refixation saccades triggered after the length shift.

played at three character-spaces from the fixation target triggered a length shift after a 0, 50, 120 or 200 msec delay. The 0 msec delay corresponds to a length shift triggered simultaneously with the onset of the first saccade. Two types of length shift were designed: one which final length was 2 letters shorter than its initial length (11 to 9 letters shift) and one which final length was 2 letters longer than its initial length (9 to 11 letters shift). There were two control conditions with no length change. 1050 pairs of 9- and 11- letter strings were constructed that share the same 9 initial letters. Six subjects participated in 3 blocks.

Figure 4 (a b) displays the effect of length shift on the refixation saccade amplitude as a function of the interval between the length shift and the refixation saccade onset. The data analysis reveals that in the 9 to 11 letter sequence condition, the mean amplitude of the refixation saccades significantly increased when occurring 140 msecs after the length shift. With shorter delays, refixation saccade amplitudes were similar to the one obtained with the 9-letter string control condition. The transition region begins 130 msecs after the length shift. Our results also indicate that, in 11 to 9 letter sequences, refixation saccades starting less than 190 msecs after the length shift had the same amplitude as the one observed in 11-letter strings whereas they decreased abruptly to reach amplitude values corresponding to 9-letter strings after this delay. Possibly, the observed difference in the ability to reduce or prolong the saccade amplitude may be due to the difference in visual feedback between the two types of length shift. Indeed, subjects reported they perceived the length shift more frequently in the case of a the letter string lengthening. An interesting pattern of results emerged in the case of a length shift triggered during the onset of the first saccade for three subjects who performed two different types of first fixation duration. Typical distributions of refixation amplitudes are shown in Figure 5 (a-b) for one of these subjects. Following short fixation duration, refixation amplitude was similar with that produced in letter sequences similar in length with that displayed before the first saccade. Such finding supports the hypothesized preprogrammed mode of operation. Only refixation saccades produced 160 msec after the first fixation onset had an amplitude appropriate to that displayed at the first fixation onset. These pattern of data could not be observed for the three remaining subjects whose first fixation duration lasted 200 to 350 msecs. Following long first fixations, an initially preprogrammed amplitude can be adjusted during the first fixation based on new visual information given to the reader.

4. CONCLUSION

Eye movement elicited by a target letter string that jumps or shifts in length reveal some interesting properties of the saccadic control in reading. First, our first experiment

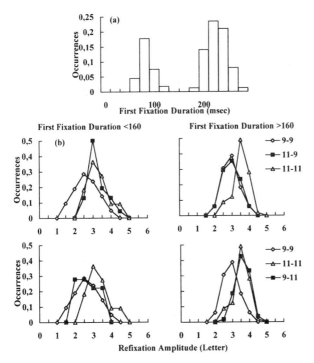

Figure 5. (a) Histogram showing distributions of first fixation duration for one subject in the 0-msec Delay condition. (b) Distributions of refixation amplitudes for first fixation duration less and more than 160 msec. Open symbols represent the control conditions, and filled squares the length shift condition.

shows that the saccadic system does not compute the refixation saccade on the basis of the target position shift. Saccades are only modified by target letter string shifts that causes strong overshoots of landing positions. Flexibility of the saccadic behavior during initial fixation is implemented by a modification of the word-object as the target for the next saccade. Initial landing positions very near or beyond the center of a word are generally followed by a saccade directed towards the following word. This favours the view that the word-object as the target for the ongoing saccades in reading could be modified rapidly by new visual information integrated during the first fixation whereas the precise adjustment of the saccade amplitude is not precisely re-computed. Along with this view, personal observations made in the lab showed an effect of the word frequency on the probability of refixation whereas the amplitude of the refixation saccade in the two-fixation cases was never found to be affected by lexical information integrated during the first fixation. This suggests that information integrated during the first fixation on a word can modify the word-object as the target for the following saccade.

Second, the data from these two experiments can be comprised in a model of eye movement control in reading which incorporates the planning of successive saccades. Programming of successive saccades can partially overlap in time. At the time a first saccade to a target letter string is planned, a second saccade is preprogrammed based on visual inputs. The global visual characteristic of a target letter string, such as its length, is coded in a movement of a given amplitude. This finding argues for the notion that refixation saccade amplitude is mapped in motor space coordinates calculated on the basis of the string length. Encouraging physiological evidence for the validity of this interpretation comes from Goldberg and Bruce (1990) that found that the critical signal from frontal eye fields is neither retinal location of a saccade target, nor its spatial location, but rather the saccadic movement the target will evoke. Further indications for a mapping in motor coordinates in reading comes from text reading studies that shows a tendency to sent the eyes at a particular distance (McConkie et al.1988) for different length words.

REFERENCES

Beauvillain C (1996) The integration of morphological and whole-word form information during eye fixations on prefixed and suffixed words, J. of Mem. and Lang 35 : 967–983.

Becker W, Jürgens R. (1979) An analysis of the saccadic system by means of double step stimuli. Vision Res19: 967–983.

Deubel H, Wolf W, Hauske G (1982) Corrective saccades: Effect of shifting the saccade goal. Vision Res 22: 353–364.

Goldberg ME, Bruce CJ (1990) Primate frontal eye fields. III. Maintenance of a spatially accurate saccade signal. J. of Neur. 64 : 489–508.

McConkie GW, Kerr PW, Reddix MD, Zola D (1988) Eye movement control during reading : I. The location of initial eye fixations on words. Vis. Res. 28 : 1107–1118.

McConkie GW, Kerr PW, Reddix MD, Zola D, Jacobs AM (1989) Eye frequency control during reading : II. Frequency of refixation a word. Percept.. Psych. 46 : 245–253.

O'Regan JK, Lévy-Schoen A, Pynte J, Brugaillère B. (1984) Convenient fixation location within isolated words of different length and structure. J. of Exp. Psyc : H.P.P. 10 : 250–257.

Pynte J (1996) Lexical control of within-word eye movements, J. of Exp. Psyc : H.P.P. 22: 958–969.

Vitu F (1991) The influence of parafoveal preprocessing and linguistic context on the optimal landing position, Perc. And Psych. 50 :58–75.

48

EYE MOVEMENTS IN READING

Are Two Eyes Better Than One?

Dieter Heller and Ralph Radach

Technical University of Aachen
Institute of Psychology
Jaegerstr. 17-19, D-52056 Aachen.

1. CURRENT RESEARCH ON EYE MOVEMENTS IN READING

The last 25 years have seen impressive advances in reading research, based on eye movement recording, with respect to both theory and methodology. An important milestone at the beginning of recent developments was the work of McConkie and Rayner on the perceptual span (see summaries in Rayner 1984; McConkie 1983). Here, for the first time, registration devices and computers were combined in a way that allowed to introduce a new dimension into reading research: the manipulation of the useful field of view under dynamic conditions.

Another influential line of research started with the discovery that fixation positions are not randomly distributed over words within a line of text but cluster at positions left of the word center (Dunn-Rankin 1978). Research around the notions of the "preferred viewing position" (Rayner 1979) and "optimal viewing position" (e.g. O'Regan and Levy-Schoen 1987) has led to the common view that eye movement control in reading is word-based (McConkie et al. 1988). At the same time it became clear that the decision to move the eyes can be made on-line, based on information acquired within a given fixation (Rayner and Pollatsek 1981).

An important base for current thinking on eye movement control in reading has also been the introduction of ideas from basic oculomotor research. The "global effect" as described by Findlay (1982) plays an essential role in O'Regan's (1990) "strategy and tactics" theory. McConkie et al. (1988) were influenced by Kapoula and Robinson's (1986) findings on the saccadic range effect. Similarly, the keystone paper by Becker and Jürgens (1979) on double-step saccades provided a theoretical base for Morrison's (1984) model of saccade control in reading.

Taken together, the central development of the last 20 years has been a shift from early "global" or "indirect" models of eye movement control to theories of direct control, where a moment-to-moment relation between eye movements and information processing is assumed.

Current Oculomotor Research, edited by Becker *et al.*
Plenum Press, New York, 1999.

Much of current research in reading is centered around the question whether there is a permanent direct control of eye movements, operating on every saccade within a text, and which properties of the text - basic visual vs. cognitive – provide the targets for saccades.

Certainly, saccade programming can be under cognitive control, as for example many regressions are caused by text processing problems (Vitu and McConkie 1998). An alternative to the currently dominating idea of permanent lexical control (e. g. Rayner et al. 1998) could involve a switching between an automatic (low level) default mode and a more controlled mode of eye guidance whenever processing resources make this possible or comprehension problems demand it. Some evidence for this dichotomy of control modes is provided by the recent finding of qualitative differences in saccade parameters for inter-word progressions vs. inter-word regressions (Radach and McConkie 1998).

We believe that the common alternative between high and low level control is of limited value, as, in reality, both cases may always co-exist. A similar argument can be made for the related alternative between direct vs. indirect control. This seems appropriate not only because some results do not fit into one or another model (see e. g. O'Regan et al. 1994; Rayner et al. 1996) but also because both types of theories do not sufficiently reflect the real complexity of the reading process.

One essential ingredient of this complexity is the type of *reading intention* present in a particular situation. Looking only at the situation of silent reading, there are several possibilities: We can skim over text with the only intention to find out whether some of the content is relevant or not. We can read a newspaper or a book with interest casually directed towards the content. Or, alternatively, we can read a difficult scientific text trying hard to understand it word by word.

The profound consequences of different types of reading intention on eye movement parameters can be demonstrated when reading under different instructions is compared (Heller 1982). Furthermore, as a result of reading intention, there can also be a variation in eye-mind span, just as there is a variable eye-voice span when reading aloud. In other words, the semantic analysis can coincide with the current fixation position. It can also go further ahead when predictions are easy or it can lag behind. An extreme form of the latter would be to realize that the eyes are already within the next line while cognition is still operating at a previous location.

Expressed in terms of the theoretical alternatives discussed above: Within the same subject and even within the same experiment, reading can include a lower or higher degree of oculomotor vs. cognitive control. The hope that some short comprehension question at the end of a text will induce the type of reading that we think it does, may be delusive.

2. BINOCULAR COORDINATION IN READING

Apart from the substantial variance in eye movement data due to instruction and intention, there is one further widely neglected aspect: Reading is, among many other things, also a result of the oculomotor and perceptual works of *two* eyes. Although the first paper on this subject appeared already in 1917 (Schmidt 1917), there are only a few recent publications (e.g. Bassou et al. 1993; Ygge and Jacobson 1994; Hendriks 1996) and normative data do virtually not exist. This is quite surprising, given the general theoretical and methodological importance of the problem and the obvious relevance for many applied questions. For example, vergence control and fixation stability have become a topic of central importance in eye movement research on dyslexia (Cornelissen et al. 1993).

The starting point of our own research was provided by the existing literature on binocular coordination in simple scanning paradigms (e. g. Collewijn et al. 1988; Zee et al. 1992). Collewijn et al. asked their subjects to look back and forth between LED's located on an iso-vergence plane with target distances between 1.25 and 80 deg. of visual angle. They found marked differences in the saccades made by the abducting (temporally moving) vs. adducting (nasally moving) eye. The saccades of the abducting eye had a larger amplitude, a higher peak velocity and a shorter duration. As a result of this, the eyes transiently diverged to a considerable extent during the saccade (about 0.3 deg for a 5 deg saccade). After the saccade, there was a vergence drift movement that had usually corrected the fixation error after about 300 ms.

One of the very few studies so far in which binocular parameters (vergence velocity) were included into an analysis of eye movements in reading was carried out by Hendriks (1996). In one experiment, she had subjects read short passages of text from a stimulus card with a viewing distance of 20 cm and letters subtending 0.6 deg. of visual angle. She found that in more than 74 percent of all observations there were convergence movements during reading fixations (as compared to divergence movements in about 17 percent of cases) and that vergence velocity was increased for larger saccades.

In the remainder of this chapter we will present results of three recent experiments on different aspects of binocular coordination in reading. We will first look at the influence of fixation position on a page of text on the binocular fixation error. We will then explore differences between binocular and monocular reading and finally discuss possible influences of task variables on binocular parameters. Before we get to the data, we will briefly describe our general methodology.

2.1. General Methods

We collected eye movement data using an AmTech ET3/4 infrared pupil reflection eyetracking system (relative accuracy < 0.1 deg., sampling rate 400/500Hz). The system consists of two independent eye trackers with data for each eye collected and calibrated separately. Extensive testing with an artificial eye indicated that both eye trackers produce identical output signals in response to identical optical input. Saccades are identified on the basis of two criteria: a velocity difference for consecutive data points of at least 15 deg/sec and a minimum saccade amplitude of 0.25 deg. In order to prevent contamination with dynamic overshoots, amplitude and velocity of postsaccadic vergence movements were computed for intervals beginning 10 ms after the onset of the current fixation. To achieve maximum convergence during calibration, calibration targets were presented for at least 2000 ms. Text was presented on a 21inch GDM 2040 Sony Monitor with black text on light grey background presented in standard courier font, one letter subtending about 1/3 deg. of visual angle. In all studies participants had normal visual acuity and no abnormalities of binocular vision.

2.2. Binocular Coordination: The Role of the Fixation Position within a Page

In a first series of experiments we obtained a detailed description of the temporal and spatial dynamics of binocular coordination during reading and other complex visual tasks. We found that the saccade amplitude asymmetries described by Collewijn et al. for a simple scanning paradigm are present in reading as well. The magnitude of amplitude differences is quite remarkable. Means are in the order of 5 percent of total movement am-

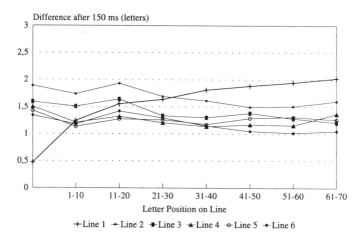

Figure 1. Mean absolute fixation position difference between both eyes at 150 ms after fixation onset as a function of the averaged (binocular) fixation location within a line of text for lines 1 to 6. Letter position value 0 on the abscissa refers to the first fixation on the line. Data from 7 subjects reading 120 lines of a popular science text.

plitude when large (10–12 letter) saccades are considered and of approximately 15 percent when small (2–3 letter) saccades are considered. During fixation, the initial disparity is reduced - but generally not offset - by a relatively uniform convergence shift. This convergence movement can be found in well over 80 percent of all fixations in most subjects. In contrast to scanning data of Collewijn et al., vergence movements in reading are considerably slower (about 1 deg./sec.) and there is usually a residual disparity at the end of each reading fixation (Heller and Radach 1995, Radach et al. 1996; see also Hendriks 1996).

We were interested in the question whether this residual disparity would lead to an accumulation of fixation error over lines of text. To investigate this problem, we asked 7 normal subjects to read a text of 120 lines in pages of 6 lines each without resting at the beginning of each new line (as it is often the case in other binocular studies). Figure 1 shows the disparity at the end of each fixation as a function of the ordinal number of the fixation on the line and the line number within the page.

Figure 1 demonstrates that during the reading of the first line there is indeed a steady accumulation of the mean fixation error up to an average value of about 2 letters. Later on, this trend is slowed and then reversed, leading to a mean fixation error of about 1.5 letters. Obviously, the visual system is not tolerating the accumulation of disparity building up as a result of properties of the oculomotor plant, if it exceeds a certain value (see the hypothetical mechanisms discussed by Collewijn et al. to account for the saccade amplitude asymmetry). Although this finding leaves open theoretical questions, it is of apparent methodological importance.

2.3. A Comparison of Eye Movements in Monocular vs. Binocular Reading

In this experiment, 8 subjects were asked to read 200 lines of text under normal binocular conditions. Then they read 200 lines with one eye covered and 200 lines with the

Table 1. Basic eye movement parameters for reading with both eyes,
with the left eye only and with the right eye only.
Saccade amplitudes are given in letters.

	Both eyes reading	Left eye reading	Right eye reading
Fixation duration (ms)	247 (121)	262 (124)	263 (134)
Saccade amplitude (progress.)	8.32 (3.56)	9.07 (4.29)	8.85 (4.32)
Saccade amplitude (regress.)	4.89 (3.01)	6.20 (4.48)	5.78 (3.29)
Proportion of regressions	16.55	19.23	18.23
Number of fixations per line	11.81 (3.52)	13.02 (3.32)	12.83 (3.17)

other eye covered. Table 1 shows a comparison of basic eye movement parameters for these conditions.

As it is evident from the table, in monocular reading fixation duration, the proportion of regressions and the number of fixations per line are increased. This is evidence for reading with one eye being more difficult; a result that is in line with comparisons of monocular vs. binocular performance in other visual tasks (Jones and Lee 1981). However, the most salient and unexpected difference is a substantial increase in the amplitude of progressive saccades under monocular viewing. A tentative hypothesis to account for this finding could be that under monocular conditions the field of view is somewhat reduced and that the saccadic system does not readily adapt to the changed spatial reference system.

The lack of difference between saccade amplitudes for monocular left and right eye saccades is in line with Collewijn et al. (1988), who did also not find such a difference, despite the binocular asymmetries described above. They also found no differences for slow movements during the fixation; a result that we can confirm for our reading data. As an illustration, for one typical subject figure 2 shows a comparison of the net drift movements of the left and right eye in monocular vs. binocular reading.

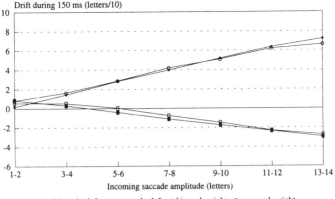

Figure 2. Net drift movements of the left and right eye during the first 150 ms of fixations as a function of incoming amplitude of progressive saccades. Data for one subject reading 200 lines with both eyes, 200 lines with the left eye covered and 200 lines with the right eye covered. Unequal contributions of both eyes to convergence are related to version drift (see Collewijn et al. 1988 for a discussion).

The figure indicates that, although one eye is covered, the movement amplitude of the seeing eye during the fixation remains about the same. There clearly is a strong relation between the drift and the amplitude signal of the saccade. If the slow movements during fixations are indeed reflex-like and preprogrammed as suggested by these results, the question arises whether they can still be sensible to task demands.

2.4. Influence of Reading Material

A first attempt to investigate influences of task variables on vergence movements during reading was made by Hendriks (1996). She compared postsaccadic vergence velocity under two conditions: reading short texts vs. reading a list of unrelated words. She found slower vergence velocities in the word list task, and concluded, that when the extraction of visual information is more difficult, vergence velocity slows down. This result seems counterintuitive, since one would assume that under more difficult conditions, if anything, vergence velocity should increase.

To shed light on this issue we did an experiment that involved a comparison between reading normal text and mixed case text. There can be no doubt that visual information extraction is more difficult in mixed case reading (e.g. Coltheart and Freeman 1974). In our experiment, this increased difficulty is clearly reflected in all general eye movement parameters. The result of central importance to our question, convergence velocity as a function of saccade size and reading task is shown in figure 3 (left panel).

Velocities range from 0.4 to 1 deg./sec. as a function of saccade size. The most interesting result, with respect to our question, is the vertical displacement of the curves for the two reading conditions. Clearly, vergence velocity is slower in the mixed case condition, and this holds over the entire range of saccades. These data provide a replication of Hendriks' results. Our next question was, whether the different convergence velocity is directly triggered by the visual input during fixation, or whether it is already inherent in the saccadic signal itself. This question can be answered by comparing the mean absolute difference in saccade size, for normal- vs. mixed case reading, as this is the main factor generating the fixation error.

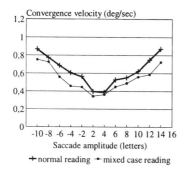 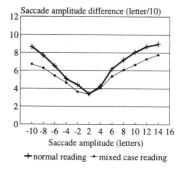

Figure 3. Left panel: Mean convergence velocity during fixations as a function of prior saccade amplitude for reading 200 lines of normal text vs. 200 lines of mixed case text (n=6). Right panel: mean absolute saccade amplitude difference as a function of averaged (binocular) amplitude of the incoming saccade. Observations in both panels are identical.

It is obvious from figure 3 (right panel) that saccade differences are larger in normal reading compared to the mixed-case condition. Accordingly, binocular fixation errors increase, and as a result of this, convergence motion is somewhat faster. In other words, in normal reading conditions the visual system is obviously able to tolerate a larger binocular fixation error than under more difficult visual conditions. In a more general context, this can be seen as a further example for the influence of reading material and reading task on local oculomotor activity (in this case binocular coordination), just as discussed in the introductory section on a more theoretical level.

3. CONCLUSIONS

One important result of binocular eye movement registration in reading is the considerable disparity between the two eyes, ranging to up to 1–3 letters. This fixation error increases during the course of successive fixations within a line. When reading more then one line, the fixation error levels off and is reduced to an average of about 1.5 letters. Our fixation errors are substantially larger than those reported by Cornelissen et al. (1993) for adult readers. This difference may be due to the fact that in their study participants were asked to fixate items on a short word list, whereas our experimental conditions are much closer to the natural dynamics of reading continuous text.

Our finding that postsaccadic drift movements are identical for binocular vs. monocular reading indicates that fixational vergence is basically reflexive and not based on specific visual input. In good agreement with this, the results of our comparison of reading normal vs. mixed case text suggest that top-down influences as induced by task demands operate primarily on saccade coordination rather then convergence movements.

Finally, to the question "are two eyes better than one?" What can be concluded from the results that have been reported? Reading involves processing two-dimensional objects - text on a flat screen. The visual system, however, is designed to analyze a three-dimensional world, in which binocular coordination plays an essential, though relatively sluggish, role. Theoretically, this should present a problem for reading, because the spatial dimensions of the text provide no functional advantages for binocular eye movements. On the other hand, there are no double images during reading; despite the observed disparity the system yields a single percept. How this arises, whether through suppression or by means of other processes, remains thus far unknown.

If one addresses the problem from a methodological viewpoint, then the answer to the question "Are two eyes better than one?" takes on a different aspect. In most of the current studies in reading research, fixation position differences are determined on the level of one letter position. This may not be a problem as long as the argument is restricted to relative comparisons between carefully controlled experimental conditions.

However, with respect to absolute fixation positions, one is tempted to say, "one eye is better than two", because disparity between the two eye positions is such that in binocular reading, no adequately precise definition of the "real" fixation position after a saccade can be given. The retinal coordinates, provided by monocular measurements in binocular reading, may not be sufficient to define the *perceptual* coordinates that are operating. And, if these perceptual coordinates are to be indicated by eye position, one should indeed ask subjects to read monocularily. Only then, there is a clear correspondence between fixation position and percept.

REFERENCES

Bassou L, Pugh AK, Granié M, Morucci JP (1993) Binocular vision in reading: a study of the eye movements of ten year old children. In: d'Ydevalle G, van Rensbergen J. (eds) Perception and Cognition. Advances in eye movement research. Elsevier, Amsterdam, pp 297–308

Becker W, Jürgens R (1979) An analysis of the saccadic system by means of double step stimuli. Vision Research 19: 967–984

Collewijn H, Erkelens C, Steinman R (1988) Binocular co-ordination of human horizontal eye movements. Journal of Physiology 404: 157–182

Coltheart M, Freeman R (1974) Case alternation impairs word identification. Bull. Psychon. Soc. 3: 102–104

Cornelissen P, Munro N, Fowler S, Stein J (1993) The stability of binocular fixation during reading in adults and children. Developmental Medicine and Child Neurology 35: 777–787

Dunn-Rankin P (1978) The visual characteristics of words. Scientific American 238: 122–130

Findlay JM (1982) Global processing for saccadic eye movements. Vision Research 22: 1033–1045

Heller D (1982) Eye movements in reading. In: Groner R, Fraisse P (eds) Cognition and Eye Movements. Deutscher Verlag der Wissenschaften, Berlin, pp 139–154

Heller D, Radach R (1995) Binocular coordination of eye movements in complex visual tasks. Perception 24, Supplement: 72

Hendriks A (1996) Vergence eye movements during fixations in reading. Acta psychologica 92: 131–151

Jones RK, Lee DN (1981) Why two eyes are better than one: The two views of binocular vision. Journal of Experimental Psychology: Human Perception and Performance 7: 30–40

Kapoula Z, Robinson DA (1986) Saccadic undershoot is not inevitable: Saccades can be accurate. Vision Research 26: 735–743

McConkie GW (1983) Eye movements and perception during reading. In: Rayner K (ed) Eye Movements in Reading. Perceptual and Language Processes. Academic Press, New York, pp 65–96

McConkie GW, Kerr PW, Reddix MD, Zola D (1988) Eye movement control during reading: I. The location of initial eye fixation on words. Vision Research 28: 1107–1118.

Morrison RE (1984) Manipulation of stimulus onset delay in reading: Evidence for parallel programming of saccades. Journal of Experimental Psychology: Human Perception and Performance 10: 667–682

O'Regan JK (1990) Eye movements and reading. In: Kowler E (ed) Reviews of oculomotor research: Vol.4. Eye Movements and Their Role in Visual and Cognitive Processes. Elsevier, Amsterdam, pp 395–453

O'Regan JK, Levy-Schoen A (1987) Eye movement strategy and tactics in word recognition and reading. In: Coltheart M (ed) The Psychology of Reading, Attention and Performance XII: The Psychology of Reading. Erlbaum, Hillsdale, NJ: pp 363–383

O'Regan JK, Vitu F, Radach R, Kerr PW (1994) Effects of local processing and oculomotor factors in eye movement guidance in reading. In: Ygge J, Lennerstrand G (eds) Eye movements in reading. Pergamon Press, New York, pp 329–348

Radach R, Heller D, Wiebories P, Jaschinski W (1996) Binocular coordination, fixation disparity and ocular dominance. Perception 25 Supplement: 87

Radach R, McConkie G (1998) Determinants of fixation positions in reading. In: Underwood G (ed) Eye guidance in reading and scene perception. Elsevier, Oxford, pp 77–100

Rayner K (1979) Eye guidance in reading: Fixation locations within words. Perception 8: 21–30

Rayner K (1984) Visual selection in reading, picture perception and visual search: A tutorial review. In: Bouma E, Bouwhuis D (eds) Attention and Performance X. Control of language processes. Erlbaum, Hillsdale, N. J.,

Rayner K, Pollatsek A (1981) Eye movement control during reading: Evidence for direct control. Quarterly Journal of Experimental Psychology 33A: 351–373

Rayner K, Reichle ED, Pollatsek A (1998) Eye movement control in reading: An overview and a model. In: Underwood G (ed) Eye guidance in reading and scene perception. Elsevier, Oxford, pp 243–268

Rayner K, Sereno SC, Raney GE (1996) Eye movement control in reading: A comparison of two types of models. Journal of Experimental Psychology: Human Perception and Performance 22: 1188–1200

Schmidt WA (1917) An experimental study in the psychology of reading. A dissertation. Supplementary educational monographs 1. The University of Chicago press, Chicago, Il.

Vitu F, McConkie G (1998) On regressive saccades in reading. In: Underwood G (ed) Eye guidance in reading and scene perception. Elsevier, Oxford, pp 101–124

Ygge J, Jacobson C (1994) Asymmetrical saccades in reading. In: Ygge J, Lennerstrand G (eds) Eye movements in reading. Pergamon Press, New York, pp 301–314

Zee DS, Fitzgibbon EJ, Optician LM (1992) Saccade-vergence interactions in humans. Journal of Neurophysiology 68: 1624–1642

49

THE RETURN SWEEP IN READING

Jörg Hofmeister,[1*] Dieter Heller,[2] and Ralph Radach[2]

[1]University of Dundee
Department of Surgery
Ninewells Hospital and Medical School
Dundee DD1 9SY, Scotland
[2]Rheinisch-Westfälische Technische Hochschule Aachen
Institut für Psychologie I
Jägerstrasse 17-19, 52056 Aachen, Deutschland

1. INTRODUCTION

A comprehensive model of eye movement control in reading will have to take into consideration not only progressive and regressive inter- and intraword saccades, but also the large return sweep saccades that bring the eyes from the end of one line of text to the beginning of another line (Suppes 1994). In normal text, about 20 percent of all fixations are preceded or followed by a return sweep and the contribution of these fixations to total reading time is substantial. From the perspective of text design, the optimal line length is assumed to depend on the reader's ability to programme and execute an accurate return sweep and to avoid the costs of additional corrective saccades (Tinker 1963, Heller 1982). Given both theoretical and practical importance, surprisingly little is known about the parameters characterising return sweeps and the factors that control them. This chapter is an attempt towards closing this gap. We will first consider return sweeps as a special case of large goal-directed saccades and briefly look at previous findings. We will then present descriptive data on return sweep landing positions and the occurrence of corrective saccades and explore the effects of line length and text justification on these variables.

1.1. The Return Sweep in Reading: A Special Case of Large Goal-Directed Saccades

For almost a century, experimental psychologists and physiologists have been interested in the characteristics of saccadic eye movements. Many recent studies have focused

---
[*] UK; e-mail: j.hofmeister@dundee.ac.uk

Current Oculomotor Research, edited by Becker *et al.*
Plenum Press, New York, 1999.

on one specific aspect: with increasing amplitude, saccades tend to undershoot their target and are frequently followed by small corrective saccades, which bring the eye close to the target. In a typical experiment, subjects are asked to fixate an abruptly appearing target displayed somewhere in the visual field. Studies using this task showed a mean undershoot of about 10 % of the required movement amplitude (e.g. Becker 1972). Much smaller amplitude errors can be observed when targets are stationary at fixed positions (e.g. Lemij and Collewijn 1987).

The latencies of corrective saccades are in the order of 120–160 ms and therefore shorter than common oculomotor reaction times. Subjects are usually not aware of the fact that they make corrective saccades, which leads to the conclusion that they represent a reflex-like behaviour (see Deubel 1994). The reason for the saccadic undershoot found in most experiments is still not clear. The limited quality of the visual signal coding target position does not seem to be the primary cause (de Bie et al. 1987). There is now consensus that corrective saccades are visually guided, but extraretinal feedback comes into play when saccade errors are large (e.g. Becker 1976). At the end of the primary saccade, the deviation of the saccade landing position from the intended goal is calculated on the basis of retinal feedback. A corrective saccade is initiated if this deviation exceeds a certain value.

The majority of results concerning the characteristics of (large) saccades were obtained using simple paradigms including sudden target onsets in an otherwise rather unstructured visual field. One might argue that this is not a typical example of every-day oculomotor behaviour, which consists mainly of saccades to stationary objects. Scanning single points is not very "meaningful" and in this respect fundamentally different from a task like reading.

Here, the goal of a saccade is not given by instructions, but by the demands of text processing. It is important to note that during reading, saccade programming is a task secondary to the primary task of visually processing text information. The co-ordination of these two tasks and the degree to which they can be carried out in parallel are currently discussed in reading research (Rayner et al. 1998, Underwood and Radach 1998). It appears that because of the dual-task nature of reading, the oculomotor system is not operating at its maximum performance and systematic oculomotor error is an inherent feature of eye behaviour (Radach and McConkie 1998). Given these considerations, return sweeps may be an appropriate model of large goal-directed saccades in a visually well structured environment. Their analysis may lead to insights into the programming of large saccades, which might not be obtained by using simple laboratory tasks that require only little cognitive effort.

1.2. The Return Sweep in Reading: A Review of Previous Findings

Early investigations into the return sweep were motivated by applied questions. Tinker and co-workers analysed the influence of typographical factors on the readability of text (Tinker 1963). They found an increase in reading time for text with lines exceeding a certain length. The authors attributed this to a substantial increase in the occurrence of regressive saccades after the return sweep (Paterson and Tinker 1940). Heller (1982), who varied line length between 13 and 28 degrees, obtained similar results. For the shortest lines he observed corrective saccades in 10 % of all cases, increasing to 53 % for the longest lines. Mean latencies of corrective saccades were 138 ms. He also reported large interindividual variations for the probability of making corrections. For texts which were rated as difficult, he found slightly more corrective saccades following return sweeps as compared to easy texts. This relation also held when the number of fixations on the lines was taken as an indicator of text difficulty. The number of corrections also appeared to be a function of reading instruction: when asked to search for typing errors, subjects made more corrections after return sweeps than in normal reading (Heller 1982).

Netchine, Guihou, Greenbaum and Englander (1983) compared the characteristics of the return sweep for different age levels. Compared to adults, children showed considerably more corrective saccades. In many cases, they needed two or more corrective saccades to reach the left text margin. With increasing age, the frequency of corrective saccades decreased. When reading text in a foreign language they started to learn, children showed much more corrective saccades at line beginnings compared to reading in their native language. A similar result was observed for adults: native French readers with average English knowledge made significantly more corrections when they read English texts. Netchine et al. interpret their results in terms of the representation of the text layout. Since children make much more fixations during reading than adults (and adults make more fixations when reading text in a foreign language), this could hamper the representation of the spatial position of the text, thus making the programming of accurate saccades more difficult. A different explanation for the effects of text difficulty and reading skill was put forward by Heller (1982). He argues that both factors might lead to a narrowing of the perceptual span, thus decreasing the size of the visual field for which a correct return sweep can be programmed.

The last fixation on a line tends to be shorter than average fixation durations in reading. Abrams and Zuber (1972) reported mean latencies of 178 ms compared to 250 ms for reading fixations. They argue that the last fixation on a line does not have the primary purpose to gather text information, but to programme the return sweep. This view was supported by results from our laboratory: degrading text by removing about 50 % of all pixels on a CRT display led to an increase of average fixation durations of more than 20 ms, while the latencies of the return sweep remained the same (Hofmeister 1997).

If the return sweep is followed by a progressive saccade, the first fixation on the new line is of longer duration than average reading fixations (Dearborn 1906, Heller 1979). Explanations put forward for this phenomenon include extra time for establishing a mode of "grouped saccade programming" (Rayner 1978), vergence movements and a "period of orientation" after the return sweep, while the first unit of information is taken in and processed (Stern 1981).

Heller and Radach (1992) analysed return sweeps in 4 subjects reading a classic novel of about 48.000 words. On the basis of eye movement patterns and fixation duration distributions at the line beginning they estimated the optimal landing position for return sweeps at about letter position 3 to 4. Actual landing position distributions had their peaks significantly further to the right. This extends the common dissociation of preferred and optimal viewing position (see Radach and Kempe 1993, Vitu and O'Regan 1995, Rayner et al. 1998 for discussions) to the case of return sweeps. Radach and Heller (1993) showed that the landing position of the return sweep is independent of the length of the first word on the new line. Within the range of return sweep launch distances present in their left justified text format (55–72 letters), the frequency of corrections was a function of landing position (position error), irrespective of the actual return sweep amplitude.

2. GENERAL METHODS

Text was presented in black letters on a light grey background using a non-proportional font (Courier new). It was displayed on a 20" ELSA (Sony) GDM 2040 computer

Table 1. Return sweep and corrective saccade parameters as a function of line length. Fixation positions and saccade amplitudes are given in letters. Return sweep launch sites are calculated from the end of a line. Undershoot in % refers to the contribution of corrective saccades to the whole leftward movement. The table shows means and standard deviations

Line length	Return sweep launch position	Return sweep landing position	Frequency of corrections in %	Amplitude of corrections in letters	Undershoot in %
10 deg. (37 letters)	3.9 (2.5)	6.0 (2.1)	33	3.4 (1.4)	12.9
16 deg. (59 letters)	4.2 (3.2)	7.8 (2.9)	50	4.6 (2.0)	9.8
22 deg. (81 letters)	4.7 (3.4)	10.1 (3.9)	68	6.1 (2.4)	9.5

monitor refreshed at 75 Hz. An ELSA WINNER 2000 graphics card provided a resolution of 1024 * 768 pixels. Viewing distance was set to 77 cm. One letter equalled about 0.275 deg. of visual angle. Each text page consisted of 6–8 lines, which were presented approximately double-spaced. Eye movements were recorded with an AMTech pupil reflection eye tracker version 3 (exp. 1, sampling rate 200 Hz) and 4 (exp. 2, sampling rate 500 Hz). Earlier studies have shown that the absolute accuracy of recordings is better than 0.25 degree, which roughly corresponds to one character width in the current experiments. To minimise head movements, a bite board and a forehead rest were used. Measurements were monocular from the left eye. Before every 8–9 pages, a calibration routine was run. To encourage subjects to read the text properly, comprehension questions were asked after each experimental session.

Before averaging data across subjects, means for individual subjects were calculated. Reported standard deviations are averaged individual standard deviations. To exclude regressive saccades with large latencies after the return sweep (which might not be corrective saccades but regressive reading saccades), the following procedure was applied: minimum latency was set to 60 ms. At the right end of the latency distribution, all values beyond two standard deviations were rejected. This procedure was repeated until no more values had to be excluded.

3. EXPERIMENT 1: THE FREQUENCY OF CORRECTIVE SACCADES

The purpose of experiment 1 was twofold: to replicate and extend earlier results on return sweep amplitudes (landing positions) and to examine independently the influence of amplitude (line length) and landing position on the frequency of corrective saccades.

Text was presented in line length 10, 16 and 22 deg., corresponding to 37, 59 and 81 letters. 9 subjects took part in the experiment. Each participant read 50 pages of text in each condition, leading to about 300 return sweeps per line length. Table 1 shows return sweep and corrective saccade parameters as a function of line length.

Increasing line length leads to a substantial rightward shift of landing positions ($F[2;16] = 20.8$, $p < 0.001$) and the frequency and amplitudes of corrective saccades increase ($F[2;16] = 49.4$, $p < 0.001$; $F[2;16] = 24.5$, $p < 0.05$). Confirming earlier results (Heller 1982), the contribution of correctives saccades to the whole leftward movement was about 10 %. Table 2 compares fixation positions before and after corrective saccades with landing positions for return sweeps without corrections. Viewing positions after corrective

Table 2. Viewing positions after corrective saccades, return sweep landing positions for cases without following corrective saccades, and return sweep landing positions for cases with one or more following corrective saccades. The table shows means and standard deviations in letter positions

Line length	Viewing position after corrective saccades	Return sweep landing position - no corrections	Return sweep landing position - 1 or more corrections
10 deg. (37 letters)	3.9 (1.3)	5.1 (1.7)	7.4 (1.9)
16 deg. (59 letters)	4.4 (1.4)	5.7 (1.9)	9.3 (2.7)
22 deg. (81 letters)	4.4 (1.5)	6.1 (2.9)	11.1 (3.4)

saccades are nearer to the left line margin than uncorrected return sweep landing positions (F[1;8] = 25.6, p < 0.001). Few return sweeps were followed by more than one corrective saccade. The values are 6% for line length 10 deg., 8% for 16 deg. and 13% for 22 deg.

While it is evident that the frequency of corrective saccades increases with increasing line length and for rightward shifted return sweep landing positions, it is a different question if there are differences between lines of different length for a given landing position. If the only factor influencing the decision to make a correction is retinal feedback, it should make no difference whether return sweeps landing e.g. at letter position 6 originate from a relatively near or relatively far starting position. To answer this question, we determined the frequency of corrective saccades as a function of line length for identical landing positions. Figure 1 shows these frequencies for subjects and return sweep landing positions for all cases where at least 15 observations for each line length were available. The figure shows that the frequency of corrective saccades tends to be higher for longer lines. Clearly, the decision to make a corrective saccade is not only a function of the magnitude of the undershoot, but also depends on target distance.

4. EXPERIMENT 2: EFFECTS OF TEXT JUSTIFICATION

This study aimed at determining the nature of the visuospatial information used to programme the return sweep. It can bee seen as a specific aspect of the more general ques-

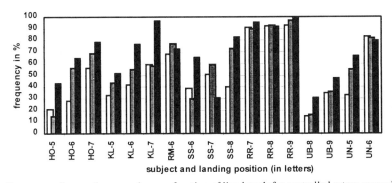

Figure 1. Frequency of corrective saccades as a function of line length for controlled return sweep landing sites. As an example, the leftmost 3 bars show the frequency of corrective saccades for subject HO for return sweep landing sites at letter position 5 for line length 10 (open boxes), 16 (grey boxes) and 22 (black boxes) degrees. The figure includes only cases in which at least 15 observations were available per subject and landing position.

tion of what type of reference system is used to navigate across a page of text (Kennedy 1992). One theoretical position states that a representation of the spatial text coordinates (e.g. left and right margins) is build up during the initial phase of reading, which is subsequently used to make pre-programmed return sweeps. This position was advocated by Leisman (1978), who proposed a relatively quick transition from *position anticipation*, the programming of sequential saccades to *position expectation*, the establishment of a set of spatial locations used to execute a fixed, reoccurring saccade program. We will call this proposal the spatial map hypothesis. The opposite theoretical position would be that each return sweep is programmed separately on the basis of visual information acquired during the last fixation on each line. The spatial map hypothesis can be tested by varying text justification. Position expectation should work best when text is left and right justified. At the other extreme, when text is right justified, but left unjustified, the spatial map hypothesis predicts difficulties, including an increase of return sweep latency and increased amplitude variability and error, perhaps with a tendency to execute saccades towards the average line beginning.

Text was formatted in four different layouts. Right justified text with a line length of 59 letters (16 deg.) was compared to two unjustified layouts, presented with a maximum deviation of ± 3 and ± 6 letters, respectively, from the line length of the justified text. Additionally, text was formatted right justified but left unjustified. Mean line length was 59 characters for all formats. Figure 2 shows an example of the different layouts. 9 subjects

1) left and right justified

In der Ethologie wird zur Zeit eine interessante Diskussion
darüber geführt, ab welchem Punkt man Lebewesen wohl Denken
und Bewußtsein zubilligen darf. Ganz bestimmt ist dafür die
...

2) right unjustified ±3 letters

Die Puppen des Katzenflohs benutzen Bodenvibrationen auf
ziemlich hinterhältige Weise. Sie liegen regungslos im Teppich
verborgen, bis ein schwaches Zittern ihnen anzeigt, daß ihr
anvisierter Wirt, die Katze, nun in Anmarsch ist. Sie springen
das ahnungslose Opfer an, wobei die letzte Phase von der
Körperwärme und vom Kohlendioxyd in seinem Atem gesteuert wird.

3) righ unjustified ±6 letters

Die Papillen im mittleren Bereich tragen dagegen nach
hinten gerichtete Härchen und stehen mit einer chemischen Analyse
der Nahrung nicht in Zusammenhang. Sie geben der Oberfläche
der Zunge die Struktur eines Reibeisens; und sie sind
von Nutzen, um das Fell zu pflegen, Flüssigkeit aufzunehmen
und das Fleisch von den Rippen der Beute zu schaben.

4) left unjustified

Diesen Zelltyp gibt es ausschließlich in der Nase, und er wird
im Mittel ungefähr alle dreißig Tage erneuert. Auch dadurch
unterscheidet er sich ganz eindeutig von allen sonstigen
Nerven- oder Rezeptorzellen des Körpers, die nie mehr erneuert
werden, falls sie einmal den Geist aufgegeben haben. Das
Riechfeld ist gelb, feucht und enthält fetthaltige Stoffe.

Figure 2. Example of the different text formats.

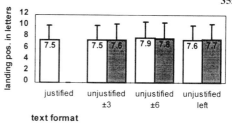

Figure 3. Return sweep landing positions in letters for the different text formats. Results are given for lines with 59 characters (open boxes) and for all lines (grey boxes). Error bars represent standard deviations.

took part in the experiment. Each participant read 25 pages of text in each condition, leading to about 150 return sweeps for each layout.

Figure 3 shows the mean return sweep landing positions for the four layouts (separately for lines with 59 characters and for all lines). Standard deviations are depicted as error bars. Apparently, text format has only very small and non-significant effects on return sweep landing positions (F[3;24] < 1). More importantly, the same accounts for the variability of return sweep endpoints (standard deviations), which show no effect of text layout (F[3;24] < 1). In the case of left unjustified text, no overshoots to the left of the line margin were found, indicating that these saccades were programmed individually on the basis of visual information. Similar results were found for the frequency of corrective saccades. Figure 4 shows small, non-significant differences, the right justified text leading to the smallest number of corrections (F[3;24] = 1.07, n.s.).

Even if the accuracy of the return sweep is not influenced by text justification, it may still take more time to programme the return sweep for unjustified text compared to the justified format. Figure 5 shows the fixation durations preceding the return sweep. The durations are shortest for the right justified text, however, the differences are not statistically significant (F[3;24] = 2.4, n.s.). The difference between right justified and left unjustified text, for which the programming of the return sweep should be most difficult, is only 7 ms.

5. DISCUSSION

The first experiment provided evidence for two sources of influence on return sweep landing positions and the frequency of corrective saccades: First, for longer lines, landing positions shift to the right, retinal errors are increased and, hence, more corrections are made. Second, when looking at identical landing positions, there still is a higher probability for making a corrective saccade when coming from a more distant line ending.

There are two possible reasons why this line lenght effect was not found by Radach and Heller (1993). In their study, variation of line lenght was only in the order of what is usually found in left justified text as displayed by current text processors. Also, as rela-

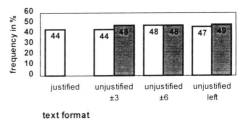

Figure 4. Frequency of corrective saccades after the return sweep for the different text formats in %. Results are given for lines with 59 characters and for all lines.

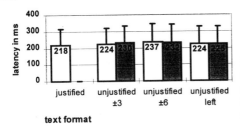

Figure 5. Duration of fixations preceding the return sweep for the different text formats in ms. Results are given for lines with 59 characters (open boxes) and for all lines (grey boxes). Error bars represent standard deviations.

tively long and short lines were mixed on the same pages, there was no opportunity for an adjustment of a general decision criterion.

In the second experiment the accuracy of the return sweep was not better for right justified text compared to different unjustified formats. Our finding of no differences between double justified and left justified text is not in harmony with Keenan (1984), who reported that when lines are broken at syntactic phrase boundaries, the resulting line legth variability leads to a decrease in reading speed. The author attributed this finding, in accordance with Leisman's (1978) hypothesis, to an increase of return sweep error and the frequency of corrective saccades. The difference in results might be attributed to the more extreme and unusual variation of line length in Keenan's experiment. We conclude from our results that right unjustified text with up to ± 6 letters variation does not impair planning and execution of return sweeps. The result of no difference in return sweep accuracy even holds for left unjustified text. For this condition, no overshoots were found, indicating that the return sweep was not programmed on the basis of the average line length. Interestingly, one subject remarked spontaneously that he did not have the impression to "see" the left line margin when reading the left unjustified text. Moreover, it is not more difficult to programme the return sweep for this rather unusual format, since mean fixation durations preceding the return sweep differed only by 7ms between the right justified and left unjustified format. Given the very small overall differences between the different text formats, the spatial map hypothesis as suggested by Leisman (1978) must be rejected. Obviously, the return sweep is programmed on the basis of visual information taken in during the last fixation(s) on a line of text.

ACKNOWLEDGMENTS

The research reported in this paper was supported by a scholarship given to the first author by the "Stiftung Volkswagenwerk". We wish to thank B. Eulenstein for programming and technical support.

REFERENCES

Abrams S G, Zuber B L (1972) Some temporal characteristics of information processing during reading. Reading Res Quart 8: 40–51
Becker W (1972) The control of eye movements in the saccadic system. Bibl Ophthalmol 82: 233–243
Becker W (1976) Do correction saccades depend exclusively on retinal feedback? A note on the possible role of non-retinal feedback. Vision Res 16: 425–427
de Bie J, van den Brink G, van Sonderen J F (1987) The systematic undershoot of saccades: A localization or an oculomotor phenomenon? In: O'Regan J K, Lévy-Schoen A (eds) Eye movements: From physiology to cognition. Elsevier, Amsterdam, pp 85–94
Dearborn W F (1906) The psychology of reading. Archives of Philosophy, Psychology, and Scientific Methods

Deubel H (1994) The anatomy of a single refixation. Unpublished habilitation thesis. Ludwig Maximilians Universität, München

Heller D (1979) Augenbewegungen bei legasthenischen und normal lesenden Kindern. (Eye movements in dyslexic and normal children.) Z. Psychol 187: 106–115

Heller D (1982) Eye movements in reading. In: Groner R, Fraisse P (eds) Cognition and eye movements. Deutscher Verlag der Wissenschaften, Berlin, pp 139–154

Heller D (1987) Typographical characteristics and reading. In: O'Regan J K, Lévy-Schoen A (eds) Eye movements: From physiology to cognition. Elsevier, Amsterdam, pp 487–498

Heller D, Radach R (1992) Returning to an unanswered question: On the role of corrective saccades in text reading (Abstract). Internat J Psychol 27: 55

Hofmeister J (1997) Über Korrektursakkaden beim Lesen von Texten und bei leseähnlichen Aufgaben. (On corrective saccades in reading and reading-like tasks.) Unpublished doctoral dissertation. Rheinisch-Westfälische Technische Hochschule, Aachen

Keenan S A (1984) Effects of chunking and line length on reading efficiency. Visible lang XVIII 1: 61–80

Kennedy A (1992) The spatial coding hypothesis. In: Rayner K (ed) Eye movements and visual cognition: Scene perception and reading. Springer, New York, pp 379–396

Leisman G (1978) Ocular-motor system control of position anticipation and expectancy. In: Senders J W, Fisher D F, Monty R A (eds), Eye movements and higher psychological functions. Erlbaum, Hillsdale N.J., pp 195–207

Lemij H G, Collewijn H (1989) Differences in accuracy of human saccades between stationary and jumping saccades. Vision Res 29: 1737–1748

Netchine S, Giuhou M-C, Greenbaum C, Englander G (1983) Retour a la ligne, age des lecteurs et accessibilité au texte. Travail hum 46: 139–153

O'Regan, J K (1990) Eye movements and reading. In: Kowler E (ed) Eye movements and their role in visual and cognitive processes. Elsevier, Amsterdam, pp 395–453

Paterson D G, Tinker M A (1940) Influence of line width on eye movements. J Exp Psychol 27: 372–377

Radach R, Kempe V (1993) An individual analysis of fixation positions in reading. In: d'Ydevalle G, van Rensbergen J (eds) Perception and Cognition. Advances in eye movement research. Elsevier, Amsterdam, pp 213–225

Radach R, Heller D (1993) Zeilenrücksprünge und Korrektursakkaden beim Lesen von Texten. (Return sweeps and corrective saccades in reading.) Paper, presented at the 36th conference of experimentally working psychologists in Münster/Germany

Radach R, McConkie G (1998, in press) Determinants of fixation positions in reading. In: Underwood G (ed) Eye guidance in reading and scene perception. Elsevier, Oxford

Rayner K (1978) Eye movements in reading and information processing. Psychol Bull 85: 618–660

Rayner K, Reichle E D, Pollatsek A (1998, in press) Eye movement control in reading: An overview and a model. In Underwood G (ed) Eye guidance in reading and scene perception. Elsevier, Oxford

Stern J A (1981) Eye movements, reading and cognition. In: Senders J W, Fisher D F, Monty R A (eds) Eye movements and higher psychological functions. Erlbaum, Hillsdale N.J., pp 145–155

Suppes P (1994) Stochastic models of reading. In: Ygge J, Lennerstrand G (eds) Eye movements in reading. Pergamon Press, New York, pp 349–364

Tinker MA (1963) Legibility of print. Iowa State University Press, Ames

Underwood G, Radach R (1998, in press) Eye guidance and visual information processing: Reading, visual search, picture perception and driving. In: Underwood G (ed) Eye guidance in reading and scene perception. Elsevier, Oxford

Vitu F, O'Regan K (1995) A challenge to current theories of eye movements in reading. In: Findlay J M, Walker R, Kentridge R W (eds) Eye movement research: processes, mechanisms and applications. Elsevier, Amsterdam, pp 381–392

50

PARAFOVEAL-ON-FOVEAL EFFECTS IN READING AND WORD RECOGNITION

Alan Kennedy

Psychology Department
University of Dundee

1. 'ATTENTION-SWITCHING' AND EYE MOVEMENT CONTROL IN READING

In this Chapter, I want to raise some questions concerning the 'attention-switching' model of eye movement control in reading first proposed by Morrison (1984). A basic assumption of this model is that after a criterion level of processing has been reached on a given word n (for example, lexical access), attention will shift discretely to the next word, $n+1$, while the eyes remain fixating n. At the same time as this attentional shift takes place, an eye movement is programmed towards word $n+1$. Thus, for a period of time, a reader may be fixating word n, preparing to make a saccade, and processing word $n+1$. If the processing of word $n+1$ is completed before the saccade takes place, a further switch of attention (to word $n+2$) may occur and a second saccade will be programmed, in parallel with the first. The way the oculomotor system deals with simultaneous programming of more than one saccade depends on their relative timing (Becker and Jurgens 1979). If the trigger commands are widely separated in time, both saccades may be executed, but the duration of the fixation following the first may be drastically reduced. If the delay is short, only the second saccade will be initiated. Between these limits, a 'compromise' saccade may be launched, to an intermediate target position.

In recent years, one or another variant of attention-switching has become the canonical model of eye movement control (Rayner et al.1996). However, the original formulation by Morrison required fairly substantial revision to deal with a number of challenges. The most obvious weakness relates to the occurrence of refixations. Since the fundamental attentional switch is between-words (in a 'forward' direction), the kind of regressive saccades commonly associated with syntactic repair operations or with the resolution of anaphor are not predicted and cannot easily be accounted for. Similarly, refixation *within* a word can only occur under rather unusual conditions, through the accident of a 'compromise' saccade falling short of its target in an adjacent word. It seems improbable that this

Current Oculomotor Research, edited by Becker *et al.*
Plenum Press, New York, 1999.

would occur often enough to produce refixation rates as high as those typically found (i.e. 10 - 14 percent of fixations). There are also difficulties accounting for the duration of successive fixations, when two or more occur on a word. Although the model makes no specific predictions about refixations, the operation of an attention-switching device suggests that, if a word is fixated twice, the first fixation should be longer than the second. In fact, the reverse is usually found (Vitu and O'Regan 1995).

A further concern relates to the role played by parafoveal processing. There is overwhelming evidence that a word which has been previewed in parafoveal vision is processed faster when it is eventually fixated (see Rayner and Pollatsek 1989, for a review). At first sight, this seems to arise quite naturally from the proposed de-coupling of attention and eye position. Word $n+1$ will be allocated covert attention (and hence processed to some degree) while the eyes remain fixated on word n, and it is not unreasonable to expect this processing to be cashed in when word $n+1$ eventually shifts into the fovea. The problem is that any preview advantage secured this way should simply be a function of the time to prepare an interword saccade. That is, it should be more or less constant and unaffected by properties of word n itself. As Henderson and Ferriera (1990) showed, this is not the case: preview advantage is greatly reduced, or even eliminated, if the foveal stimulus is difficult. There have been various attempts to deal with this problem, while preserving the overall integrity of the theoretical approach. Henderson and Ferriera themselves postulated a processing deadline, beyond which an eye movement must inevitably occur. With this addition, and by the exercise of some theoretical ingenuity, it becomes possible to predict effects of foveal load on the size of preview advantage The argument is as follows: if a fixated word is particularly hard to process, the deadline will expire before attention shifts and a saccade will be launched, but with a target within the current word, since that is where attention remains directed. Crucially, on those occasions where this refixation is cancelled, the time taken to programme the second saccade will not be available for parafoveal processing.

There is, in fact, not much empirical evidence that the operation of a saccade programming deadline is responsible for the obtained foveal-on-parafoveal interaction. As Schroyens et al. (1998) point out, the reduced preview benefit should only be associated with 'cancelled refixation' cases, where there is a single fixation of word n. If a word is actually refixated, the preview advantage should return to its predicted value, equivalent to the normal saccade programming time, and no interaction with foveal load should be found. Although Schroyens et al. replicate the finding that the preview advantage is smaller for difficult foveal words, the effect was not restricted to 'single-fixation' cases. Much the same conclusion was drawn by Kennison and Clifton (1995) who failed to show any hint of bimodality in the distributions of single fixation durations on word n, such as would be found if a deadline were operating.

Reichle et al. (1998) have recently suggested that this failure to offer a convincing account of foveal-on-parafoveal effects is symptomatic of a more general difficulty, arising from the proposal that the trigger for an attentional shift is completion of processing on the currently-fixated word. There is something inherently implausible in a model which allows for no spillover effects, difficulty processing word n being inherited as part of the processing load on word $n+1$. Reichle et al. make the alternative suggestion that the trigger for an eye movement and the trigger for an attentional shift are not be the same cognitive event. In their 'E-Z Reader' model, an eye movement is programmed as soon as a pre-lexical 'familiarity check' on the fixated word is completed. The crucial attentional shift to word $n+1$ occurs later, on completion of lexical access. The E-Z Reader model represents the most sophisticated incarnation to date of the attention-switching approach. It produces a reasonably good fit to observations of fixation duration and refixation rate as a function of word frequency and elegantly handles most of the difficulties noted above. In addition, the model predicts the occurrence of both 'word-skipping' and short-duration fixations. To the degree that it is quantitative (i.e. implemented as a form of transition network in a computer model) it also has distinct advantages over purely qualitative models, such as that of O'Regan and Levy-Schoen (1987). It is nonetheless, not immune from two general criticisms which fall on all attention-switching models. I will consider these in turn.

First, making an attentional shift no longer contingent on completion of lexical access is a clear improvement and leads to a more satisfactory treatment of refixations. But a great deal still hinges on the concept of 'attention' itself, which is notoriously vague. Reichle et al. discuss, and reject, the idea that some form of 'process monitoring' might play a role in eye movement control, stating "[we]...assume that the signal to move the eyes is the successful completion of a psychological process (such as lexical access). In particular, we wanted to avoid having to posit that decisions to move or not the eyes are based on noticing that one is having difficulty in extracting information". But the question arises as to whether the operation of 'attention' has actually achieved this degree of processing autonomy, or whether, in fact, it has simply smuggled in much the same sort of cognitive work under another name. Until it is clear *how* action flows from the output of an attentional device, it remains seriously under-specified. Second, it is far from clear whether the terms 'foveal' and 'parafoveal' actually support the processing distinction asked of them. Eye movement control in reading is relatively invariant over viewing distance (O'Regan 1990) and it could plausibly be argued that the terms simply denote the trivial distinction between 'currently fixated' and 'to-be-fixated' words. But acuity varies continuously across the visual field and the influence of this fact on processing efficiency is far from trivial (Bouma 1971,1973; O'Regan 1989). For example, information from two degrees to the right of fixation becomes available 90–100 msec later than information one degree to the right (Schiepers 1980), raising the question as to whether it is sensible to characterise 'attention-switching' as essentially discrete? The fact is, each fixation is followed by a train of events in which stimulus information becomes available, over time, across the visual field. Thus, even if some early familiarity check at the point of fixation *permits* an eye movement to be programmed, the specification of its target will be a function of the duration of the current fixation. Considerations such as these have drawn several research groups to reconsider the process of attention-switching and question some of its fundamental assumptions. For example, do 'word objects' constitute the primary visual stimulus in reading and, if so, are they necessarily processed serially? Is the search for the critical cognitive event (pre-lexical check, lexical access etc.), which triggers the switch of attention well-motivated or are we simply chasing yet another elusive 'magic moment' (Balota 1990)?

2. PARALLEL PROCESSING?

A defensible alternative view is that processing occurs across the visual field as a whole and in parallel. This is not to deny the privileged status of the fovea, since it is over this region that high-quality feature information becomes rapidly available. But information from other regions of the visual field is also available, with varying degrees of specificity, and may influence processing throughout each fixation (Schiepers 1980). By abandoning the notion of processing as an autonomous serial process, we open up the possibility that mutual processing interactions take place between successive words. Up to the present, the evidence for this kind of "cross-talk" has been rather unclear. Carpenter and Just (1983) used linear regression techniques to partition variance in gaze duration between a number of measures, including length and word frequency, and concluded that features of word $n+1$ had negligible effects on fixation times on word n. The problem with this conclusion, however, is that they also failed to show the well-established modulation of preview effect, in the form of n and $n-1$ interactions, as reported by Henderson and Ferriera (1990). It is possible that the regression technique is simply too insensitive to address this issue. A more systematic laboratory study was carried out by Henderson and Ferreira (1993), who manipulated the frequency of successive words embedded in short sentences. The results showed that foveal inspection time was actually (non-significantly) *shorter* for a low frequency parafoveal word than for a high frequency one (244 vs. 252 msec). The experiment showed a clear preview effect, so there was little doubt that parafoveal words were processed during foveal inspection, but it appeared that the parafoveal information was only extracted *following* processing of a foveal word. On the other hand, it could be argued that the obtained modulation in foveal inspection time provided poor support for the null hypothesis, since a parallel processing account actually predicts a processing trade-off, consistent with the obtained 'inverted' outcome.

3. THE 'LOOKS-MEANS' TASK

I have recently revisited this question of parafoveal-on-foveal effects, using a laboratory task and manipulating both lexical and sub-lexical properties of target words (Kennedy 1998). The experimental task was the 'looks-means' decision task described by Kennedy and Murray (1997). In this, participants viewed a fixation marker which was then replaced by a string of three words, the marker ensuring initial fixation on the third letter of the initial 'prompt' word, which was invariably either the word 'looks' or the word 'means'. Depending on which of these two prompt words was presented, participants judged whether the following two words had the same spelling or the same meaning. Properties of the second word were systematically manipulated, crossing word frequency, initial trigram 'informativeness' (defined by the number of words sharing the initial trigram), and trigram token frequency, or 'familiarity', (for further discussion of these terms see Pynte et al. 1995). For example, 'arena' is a word of low frequency, with few other words sharing its initial trigram, but with very 'familiar' initial letters. These three factors were systematically manipulated for targets either five- or nine-letters in length.

Even for this simple experimental task, eye movement behaviour was remarkably complex. The most notable feature was that refixations of the prompt word occurred and these were directly related to properties of the parafoveal target word. The direction of the effects was unexpected in some respects: there was a (non-significant) tendency for more prompt refixations if the target was a short, low frequency, word (high frequency = 0.15; low frequency = 0.18). This could be considered a conventional frequency effect, albeit relating to an as-yet unfixated word. But for long targets, there were significantly more refixations with high frequency words (high frequency = 0.17; low frequency = 0.13) [*]. This pattern of results attaches a special significance to long, low frequency, targets, where the probability of refixating the prompt was unexpectedly low. The measure of gaze duration on the prompt answers the question as to whether a low refixation rate was compensated

---

[*] unless otherwise stated, all differences reported were significant (p < 0.05) for F1 and F2

by longer inspection time. This is quite clearly not the case: prompt gaze associated with long, low frequency, targets was significantly shorter than in other conditions. Obviously, we have here *prima facie* evidence that the frequency of an unfixated word $n+1$ can influence behaviour on word n, but the measure of gaze duration is difficult to interpret, since refixations act to bring the eyes very close to the target word, drastically changing its visibility. This point can be met by analyses restricted single fixations on the prompt (around 85 percent of the data). In this case, no significant effects of target word frequency were evident, but there was significant effect of both the length and the 'informativeness' of the unfixated target. Long targets continued to be associated with shorter prompt fixation duration than short targets (266 msec vs 258 msec). In addition, targets with 'uninformative' initial letters were associated with short prompt fixation, although this was only the case for long words (high initial trigram frequency = 244 msec; low = 272 msec). In the case of short words, there was no difference (265 msec vs 267 msec). There were no effects of target 'familiarity'.

This pattern of results can be interpreted in terms of a single mechanism: time spent fixating a word is modulated by the difficulty of an adjacent word. 'Difficulty' can be defined in terms of visibility (long words are less readily perceived in parafoveal vision), frequency, or informativeness. A difficult stimulus configuration at $n+1$ is associated with a reduced inspection time at n. In contrast, if information relating to $n+1$ can be acquired rapidly, the pattern of results suggests an inflated inspection time or a within-word shift, inching the reader closer to the parafoveal stimulus without actually triggering an inter-word saccade. In looking for the critical trigger for an inter-word saccade it is difficult to avoid a process-monitoring account, with inspection time on n modulated by the rate of acquisition of parafoveal information (either lexical or sublexical) from $n+1$. The effects are quite small (which may be another reason why Carpenter and Just (1983) did not find them), but are statistically reliable. They are not compatible with the notion of attention-switching, but can be readily accommodated by a model in which foveal and parafoveal processing occurs in parallel. Analyses of fixation times on the target word itself support this conclusion, with clear evidence of a processing trade-off. Extended time processing the prompt was reflected in shorter foveal target processing time and vice-versa, with a significant negative correlation between fixation duration on the prompt and target words.

This interpretation of the results is plausible, but before it can be accepted, it is necessary to consider two significant objections. First, the experimental task is simply not a convincing analogue of normal reading. It is ominous that some of the more robust and reproducible eye movement effects found in studies of words viewed in isolation (e.g. the effects of word frequency on fixation duration or the effect of initial landing position on gaze or refixation rate), become diluted, or at least statistically much less reliable, when examined in the context of normal reading (Rayner 1995). It follows that a question mark inevitably hangs over any claims regarding eye movement control in reading which rest on the use of highly simplified laboratory tasks. A second, more technical objection, relates to the low foveal load in the task. It might be more accurate to describe the prompt as presenting a zero load, in that a decision could be made, in principle, without even reading it. There are theoretically plausible counters to this, in particular, the claim that word-identification is mandatory (Murray 1982), but it remains true that generalising to normal reading from a task in which the same word n is seen over a hundred times is questionable. I will conclude this Chapter by addressing this issue in two ways. First, by an examination of parafoveal-on-foveal effects in a large corpus of eye movement data derived from normal reading; and second, by a modification of the laboratory task.

4. PARALLEL PROCESSING IN NORMAL READING: A CORPUS ANALYSIS

The most direct way of responding to objections based on claims regarding the low ecological validity of the laboratory task is to examine word-on-word interactions in normal reading. I have recently undertaken this task in collaboration with Ralph Radach[*] using his corpus of eye movement recordings derived from four native German-speakers as they read about half of *Gulliver's Travels*. The corpus (Radach 1996) comprises around 50,000 fixations and saccades for each reader, together with letter and word frequency information generated from the text itself and also from the German CELEX corpus (Celex 1995). Cases were identified in which a word (n) received a single fixation and its fixation duration was then computed as function of the length, word frequency and trigram informativeness of the word lying immediately to its right ($n+1$). Data were entered into the analyses for words 5–8 letters in length, with a frequency greater than 100 per million. Launch position into n was never greater than 15 characters to its left and data were restricted to cases where landing position on n was more or less centred. Since word frequency and word length were highly correlated, word and trigram frequency data were computed as quartiles for each word length separately. To assess the validity of the experimental data reported above, fixation time on a given word n (restricted to cases receiving a single fixation) was examined as a function of three properties of $n+1$: its length, its word frequency and its 'informativeness'.

There was clear evidence that fixation duration on word n was modulated by the length of $n+1$, with an 'inverted' effect similar to that found in the laboratory task. Fixation duration on n was shorter when $n+1$ was long and this was true regardless of the length of n itself. Thus, fixation duration on a short word was 248 msec when the next word was long (7 - 10 letters) and 264 msec when the next word was short (4 letters). For cases where n was longer, the same influence was evident (long $n+1$ = 274 msec, short $n+1$ = 284 msec). There were insufficient cases to allow word frequency and initial trigram frequency to be crossed in the design and analyses of these were carried out independently, using a total of approximately 5200 cases in each case. There was an overall word frequency effect, with current fixation duration modulated as a function of properties of an adjacent parafoveal word (low = 277 msec, high = 263 msec). It will be recalled that a trend in this direction was only found in the laboratory task data when the target was short and refixations might have brought the eyes very close to it. Unfortunately in a corpus analysis attempts to partition the data to address such questions leads to a rapid loss of cases. Turning to the question of the effects of trigram frequency, the duration of single fixations on a given word n also changed as a function of the frequency of the initial trigram of word $n+1$. Frequent trigrams were associated with shorter fixation duration (low = 277 msec, high = 266 msec). This outcome accords with the results of the experimental data for long targets, where possibly only the initial letters would be clearly visible, and further supports the suggestion that fixation duration on word n is modulated by sub-lexical properties of word $n+1$. The direction of the effect suggests that an inter-word saccade may be launched earlier if the number of lexical 'candidates' for the next word is relatively large. Clearly, parallel processing of this form cannot be accounted for in terms of

---

[*] I am grateful to Ralph Radach for making available his corpus of eye movement data and for many insightful comments on the analyses

an attention-switching model, if it is assumed that processing on word n is wrapped up before work on $n+1$ commences.

5. PARALLEL PROCESSING IN A SEARCH TASK

The corpus data answer doubts about the ecological validity of the laboratory task quite satisfactorily, but have limitations. It is only possible to estimate statistical significance by items and a factorial analysis of the relevant variables (i.e. length, word frequency and informativeness) is not feasible. In an attempt to address these issues, a further laboratory study has been completed, attempting to eliminate problems caused by continual repetition of a single prompt word. The experimental task employed *different* prompt words on each trial. The procedure made use of the 'clothing-search' task used by Schroyens et al. (1998). As before, each trial began with a fixation marker, followed by a display of three words, initial fixation being located at letter-position three of the first word. Participants were instructed to make a series of eye movements from word to word and to press a button if they detected an article of clothing. The first (prompt) word was a randomly selected, high-frequency, five-letter word. The crucial experimental items were displayed as the second stimulus word, using the same set of five-letter and nine-letter targets. A completely different random allocation of prompt words to experimental targets was used for each participant. Words classed as articles of clothing were very rare and were distributed randomly between the three display positions.

There was again a highly significant effect of the length of the target word ($n+1$) on prompt (word n) fixation duration, with shorter fixation times on the prompt (272 msec) when the target was long than when it was short (293 msec). The effects of word frequency and trigram informativeness were more complex and are summarised in Table 1.

Although the prompt was refixated around 10 percent of the time, refixations in this task were not significantly associated with any of the manipulated variables. Nonetheless, Table 1 shows 'single fixation' data to allow comparison with the 'looks-means' decision task. Each of the measures in Table 1 showed a significant interaction between word frequency and trigram informativeness (there were no effects of target 'familiarity'). In the case of prompt inspection time (gaze), the Table shows a single value significantly shorter than the other three: low frequency targets with rare initial trigrams were associated with relatively short prompt inspection time. The form of this frequency effect is again 'inverted', with shorter duration associated with the low frequency items. Interestingly, the difference is of the same order of magnitude as the, non-significant, effect reported by Henderson and Ferreira (1993). Inspection of behaviour on the target itself also suggests a trade-off, since gaze duration was longer in the equivalent cell. Overall, the effect of low

Table 1. Fixation duration (msec) on the prompt word ('single fixation' cases) as a function of the word frequency (WF) and initial trigram frequency (TF) of the target word. High initial trigram frequency equates to an 'uninformative' initial letter sequence. First fixation duration and gaze duration on the target are also shown

	Prompt gaze duration		Target first fixation duration		Target gaze duration	
	High TF	Low TF	High TF	Low TF	High TF	Low TF
High WF	289	292	256	253	289	278
Low WF	288	281	255	262	295	303

word frequency appeared the dominant variable influencing prompt gaze duration. The main effect of Trigram Informativeness, which runs against the trends evident in both the 'looks-means' task and the corpus analysis, was not significant. It is the case, of course, that an effect of word frequency is implausible for long target words and, although there was no statistical interaction with Target Length, separate analyses of the two lengths confirmed that the effect was confined to short target words, with no effects attributable to long targets.

6. CONCLUSIONS

The data reveal a significant effect of the length of a parafoveal target $n+1$ on inspection time on n. Although this outcome has not previously been reported, it was present in all three tasks under consideration, and appears ubiquitous. The direction of the effect suggests an inflation of inspection time if $n+1$ is short and, consequently, more likely to be identified. The effects of word frequency and informativeness of $n+1$ were less consistent, but conform to a pattern. If a parafoveal word $n+1$ is 'difficult', inspection time on word n is also reduced. For short targets, the most potent influence here is not the token 'familiarity' of word $n+1$, which exerted little or no influence, but its frequency. When word $n+1$ is of low frequency, time on word n is slightly shorter. The data also suggest that sub-lexical properties play the same role, but only if the target is long. In this case, targets with many neighbours (when identification may be difficult) induces an inter-word saccade earlier than targets with few.

REFERENCES

Balota D A (1990) The role of meaning in word recognition. In: Balota D A, Flores d'Arcais G B, Rayner K (eds) Comprehension processes in reading. Erlbaum, Hillsdale N.J., pp 9–32

Becker W, Jürgens R (1979) An analysis of the saccadic system by means of double-step stimuli. Vision Res 19: 967–983

Bouma H (1971) Visual recognition of isolated lower case letters. Vision Res 11: 459–474

Bouma H (1973) Visual interference in the parafoveal recognition of initial and final letters of words. Vision Res 13: 767–782

CELEX German database (1995) Release D25. Nijmegen Centre for Lexical Information

Henderson J M, Ferreira F (1990) Effects of foveal processing difficulty on the perceptual span in reading: Implications for attention and eye movement control. J Exp Psychol Learn Mem Cognit 16: 417–429

Henderson J M, Ferreira F (1993) Eye movement control during reading: Fixation measures foveal but not parafoveal processing difficulty. Can J Exp Psychol 47: 201–221

Kennedy A (1998) The influence of parafoveal words on foveal inspection time: evidence for a processing trade-off. In: Underwood G (ed) Eye guidance in reading, driving and scene perception. Oxford, Elsevier (in press)

Kennedy A, Murray W S (1996) Eye movement control during the inspection of words under conditions of pulsating illumination. Eur J Cognit Psychol 8: 381–403

Kennison S M, Clifton C (1995) Determinants of parafoveal preview benefit in high and low working memory capacity readers: Implications for eye movement control. J Exp Psychol Learn Mem Cognit 21: 68–81

Morrison R E (1984) Manipulation of stimulus onset delay in reading: Evidence for parallel programming of saccades. J Exp Psychol Hum Percept Perform 10: 667–682

Murray W S (1982) Sentence matching: The influence of meaning and structure. Unpublished PhD Thesis Monash University, Australia

Murray W S, Rowan M (1998) Early, Mandatory, Pragmatic Processing. J Psycholing Res 27: 1–22

O'Regan J K (1989) Visual acuity, lexical structure and eye movements in word recognition. In: Elsendoorn B, Bouma H (eds) Working models of human perception. London, Academic Press, pp 261–292

O'Regan J K (1990) Eye movements and reading. In: Kowler E (ed.) Eye movements and their role in visual and cognitive processes. Amsterdam, Elsevier, pp 395–453

O'Regan J K, Levy-Schoen A (1987) Eye movement strategy and tactics in word-recognition and reading. In: Coltheart M (ed) Attention and performance XII: The psychology of reading. Hillsdale, Erlbaum, pp 363–383

Radach R (1996) Blickbewegungen beim Lesen: Psychologische Aspekte der Determination von Fixationspositionen (Eye movements in reading). Münster, Waxmann

Rayner K (1995) Eye movements and cognitive processes in reading, visual search, and scene perception. In: Findlay J M, Walker R, Kentridge R W (eds) Eye movement research: mechanisms, processes and applications. Amsterdam, North-Holland, pp 3–22

Rayner K, Pollatsek A (1989) The psychology of reading. Englewood Cliffs, N.J., Prentice-Hall

Rayner K, Sereno S C, Raney G E (1996) Eye movement control in reading: A comparison of two types of models. J Exp Psychol Hum Percept Perform 22: 1–13

Reichle E D, Pollatsek A, Fisher D L, Rayner K (1998) Towards a model of eye movement control in reading. Psychol Rev 105: 125–157

Schiepers C (1980) Response latency and accuracy in visual word recognition. Percept Psychophys 27: 71–81

Schroyens W, Vitu F, Brysbaert M, d'Ydewalle G (1998) Visual attention and eye movement control during reading: The case of parafoveal processing. In: Underwood G (ed) Eye guidance in reading, driving and scene perception. Oxford, Elsevier (in press)

Vitu F, O'Regan J K (1995) A challenge to current theories of eye movements in reading. In: Findlay J M, Walker R, Kentridge R W (eds) Eye movement research: mechanisms, processes and applications. Amsterdam, North-Holland, pp 382–392

51

FIXATION CONTROL AND ANTISACCADES IN DYSLEXIA

Monica Biscaldi, Stefan Gezeck, and Burkhart Fischer

Brain Research Unit
Hansastr. 9
79104 Freiburg, Germany

1. INTRODUCTION

While we are reading our eyes are driven by a combination of visual and linguistic properties of the text and by shifts of attention along the text. These cognitive factors influence the cortical-subcortical brain circuitries that basically control saccade programming. Cognitive strategies and saccade programming determine together how intensively a target is fixated, how efficiently attentional selection processes are working, and where and when the eyes will move next (Vitu et al. 1995). The hypothesis of a basic dysfunction in eye movement control in dyslexia independent of linguistic difficulties has been controversely discussed during the past (Stark et al. 1991). Our studies, however, have shown that the reflexive component of the saccadic system (measured in tasks requiring saccades to suddenly appearing targets) is underdeveloped in many dyslexic subjects (Biscaldi et al. 1998). Since fixation control, i.e. the ability of suppressing reflexive saccades, and voluntary saccade generation were found to develop with different speed in a standard population between 8 and 20 years of age (Fischer et al. 1997), we investigated the control of voluntary vs. reflexive saccades in dyslexics.

2. METHODS

One-hundred-fifty-four subjects (age between 9 and 20 years) were included in the statistical analysis. After performing various intelligence, cognitive, and achievement tests, 99 subjects were categorized as dyslexic if their reading or spelling achievement was below the 25% level relative to a standard population of the same school grade and at least one standard deviation below their IQ level. The remaining 55 subjects formed the control

Current Oculomotor Research, edited by Becker *et al.*
Plenum Press, New York, 1999.

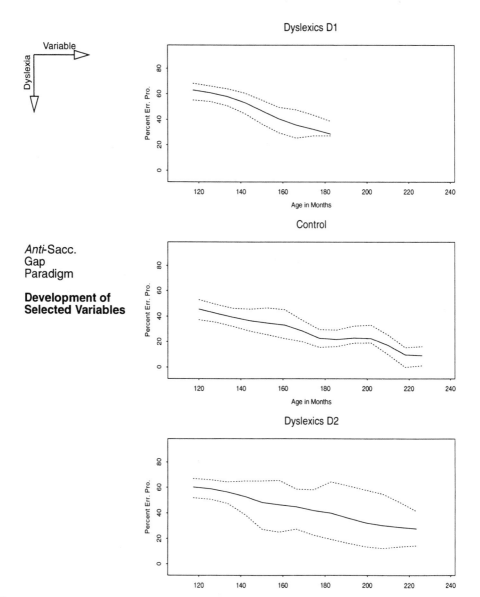

Figure 1. Estimated developmental course of two variables (percent errors and percent corrected errors vs. age in months) from the antisaccade task.

group. Dyslexic subjects that, in spite of average intelligence level, scored below average in tasks measuring phonological discrimination, sequential short-term memory, and attentional loading were grouped together as D1 (62 subjects). The remaining dyslexics, called D2 (37 subjects) performed above average in all kinds of cognitive tests used in this study. In the overlap prosaccade task, the fixation point remained visible throughout the trial and the subject, after fixating at the central stimulus for 1.4 s, had to look at a peripheral target appearing randomly to the left or right at 4° eccentricity and remaining visible for 800 ms.

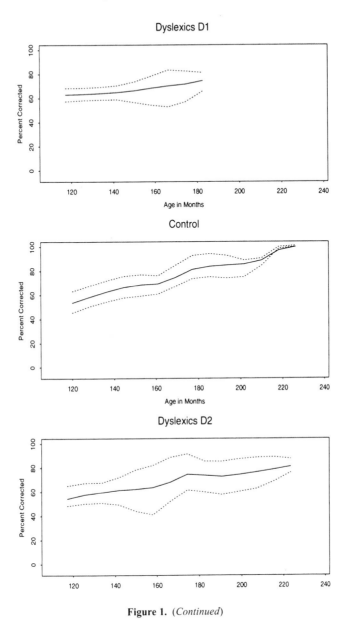

Figure 1. (*Continued*)

In the gap antisaccade task a gap of 200 ms (which implies an extra fixation effort) was introduced between fixation-point offset and stimulus onset. The subjects were instructed not to look at the appearing stimulus but to make a saccade to a symmetrical position on the side opposite to the stimulus. Two-hundred trials were presented in each task. To take into account the saccadic development, individual means of saccadic variables were normalized on the basis of eye movement data collected from a standard population of the same age.

3. RESULTS

The standard deviation of the SRT, the number of late (SRT > 400ms) and anticipatory (SRT < 80) saccades in the overlap prosaccade task significantly differentiated between control subjects and the two types of dyslexic subjects (Biscaldi et al. 1998). In the antisaccade task, the number of errors (saccades erroneously directed to the stimulus) was significantly increased both in D1 and D2 dyslexics. Differences in the saccadic performance of the two types of dyslexics were found in the number of express saccades from the overlap prosaccade task and in the mean SRT of the correct antisaccades. Both were increased only in the D2 subjects as compared to the control group.

Control subjects improved their performance with age reducing their error rate from about 45% to less than 20% and increasing the correction rate of the errors from 50% to 100%, at age 9 and 18 respectively. Although the dyslexic subjects improved their ability of suppressive involuntary saccades too, their performance remained worse than in normal subjects at all ages. This indicates that the neural systems controlling saccade programming are not definitively impaired but rather underdeveloped. To estimate the frequency of saccadic eye movement dysfunctions in dyslexics the quality of individual saccadic performances was judged by the deviation of individual means of saccadic variables from the means of age-matched standard subjects. About 60% D2, 50% D1, and less than 20% control subjects showed significant deviations of variables related to the "voluntary" saccadic control.

4. DISCUSSION

In about 50% subjects of a dyslexic population the ability of suppressing involuntary glances to a suddenly appearing visual stimulus in an antisaccade task is significantly reduced as compared to age-matched normally reading control subjects. The deficit seems to occur more frequently in so-called D2 dyslexics. The neural circuitry involved probably goes through the frontal cortex, maybe mostly through prefrontal structures (Rivaud et al. 1994). The circuitry could use neurons whose activity is related to fixation and suppression of involuntary, reflexive saccades. Similar findings were obtained in ADHD children (Munoz et al. 1997) and schizophrenic subjects (McDowell & Clementz 1997). At present we cannot claim a direct influence of the saccadic dysfunction on the reading performance. It could also be that the developmental lag in saccadic control is partly a consequence of the reading difficulties. In any case, children with developmental deficits in saccade control may have difficulties in acquiring reading skills as perfect as required by their age.

REFERENCES

Biscaldi M, Gezeck S, Stuhr V (1998) Poor saccadic control correlates with dyslexia. Neuropsychologia, in press
Fischer B, Biscaldi M, Gezeck S (1997) On the development of voluntary and reflexive components in human saccade generation. Brain Res 754: 285–297
McDowell JE, Clementz BA (1997) The effect of fixation condition manipulations on antisaccade performance in schizophrenia: studies of diagnostic specificity. Exp Brain Res 115: 333–344
Munoz DP, Goldring JE, Hampton KA, Moore KD (1997) Control of purposive saccadic eye movements and visual fixation in children with attention deficit hyperactivity disorder. Proceedings of the 9th ECEM in Ulm, p 80

Rivaud S, Müri RM, Gaymard B, Vermesch AI, Pierrot-Deseilligny C (1994) Eye movement disorders after frontal eye field lesions in humans. Exp Brain Res 102: 110–120

Stark LW, Giveen SC, Terdiman JF (1991) Specific dyslexia and eye movements. In: Stein JF (ed) Vision and visual dyslexia (Vision and visual dysfunction, Vol. 13). Macmillan, London pp 203–232

Vitu F., O'Regan J.K., Inhoff A.W., Topolski R. (1995) Mindless reading: Eye-mevement characteristics are similar in scanning letter strings and reading text. Perception & Psychophysics 57: 352–364

52

RELATIONSHIP BETWEEN VISUAL ATTENTION AND SACCADE TARGET SELECTION IN READING

Karine Doré and Cécile Beauvillain

Laboratoire de Psychologie Expérimentale, URA 316 CNRS
Université René Descartes and EPHE, Paris, France

1. INTRODUCTION

While reading, periods of fixations are interrupted by fast movements of the eyes, the saccades. These saccadic eye movements provide a rapid means of bringing the fovea on the « interesting objects » present in the text line. There has been considerable interest in the processes associated with how readers select where to look next, and there is evidence suggesting that readers select the word-object to the right as subsequent eye movement target. The length of a yet-to-be fixated word strongly influences where a reader fixates in that word (Rayner, 1979). Moreover, where to move the eyes does not depend exclusively on word boundary information. Research made in the laboratory showed that letter groupings that are unusual for a reader of a given language provide a salient signal that « attracts » the next saccade (Beauvillain, Doré, and Baudouin, 1996; Doré and Beauvillain, 1997; Beauvillain and Doré, 1998). Therefore, a selection process that delivers coordinates of the next movement should be influenced by information acquired from the word to which the eyes are directed prior to the eye movement. It has been suggested that this process is carried out through a spatial attention mechanism (Henderson, 1992). According to this hypothesis, a common attentional mechanism selects objects for recognition as well as provides the future saccade target location. More recently, other researchers have proposed the notion of an obligatory and selective coupling of saccade programming and visual attention (Deubel and Schneider, 1996; Hoffman and Subramaniam, 1995).

Since no explicit target into the words are given to readers, we need to assess the strength of the relation between saccade programming and attentional focusing. Indeed, it is possible that the two selection mechanisms are not strictly coupled. Visual attention may be allocated to abstract subword units that are likely to be active units of integration while a saccade is programmed to a location that corresponds to the center of gravity de-

Current Oculomotor Research, edited by Becker *et al.*
Plenum Press, New York, 1999.

fined by low-level properties of the target letter string. On the other hand, visual attention should be spatially allocated to locations where the saccade will be directed.

We present an experiment which investigates how visual attention is distributed in a letter string that is the target for the subsequent saccade. We intended to examine how different initial letters composing a target letter string are discriminated during saccade preparation. Participants were instructed to saccade to an isolated nonsense letter string displayed on a computer screen at a visual angle of 2°30 from fixation point. After a 100 ms delay, one of the letters was replaced by another letter during 50 ms for half of the trials. Next, the letters were removed from the screen and immediately replaced by dashes on which the eye movement finally occurred. Participants had to indicate whether they had detected that one of the letters had been switched. The exchanged letter could be in the 2nd, 3rd, or 4th position in the string.

The distribution of visual attention allocation in the target string is reflected by the letter change detection performance. Two different types of 6 and 10 letter strings were used that differed only by the nature of their initial bigram (i.e., the two initial letters): Orthographically Illegal-Beginning and Orthographically Legal-Beginning strings. The orthographic legality was measured by the positional frequency of occurrence of bigrams in French.

2. RESULTS

Figure 1 presents detection performances for each of the 4 subjects (thin lines) as well as mean performance of all subjects (thick line), measured as percentage of accurate detection. Globally, there was a strong effect of letter position, as performance decreased with eccentricity ($p < .05$). Interestingly, in the legal letter strings condition, this letter position effect was influenced by the length of the letter string. For 6-letter Legal Strings (Fig. 1a), detection performance dropped significantly from 70% to 58% for the 3rd and 4th letter, respectively, whereas results remained roughly the same in the 10-letter letter Legal Strings (Fig. 1b). Consequently, performance on the 4th letter was significantly better for 10-letter strings (66%) than for 6-letter stings (55%). This pattern of data differs for 6- and 10-Illegal strings. In this condition, detection performance is good for the 2nd letter (M =81%) but drops to 63% for the 3rd and 4th letter (Fig. 1c and 1d).

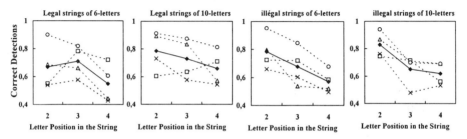

Figure 1. Mean Correct Detection for each subject (thin lines) and for all subjects (thick line) as a function of Letter String Length (6-letter vs. 10-letter strings), Letter Position in the String (the 2nd, 3rd, 4th letter) and Orthographic Structure of the String Beginning (Legal vs. Illegal).

3. RELATIONSHIP BETWEEN DETECTION PERFORMANCE AND LANDING POSITION

Figure 2 shows detection performances as a function of landing position for the three letter positions in 6- and 10-letter (legal and illegal) strings. The mean landing position in the 6- and 10-letter strings were 2.8 and 3.5, respectively. For legal strings, landing positions did not affect detection performances when letter switch occurred in locations where the eye usually landed, that is 2nd and 3rd letter for 6-letter strings (Fig. 2a) and 3rd and 4th letter for 10-letter strings (Fig. 2b). Interestingly, detection performance was influenced by landing position when the exchange occurred far from it, that is 4th letter in the 6-letter strings (Fig. 2a) and, to some extent, 2nd letter in the 10-letter strings (Fig. 2b). This finding may indicate that attention is mainly allocated to a specific landing position.

In the illegal string condition, the best performances, obtained when the 2nd letter was switched, did not depend on landing position, as it was the case for 3rd and 4th letter. This result may show that illegal initial bigrams best focus readers' attention allocation,

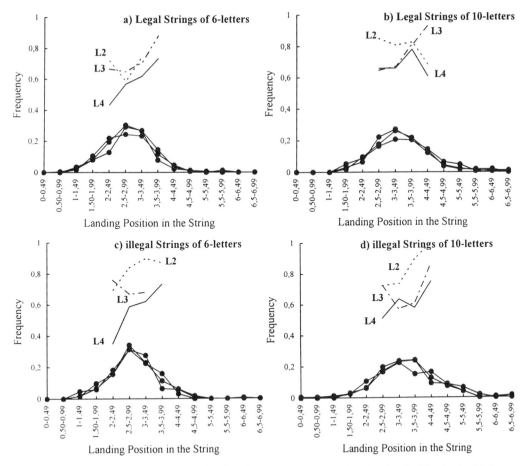

Figure 2. Mean Correct Detection on the 2nd, 3rd or 4th letters as a function of the Landing Position for the 6-letter Legal Strings (a), the 10-letters Legal Strings (b), 6-letter Illegal Strings (c) and the 10-letters Illegal Strings (d) and Respective Landing Position Distributions.

because a letter change inside the illegal initial bigram resulted in the best detection performance, regardless of the string length and effective landing position. Outside this attentional window determined by the illegal initial bigram, detection performances depends on
landing position (Figures 2c and 2d).

4. CONCLUSION

Our experiment revealed a close relation between saccade target selection and letter
recognition. Letter eccentricity cannot account for the observed effect of string length on
detection performance. Our results indicate that attention is more precisely allocated in a
window that primarily depends on landing position. Generally, this window should correspond to the region around the saccade target position. Interestingly, presence of a salient
component at the beginning of the letter string focuses reader's attention. Consequently,
letter recognition within this salient structure is not fully coupled to the effective landing
position (see also Deubel and Schneider, 1996 for a discussion on this point). Interestingly, our data suggest that letter recognition and saccade programming are not strictly
coupled in reading, neither spatially nor temporally. Salient objects receive some priori-
tized visual processing even if they do not stand in the precise location where the eye
lands.

REFERENCES

Beauvillain C, Doré K (1998) Orthographic codes are used in integrating information from the parafovea by the
    saccadic computation system. Vision Res 38: 115–123
Beauvillain C, Doré K, Baudouin V (1996) The "center of gravity" of words: Evidence for an effect of the word-
    initial Letters. Vision Res 36: 589–603
Deubel H, Schneider WX (1996) Saccade target selection and object recognition: evidence for a common atten-
    tional mechanism. Vision Res 36: 1827–1837
Doré K, Beauvillain C (1997) Latency dependence of word-initial letter integration by the saccadic system. Per-
    cept Psychophys 59: 523–533
Henderson JM (1992) Visual attention and eye movement control during reading and picture viewing. In Rayner K
    (Ed.), Eye movements and visual cognition. Berlin : Springer
Hoffman JE and Subramaniam B (1995) The role of visual attention in saccadic eye movements. Percep Psycho-
    phys 57: 787–795
Rayner K (1979) Eye guidance in reading : fixation location within words. Percept 8: 21–30

53

READING

Influence of Letter Size, Display Quality, and Anticipation

C. C. Krischer,[1] J. Zihl,[2] and R. Meissen[1]

[1]Forschungszentrum Jülich
[2]Universität und Max-Planck Institut für Psychiatrie, München

Measurements of reading speed (WPM) serve to study how visually degraded input - as found in computer work - affects the speed of information processing. We observe for each of the different qualities (v) of display we used characteristic WPM-letter size dependencies. Maximal reading speeds (WPM_{max}) were reached for letters magnified about five times the threshold size. For blurred and dimmed display WPM_{max} changes characteristically with v and can be described by a simple equation with one constant characterizing the difference in function for blur or dim. By analyzing reading speed in terms of eye jumps (saccades) occuring at intervals of about 250 ms (fixation durations) it is calculated that saccade size is chosen to render well resolvable fixated letters. Based on results of other authors of eye movement recordings and neuro-networking we derive a working hypothesis in which saccadic eye movement (progress in reading) depends on the quality of the retinal images and on cognitive anticipation of images, both being closely related to the structure of the retina and visual cortex.

WPM (words per minute), the speed of reading „easy" texts is measured by accounting both, for the influence of letter size and display quality (v, effective visual acuity, range 0.05–1). A new variable is introduced, the "threshold-normalized letter size" s_{th}. For the same values of s_{th} subjects are faced with comparable difficulties in letter recognition. We change the threshold sizes by degrading the input quality with blurring film or dimming neutral density filters. The resulting effective visual acuity v (its reciprocal is the threshold size) is measured prior to each reading measurement with a horizontally moving square wave grating diplayed on the text display device. This acuity measurement is the basis for the selection of the s_{th} values in the range of 1.5 - 60.

Inspite of variations of v in the wide range of 0.05 - 1 a maximum WPM is always reached for blurred or dimmed display, near $s_{th} = 5$, Fig. 1. By normalizing the reading speed to the maximum speed reached by each subject, all size-dependencies coincide in one curve, Fig. 1. We explain this size dependence on the basis of the special ("centro-focal") structure of the retina and visual pathway. Two opposing effects of letter size have to

Current Oculomotor Research, edited by Becker *et al.*
Plenum Press, New York, 1999.

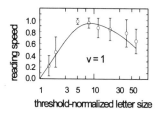

Figure 1. Dependence of oral reading speed relative to the maximal value reached by each subject on threshold-normalized letter size. Error bars are standard deviations for 14 subjects. The solid curve is calculated with Eq. 1 with parameters a = 0.47 and b = 0.0113.

be considered: a) an increase of WPM with letter size due to improved letter recognition (decisive for letters near threshold size) and b) a decrease of WPM with letter size due to reduced cortical representation and visual acuity in the retinal periphery (effective for very large letters). Assuming exponential dependencies for both effects the following equation results:

$$WPM = 1.06_*[1\text{-}exp(-s_{th*}a)]_*exp(-s_{th*}b) \qquad (1)$$

the constants a characterizing the rise and b the fall. The curves calculated with Eq. 1 fit the data quite well for normal display quality (control), for blurred or dimmed input, and for data of Legge et al 1985 (silent reading), provided WPM is normalized to maximal speed reached under each display condition; Fig. 1 gives an example.

Degrading the input yields – for optimized letter size - smaller WPM_{max} values than the 158 WPM_{max} measured for normal display conditions, Fig 2. In analogy to the size-dependence we assume that WPM increases as the density of usable receptor cells increases. We find that the hyperbolic tangent-function is capable of describing the dependence of WPM_{max} on display quality v (and hence on the resolution of the picture):

$$WPM_{max} = tanh(E_*v) \qquad (2)$$

with E being a factor called "reading expectance" that characterizes the performance for blurred or dimmed display, Fig. 2. E is also identical with the slope of the output - input quality curve near the origin (v << 1). The initial rise of the curves, being 2,4 for dimmed and 6.7 for blurred display, characterizes how much the reading output – which contains major portions of non-visual (cognitive) components - is affected by the two kinds of visual degradation.

To find out how saccadic amplitude is changed by different degrees of blurring we assume that WPM_{max} consists of saccades made every 250 ms (the average duration of one fixation). The result is that the saccades appear to be made for each display quality with such amplitudes as to allow good resolution of the fixated letters within the central region of good visual acuity (Aulhorn and Harms 1972). The much poorer performance of

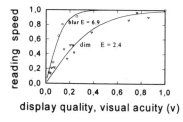

Figure 2. Mean maximal reading speeds (WPM_{max}) reached in curves of the type shown in Fig. 1 as a function of display quality v (effective visual acuity). WPM_{max} = 1 corresponds to 158 WPM, the reading speed for optimal display quality. Upper and lower curves are measured for blurred or dimmed display, respectively. The solid curves are calculated with Eq. 2 and reading expectances E are marked in the figure.

dimmed as compared to blurred display is attributed to the additional slowing of retinal function in dim light.

To explain the results in view of the outlined eye movement analysis we make use of a recent theory on neuro-networking together with special observations made in oculomotorics. A new approach suggests that in sensory processing the neuro-network is to be tuned to the pending input (Tononi et al 1996). Candidates for such a tuning process can be special non-retinal (efferent) components of eye movements (von Holst and Mittelstaedt 1954), i.e. an „internal predictive feedback pathway" (Becker and Jürgens 1979). In addition, the study of the scan paths in picture viewing revealed that "top down cognitive modelling" is a major constituent in the control of saccadic eye movement (Stark and Choi 1996).

Making use of such concepts we suggest in a working hypothesis (called "model") that the dependencies on size and display quality are a consequence of bottom up retinal images interacting with the top down non-retinal components that accompany reading (McConkie 1979). Thereby the non-retinal components are to represent the tuning of the processing cells to the pending task in the form of anticipated images, called "templates". According to familiar principles of visual perception one expects optimal performance when the image has optimal cortical representation, i.e. is of foveal size. The data of Fig. 1 and 2 confirm this. Furthermore we assume in an intuitive (yet speculative) manner that cognitive processing always yields templates of constant foveal size because the constituents are most likely imaged in a foveal standard size. Therefore, any mismatch of the image size with respect to the template (of foveal size) should result in poorer performance. Our results and many others (references on request) confirm this: Hypofoveal images cause a steep decrease of reading speed; hyperfoveal size has a much smaller effect, Fig. 1, Eq. 1.

According to the model the release of reading saccades should therefore depend on the visual resolution of the image - as seen in Fig. 2 - but also on the cognitive skill of the reader (which could be termed "cognitive resolution"). For beginners with modest cognitive skill in reading it is to be assumed that their templates contain much less information than those of normal readers. Support for this notion comes from recordings of reading eye movements showing that beginners make only one-letter saccades (Taylor 1965). The fact that all text books for beginners have large print confirms this aspect of the model.

Any slowing of retinal function - as found in dimming – should, according to the model, slow down the senso-cognitive interaction, i.e. prolong the fixation duration and thereby have - via the short term memory - also an effect on the template generation. Many saccadic eye movement results, such as in smooth pursuit or saccadic latency (van Die and Collewijn 1984, Doma and Hallet 1988) support such facets of the model being based on the findings of Fig. 2, Eq. 2.

REFERENCES

Aulhorn E, Harms H (1972) Visual Perimetry. In: Handbook of Sensory Physiology Vol VII/4 Springer, Berlin, pp 102–145

Becker W, Jürgens R (1979) An analysis of the saccadic system by means of double step stimuli. Vision Res 19: 967–983

Doma H, Hallet PE (1988) Dependence of saccadic eye-movements on stimulus luminance, and an effect of task. Vision Res 28: 915–24

Legge GE, Pelli DG, Rubin GS, Schleske MM (1985) Psychophysics of reading I. Normal vision. Vision Res 25: 239–52

McConkie GW (1979) On the role and control of eye movement in reading. In: Kolers PA Wrolstadt ME (eds) Processing of visual language. Plenum Press, London, pp 37–48

Stark LW, Choi YS (1996) Experimental Metaphysics: The scanpath as an epistemological mechanism. In: Zangemeister, Stiehl, Freksa (eds.) Visual attention and cognition. Elsevier Science B.V. pp 3–69

Taylor SE (1965) Eye movements in reading: facts and fallacies. Am Ed Res J 2 187–202

Tononi G, Sporns O, Edelman GM (1996) A complexity measure for selective matching of signals by the brain. Proc Nat Acad Sci USA 93: 3422–3427

Van Die GC, Collewijn H (1986) Control of human optokinetic nystagmus by the central and peripheral retina: effects of partial visual field masking, scotopic vision and central retinal scotomata. Brain Res 383: 185–94

Von Holst E Mittelstaedt H (1954) Das Reafferenzprinzip. Naturwissenschaften 37: 464–476

54

EYE MOVEMENT DEFICITS IN CEREBELLAR DISEASE[*]

U. Büttner[†]

Deptartment of Neurology
Ludwig Maximilians University
Munich, Germany

1. INTRODUCTION

The cerebellum is known to improve but not generate eye movements. Thus without the cerebellum all types of eye movements are still possible, an exemption being smooth pursuit eye movements (SPEM) which can no longer be performed after total cerebellectomy (Westheimer and Blair, 1973). It is also well established that certain areas of the cerebellum are more involved in oculomotor control than others. Three major cerebellar structures related to oculomotor functions have been distinguished: I. The floccular region, II. the oculomotor vermis with the underlying fastigial nucleus and III. the nodulus. However, there are certainly other structures of the cerebellum, which are also involved in oculomotor control (Ron and Robinson, 1973; Mano et al. 1991; Straube et al. 1997). In the following some recent results concerning the role of the cerebellum in oculomotor control will be presented. Emphasis will be laid on the relation of structure and function. However, in patient studies this is often not possible in detail.

2. FLOCCULAR REGION

2.1. General Considerations

The flocculus and parts of the ventral paraflocculus are part of the vestibulo-cerebellum and are referred to here as the floccular region (Büttner and Büttner-Ennever, 1988). A number of oculomotor deficits occur with lesions to these structures, including defect smooth pursuit eye movements (SPEM), impaired visual suppression of the vestibulo-ocu-

---

[*] Supported by the Deutsche Forschungsgemeinschaft (DFG)

[†] e-mail: ubuettner@brain.nefo.med.uni-muenchen.de

Current Oculomotor Research, edited by Becker *et al.*
Plenum Press, New York, 1999.

lar reflex (VOR-supp), gaze-evoked nystagmus, rebound nystagmus, downbeat nystagmus and postsaccadic drift (Leigh and Zee, 1991).

2.2. Gaze-Evoked Nystagmus, SPEM, and VOR-Suppression

From single unit studies in monkeys it is well established that neurons involved in SPEM generation also participate in VOR-suppression (Büttner and Büttner-Ennever, 1988). Accordingly, there is a high correlation between the SPEM deficit and the VOR-supp performance. With a SPEM gain (eye velocity/stimulus velocity) close to 1 the VOR-supp is nearly complete, but deteriotates with a lower SPEM gain (Dichgans et al. 1978; Büttner and Grundei, 1995). Gaze-evoked nystagmus indicates a deficit of the common neural integrator for eye movements. For horizontal eye movements this integrator has been located within the vestibular nuclei/nuclei praepositus hypoglossi-complex (Straube et al. 1991; Cannon and Robinson, 1987) but also the cerebellum, particularly the floccular region, plays a major role (Zee et al. 1981).

In 52 patients with gaze-evoked nystagmus and/or a SPEM-deficit the relation of SPEM and gaze-evoked nystagmus was studied (Büttner and Grundei, 1995). All patients with gaze-evoked nystagmus also had a SPEM deficit. Both deficits were highly correlated with a correlation coefficient of r=>0.8, a value similar to that found for the correlation of SPEM performance and VOR-supp. Although it cannot be proven for all patients, it is very likely that the gaze-evoked nystagmus and the SPEM deficit are in most instances due to a lesion of the floccular region. Twenty-five percent of the patients had a SPEM deficit without gaze-evoked nystagmus. This certainly is not due to a lesion of the floccular region (Zee et al. 1981). In the cerebellum such an eye movement pattern can be found with lesions to the oculomotor vermis/fastigial nucleus (see below). However, it can also be seen with lesions outside the cerebellum (Büttner and Büttner-Ennever, 1988). Only 4% of the patients had an isolated gaze-evoked nystagmus without a SPEM-deficit. The gaze-evoked nystagmus was always weak (Büttner and Grundei, 1995).

These results show, that any substantial gaze-evoked nystagmus is always combined with a SPEM-deficit, as seen in lesions of the floccular region (Zee et al. 1981). Basically, the SPEM-deficit could be a consequence of a malfunction of the neural integrator. However, this only manifests itself with very short time constants of the postsaccadic drift (200 - 300 msec), which up to now has only been encountered experimentally (Straube et al. 1991; Cannon and Robinson, 1987). In patients, it can be estimated that the shortest time constants of the postsaccadic drift are not below 1 sec, which is insufficient to have a major effect on SPEM gain (Büttner and Grundei, 1995). It is more likely that the close anatomical vicinity of the gaze-holding and smooth pursuit mechanisms are responsible for the combined deficit.

2.3. Centripetal Gaze-Evoked Nystagmus

Lesions of the floccular region also lead to rebound nystagmus. It occurs after extended lateral gaze when the eye returns to the midposition. With rebound nystagmus patients usually have a gaze-evoked nystagmus with the fast phase beating away from the midposition of the eye (centrifugal) and which decreases in intensity during sustained (about 30 sec) lateral gaze. On return to the midposition a nystagmus with the fast phase beating to the opposite direction for about 5–20 sec can be seen (rebound nystagmus). This rebound nystagmus can also be attributed to a failure of the neural integrator. Integration requires a null-position. For the oculomotor system it represents the eye position, at which no postsaccadic drift occurs and beyond which the postsaccadic drift reverses direc-

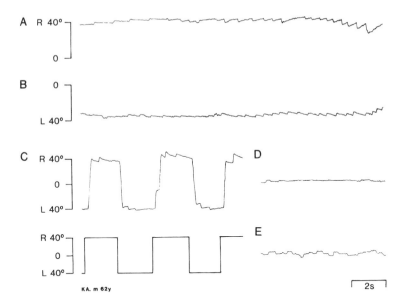

Figure 1. Centripetal gaze-evoked nystagmus in a patient with Creutzfeldt-Jacob-disease. EOG-recording of horizontal eye position. The patient has no spontaneous nystagmus in the dark (E) or light, while looking straight ahead (D). Initially, after saccades to lateral eye positions (C) the eye drifts back to the midposition of the eye (centrifugal gaze-evoked nystagmus). After sustained lateral gaze, nystagmus reverses direction (A, B) with the eye drifting away from the midposition of the eye (centripetal gaze-evoked nystagmus). The nystagmus reversal from initial right nystagmus to left nystagmus can be seen in (A). The lower half in (C) represents the position of a visual target. L = left; R = right (from Helmchen and Büttner, 1995a).

tion. The null-position usually coincides with the midposition of the eye (gaze straight ahead), but it can also differ, as has been shown experimentally (up to 35 deg, Straube et al., 1991) and in congenital nystagmus (Kurzan and Büttner, 1989). In rebound nystagmus it is assumed that the extended lateral gaze leads to a dynamic shift of the null-position towards the actual lateral eye position. Consequently the gaze-evoked nystagmus disappears and reappears as rebound nystagmus after returning to the midposition with the null-position still in lateral gaze. A dynamic shift of the null-position is also common in congenital nystagmus (Kurzan and Büttner, 1989).

Recently a patient with cerebellar signs resulting from Creutzfeldt-Jacob disease could be investigated, who presented the unusual sign of centripetal gaze-evoked nystagmus (Helmchen and Büttner, 1995 a). This patient had no nystagmus in the light or dark while looking straight ahead (midposition of the eye) (Fig. 1).

On lateral gaze to the left or to the right initially centrifugal gaze-evoked nystagmus was present, which reversed direction into centripetal nystagmus (fast phase beating to the eye position of straight ahead) after 15–30 sec. This patient in addition had rebound nystagmus, when the eyes returned from the sustained lateral fixation to the straight ahead eye position (Helmchen and Büttner, 1995 a). Centripetal gaze-evoked nystagmus is a rare clinical finding and only few reports are in the literature (Zee et al. 1976; Leech et al. 1977). These findings however strongly support present concepts on gaze-holding and neural integration in the oculomotor system. For all patients with centripetal gaze-evoked nystagmus no circumscribed cerebellar lesions have been described. A lesion of the archicerebellum is very likely. Apart from the floccular region the nodulus/uvula region are also possible candidates. Lesions here lead to periodic alternating nystagmus (PAN), which is also considered to result from interaction of a gaze holding deficit and a shifting null position (Grant et al. 1993; Rudge and Leigh, 1976).

3. OCULOMOTOR VERMIS/FASTIGIAL OCULOMOTOR REGION

3.1. General Considerations

Lobulus VI and VII are considered as the oculomotor vermis (Yamada and Noda, 1987). Lesions here lead to oculomotor deficits which will be considered below. The oculomotor vermis is immediately located posterior from the primary fissure, which separates the anterior from the posterior vermis. Whereas most lobuli of the vermis belong to the spinocerebellum the oculomotor vermis is considered as pontocerebellum, since it receives a major mossy fiber input from the pons (Yamada and Noda, 1987). The Purkinje cells (PCs) from the oculomotor vermis project to the caudal part of the fastigial nucleus (fastigial oculomotor region, FOR; Noda et al., 1990). The FOR projects to saccade related brainstem structures and the vestibular nuclei (Noda et al. 1990). The oculomotor vermis as well as the FOR contain smooth pursuit (oculomotor vermis: Suzuki and Keller, 1988 a, b; FOR: Büttner et al., 1991; Fuchs et al., 1994 b) and saccade (oculomotor vermis: Helmchen and Büttner, 1995 b; Ohtsuka and Noda, 1995; FOR: Helmchen et al., 1994; Fuchs et al., 1993) related neurons.

3.2. Saccade Deficits

Lesions of the oculomotor vermis as well as of the FOR lead to step-size error dysmetria (Leigh and Zee, 1991). With step-size error dysmetria saccades to a visual target are either too small (hypometric) or too large (hypermetric) and corrective saccades have to bring the foveal region of the eye to the visual target. It should be emphasized that visually guided saccades (externally triggered) are more affected than saccades to stationary visually targets (internally triggered) (Straube et al. 1995). Scanning saccades are generally unremarkable (Büttner and Straube, 1995).

In the monkey unilateral lesions in the FOR lead to a direction-specific deficit. Microinjections of the $GABA_A$-agonist muscimol cause hypometric saccades to the contralateral and hypermetric saccades to the ipsilateral side (Robinson et al. 1993). Bilateral injections (Robinson et al. 1993) or lesions (Optican and Robinson, 1980) cause a pronounced hypermetria. This is also seen with lesions in patients (Büttner et al. 1994). Purkinje cells (PCs) in the cerebellar cortex use GABA as an inhibitory transmitter. Consequently unilateral lesions of the oculomotor vermis (removal of inhibition) cause a reverse pattern with hypometric saccades to ipsilateral and hypermetric saccades to the contralateral side (Aschoff and Cohen, 1971). Also bilateral lesions cause a general hypometria as seen experimentally (Takagi et al. 1996) and in patients (Vahedi et al. 1995).

3.3. Smooth Pursuit Eye Movements

Lesions of the oculomotor vermis/fastigial oculomotor region (FOR) also affect smooth pursuit eye movements (SPEM). Unilateral microinjections of the $GABA_A$-agonist muscimol into the FOR lead to a reduced smooth pursuit gain (cogwheel smooth pursuit) to the contralateral side (Robinson et al. 1997). Similarly, also the fast initial rise of optokinetic slow-phase velocity is affected, which is related to smooth pursuit mechanisms

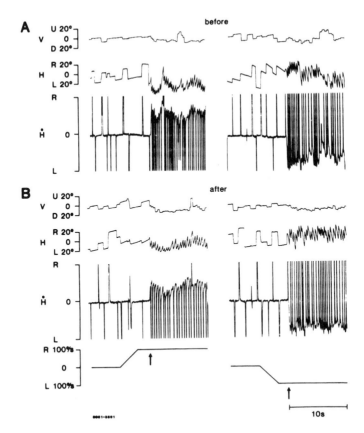

Figure 2. Optokinetic nystagmus in the monkey before (A) and after (B) a microinjection of the GABA$_A$-agonist muscimol in the left fastigial oculomotor region (FOR). Search coil recording. Traces from above: V = vertical, H = horizontal eye position, Ḣ = horizontal eye velocity. Velocity of saccades is arbitrarly clipped. The stimulus profile is shown under (B). At the upward arrow an optokinetic stimulus (100 deg/s constant velocity) is presented. This leads to a symmetrical rapid increase of slow phase eye velocity in (A). After the injection (B) this initial increase is reduced by ca. 50 % with stimulation to the contralateral (right) side, but remains unaltered with stimulation to the ipsilateral (left) side. A further gradual increase in eye velocity (velocity storage mechanism) cannot be seen during the time period shown in this figure.

(Kurzan et al. 1993) (Fig. 2). The gradual increase in slow-phase velocity during constant velocity optokinetic stimulation, reflecting the 'velocity storage' mechanism, is not affected (Kurzan et al. 1993). The use of step-ramp stimuli also clearly demonstrates that the acceleration of contralateral pursuit is reduced (Robinson et al. 1997).

In contrast, with ipsilateral step-ramp stimuli the acceleration is increased. Occasionally during sinusoidal stimuli the SPEM gain to the ipsilateral side increases, which requires back-up saccades for correction in contrast to the catch-up saccades with reduced SPEM-gain (Fuchs et al. 1994 a). The fast initial rise of OKN velocity to the ipsilateral side is not reduced (Kurzan et al. 1993) (Fig. 2) and the average gain during sinusoidal stimuli is only slightly reduced (Robinson et al. 1997). Thus in contrast to the contralateral side, the SPEM gain to the ipsilateral side is not or only slightly reduced. With bilateral FOR injections acceleration during step ramp stimuli does not alter. For sinusoidal stimuli the SPEM gain is reduced (Robinson et al. 1997). However in an earlier study normal

Table 1. Effect of unilateral and bilateral lesions in the oculomotor vermis and fastigial oculomotor region (FOR) on saccades (hyper- or hypometric) and smooth pursuit eye movements (SPEM). Downward arrow indicates reduced SPEM gain

	saccades			SPEM		
	unilateral		bilateral	unilateral		bilateral
	ipsi-	contra-		ipsi-	contra-	
oculom. vermis	hypo-	hyper-	hypo-	?	?	↓
FOR	hyper-	hypo-	hyper-	normal or ↓	↓	normal or ↓

smooth pursuit performance after bilateral deep cerebellar nuclei lesions has been reported (Optican and Robinson, 1980). Normal SPEM during sinusoidal stimulation were also seen in a patient with severe saccadic hypermetria and a lesion affecting the FOR on both sides (Büttner et al. 1994).

Lesions of the oculomotor vermis lead to a reduced smooth pursuit gain, which has been shown both experimentally (Keller, 1988) and in clinical studies (Pierrot-Deseilligny et al. 1990; Vahedi et al. 1995).

3.4. Comparison of SPEM and Saccade Deficits

Single unit recordings in the FOR during saccades support the hypothesis, that the neuronal discharge improves acceleration of saccades to the contralateral and deceleration of saccades to the ipsilateral side (Helmchen et al. 1994; Fuchs et al. 1993). Consequently a lack of these signals leads to contralateral hypometric and ipsilateral hypermetric saccades (Büttner and Straube, 1995). Similarly the neuronal data during smooth pursuit eye movements also suggest a role in contralateral acceleration and ipsilateral deceleration (Fuchs et al. 1994).

Based on this, as a rule saccade and SPEM deficits after FOR and oculomotor vermis lesions are related. Saccadic hypometria is always combined with a reduced SPEM gain (Table 1). This can be seen with contralateral eye movements after unilateral FOR and oculomotor vermis lesions (Büttner and Straube, 1995). Theoretically hypermetric saccades might be combined with an increased SPEM gain. This, however is seen only rarely (Fuchs et al. 1994). Generally hypermetric saccades are associated with largely normal SPEM, as encountered during ipsilateral movements after unilateral (Robinson et al. 1997; Kurzan et al. 1993) and bilateral FOR lesions (Büttner et al. 1994; Optican and Robinson, 1980). However, since a reduced SPEM gain after bilateral FOR lesions has also been encountered (Robinson et al. 1997) this point needs further investigation.

REFERENCES

Aschoff JC, and Cohen B (1971) Changes in saccadic eye movements produced by cerebellar cortical lesions. Exp Neurol 32: 123–133

Büttner U, and Büttner-Ennever JA (1988) Present concepts of oculomotor organization. Rev Oculomot Res 2: 3–32

Büttner U, Fuchs AF, Markert-Schwab G, and Buckmaster P (1991) Fastigial nucleus activity in the alert monkey during slow eye and head movements. J Neurophysiol 65: 1360–1371

Büttner U, and Grundei T (1995) Gaze-evoked nystagmus and smooth pursuit deficits: their relationship studied in 52 patients. J Neurol 242: 384–389

Büttner U, and Straube A (1995) The effect of cerebellar midline lesions on eye movements. Neuro-ophthalmol 15: 75–82

Büttner U, Straube A, and Spuler A (1994) Saccadic dysmetria and "intact" smooth pursuit eye movements after bilateral deep cerebellar nuclei lesions. J Neurol Neurosurg Psychiatry 57: 832–834

Cannon SC, and Robinson DA (1987) Loss of the neural integrator of the oculomotor system from brain stem lesions in monkey. J Neurophysiol 57: 1383–1409

Dichgans J, von-Reutern GM, and Rommelt U (1978) Impaired suppression of vestibular nystagmus by fixation in cerebellar and noncerebellar patients. Arch Psychiatr Nervenkr 226: 183–199

Fuchs AF, Robinson FR, and Straube A (1993) Role of the Caudal Fastigial Nucleus in Saccade Generation .1. Neuronal Discharge Patterns. J Neurophysiol 70: 1723–1740

Fuchs AF, Robinson FR, Straube A (1994 a) Preliminary observations on the role of the caudal fastigial nucleus in the generation of smooth-pursuit eye movements. In: Fuchs AF, Brandt T, Büttner U, Zee D (eds) Contemporary Ocular Motor and Vestibular Research: A Tribute to David A. Robinson. Georg Thieme Verlag, Stuttgart, pp 165–170

Fuchs AF, Robinson FR, and Straube A (1994 b) Participation of the caudal fastigial nucleus in smooth-pursuit eye movements. I. Neuronal activity. J Neurophysiol 72: 2714–2728

Grant MP, Cohen M, Peterson RB, Halmagyi GM, McDougall A, Tusa RJ, and Leigh RJ (1993) Abnormal eye movements in Creutzfeldt-Jacob disease. Ann Neurol 34: 192–197

Helmchen C, and Büttner U (1995 a) Centripetal nystagmus in a case of Creutzfeldt-Jacob disease. Neuro-ophthalmol 15: 187–192

Helmchen C, and Büttner U (1995 b) Saccade-related Purkinje cell activity in the oculomotor vermis during spontaneous eye movements in light and darkness. Exp Brain Res 103: 198–208

Helmchen C, Straube A, and Büttner U (1994) Saccade-related activity in the fastigial oculomotor region of the macaque monkey during spontaneous eye movements in light and darkness. Exp Brain Res 98: 474–482

Keller EL (1988) Cerebellar involvement in smooth pursuit eye movement generation: flocculus and vermis. In: Kennard C, Rose FC (eds) Physiological Aspects of Clinical Neuro-Ophthalmology. pp 341–354

Kurzan R, and Büttner U (1989) Smooth pursuit mechanisms in congenital nystagmus. Neuro-ophthalmol 9: 313–325

Kurzan R, Straube A, and Büttner U (1993) The effect of muscimol micro-injections into the fastigial nucleus on the optokinetic response and the vestibulo-ocular reflex in the alert monkey. Exp Brain Res 94: 252–260

Leech J, Gresty M, Hess K, and Rudge P (1977) Gaze failure, drifting eye movements, and centripetal nystagmus in cerebellar disease. Br J Ophthalmol 61: 774–781

Leigh RJ, Zee DS (1991) The neurology of eye movements. F.A. Davis, Philadelphia,

Mano N, Ito Y, and Shibutani H (1991) Saccade-related Purkinje cells in the cerebellar hemispheres of the monkey. Exp Brain Res 84: 465–470

Noda H, Sugita S, and Ikeda Y (1990) Afferent and efferent connections of the oculomotor region of the fastigial nucleus in the macaque monkey. J Comp Neurol 302: 330–348

Ohtsuka K, and Noda H (1995) Discharge Properties of Purkinje Cells in the oculomotor vermis during visually guided saccades in the macaque monkey. J Neurophysiol 74: 1828–1840

Optican LM, and Robinson DA (1980) Cerebellar-dependent adaptive control of the primate saccadic system. J Neurophysiol 44: 1058–1075

Pierrot-Deseilligny C, Amarenco P, Roullet E, and Marteau R (1990) Vermal infarct with pursuit eye movement disorders. J Neurol Neurosurg Psychiatry 53: 519–521

Robinson FR, Straube A, and Fuchs AF (1993) Role of the Caudal Fastigial Nucleus in Saccade Generation .2. Effects of Muscimol Inactivation. J Neurophysiol 70: 1741–1758

Robinson FR, Straube A, and Fuchs AF (1997) Participation of caudal fastigial nucleus in smooth pursuit eye movements. II. Effects of muscimol inactivation. J Neurophysiol 78: 848–859

Ron S, and Robinson DA (1973) Eye movements evoked by cerebellar stimulation in the alert monkey. J Neurophysiol 36: 1004–1022

Rudge P, and Leigh J (1976) Analysis of a case of periodic alternating nystagmus. Neurol Neurosurg Psychiat 39: 314–319

Straube A, Deubel H, Spuler A, and Büttner U (1995) Differential effect of a bilateral deep cerebellar nuclei lesion on externally and internally triggered saccades in humans. Neuro-ophthalmol 15: 67–74

Straube A, Kurzan R, and Büttner U (1991) Differential effects of bicuculline and muscimol microinjections into the vestibular nuclei on simian eye movements. Exp Brain Res 86: 347–358

Straube A, Scheuerer W, and Eggert T (1997) Unilateral cerebellar lesions affect initiation of ipsilateral smooth pursuit eye movements in humans. Ann Neurol 42: 891–898

Suzuki DA, and Keller EL (1988 a) The Role of the Posterior Vermis of Monkey Cerebellum in Smooth-Pursuit Eye Movement Control. I. Eye and Head Movement-Related Activity. J Neurophysiol 59: 1–18

Suzuki DA, and Keller EL (1988 b) The Role of the Posterior Vermis of Monkey Cerebellum in Smooth-Pursuit Eye Movement Control. II. Target Velocity-Related Purkinje Cell Activity. J Neurophysiol 59: 19–40

Takagi M, Zee DS, Tamargo R (1996) Effect of dorsal cerebellar vermal lesions on saccades and pursuit in monkeys. Soc Neurosci 22: 1458(Abstract)

Vahedi K, Rivaud S, Amarenco P, and Pierrot-Deseilligny C (1995) Horizontal eye movement disorders after posterior vermis infarctions. J Neurol Neurosurg Psychiatry 58: 91–94

Westheimer G, and Blair SM (1973) Oculomotor defects in cerebellectomized monkeys. Invest Ophthalmol 12: 618–621

Yamada J, and Noda H (1987) Afferent and efferent connections of the oculomotor cerebellar vermis in the macaque monkey. J Comp Neurol 265: 224–241

Zee DS, Yamazaki A, Butler PH, and Gücer G (1981) Effects of ablation of flocculus and paraflocculus on eye movements in primates. J Neurophysiol 46: 878–899

Zee DS, Yee RD, Cogan DG, Robinson DA, and Engel WK (1976) Ocular motor abnormalities in hereditary cerebellar ataxia. Brain 99: 207–234

55

THREE-DIMENSIONAL PROPERTIES OF SACCADIC EYE MOVEMENTS IN PATIENTS WITH CEREBELLAR ATAXIA

M. Fetter,[1] D. Anastasopoulos,[2] and T. Haslwanter[1]

[1]Department of Neurology
Eberhard-Karls-University
Hoppe-Seyler Str. 3, 72076 Tübingen, Germany
[2]Department of Neurology
University of Ioannina
Ioannina, Greece

1. INTRODUCTION

Eye muscles in humans are arranged such that, by appropriate activation, they allow for eye rotations with three degrees of freedom. Yet it has been known for more than a century that during fixation, while the head is stationary, the eyes do only utilize the horizontal and vertical degrees of rotational freedom while the torsional position of the line of sight is kept constant, i.e., during fixation, the eye is restricted to a two-dimensional (2-D) subspace of the three-dimensional (3-D) space of all possible orientations. This has been first described qualitatively by Donders (1847) who stated that the amount of torsion is fixed for all eye positions, independent of from where the eye has reached a particular position. The geometric consequence of this statement is that all eye positions lie in a 2-D surface. By observing the systematic tilt of afterimages in different gaze directions, Helmholtz was able to determine which 2-D subspace the eye is restricted to. He found, according to what Listing suggested, that the eye positions are not only confined to a surface but to a plane called Listing's plane. This result, cited as Listing's law (LL) by Helmholtz (1863), is most simply described if eye positions are expressed in terms of the axes of their rotational displacements from a particular eye position known as primary position and represented by *angular position vectors*. Then LL states that the eye assumes only those positions that can be reached from primary position by a single rotation about an axis in Listing's plane, which lies orthogonal to the gaze direction in primary position.

With the advent of the 3-D magnetic-search coil technique precise measurements of eye position in three dimensions with high temporal and spatial resolution became possi-

Current Oculomotor Research, edited by Becker *et al.*
Plenum Press, New York, 1999.

ble. With this method, LL could be confirmed for saccades and smooth pursuit in both monkeys and normal humans (Ferman et al. 1987; Haslwanter et al. 1991; Tweed and Vilis 1990; Tweed et al. 1992).

In recent years convincing evidences have been accumulated that LL is at least partly due to a neurally-imposed constraint on the oculomotor output that reduces the rotational degrees of freedom, since large deviations from LL can occur during vestibular stimulation where the vestibuloocular reflex (VOR) tries to stabilize the eye in space in all degrees of freedom (Crawford and Vilis 1991; Fetter et al. 1994; Henn et al. 1992; Tweed et al. 1994a; 1994b) or during sleep (Nakayama 1975). However, there is still some debate whether LL could not entirely be caused by orbital mechanics (Schnabolk and Raphan 1994; Tweed et al. 1994c). Recently, it has been shown by Demer and coworkers (1995) that there do exist pulleys and associated tissues that may act as a mid-orbital suspension, passively determining LL. These authors suggest that coordinated innervations need only be consistent with passive constraints.

If LL is based on neural mechanisms one should find central lesions that produce violations of the law. Since the cerebellum is heavily involved in ocular motor control (see Leigh and Zee 1991), we investigated visually triggered random saccades in patients with cerebellar ataxia to evaluate if the cerebellum plays a major role in the implementation of LL.

2. METHODS

2.1. Subjects

Sixteen patients with cerebellar ataxia, predominantly presenting with cerebellar symptoms, and 8 age matched normal subjects gave their informed consent to the study according to a protocol of the local ethics committee. In all cases the ataxia was progressive and possible symptomatic causes (toxic, malignancy, hypothyroidism, vitamin deficiency, inflammatory or vascular etiology) were excluded. Severity of cerebellar dysfunction was assessed by using the rating scale developed by Massaquoi and Hallett (Wessel et al. 1995). The diagnosis of ADCA (autosomal dominant cerebellar ataxia) was made if the family history was positive. It was further distinguished between ADCA-I (2 patients), when additional noncerebellar symptoms were present, and ADCA-III (almost pure cerebellar ataxia; 3 patients). With molecular genetic testing an expansion of the CAG repeat at the SCA1 locus could be demonstrated in one patient with ADCA-I. Patients with idiopathic late onset ataxia (IDCA, after the age of 25 years) were similarly classified according to the presence (MSA-C; cerebellar type of multiple system atrophy; 1 patient) or absence of additional noncerebellar signs (IDCA-C; 5 patients). The remainder of patients were classified as early onset cerebellar ataxia (EOCA, before the age of 20; 5 patients). The latter patients did not show the characteristic clinical and radiographic features of Friedreich's ataxia (Klockgether et al. 1993; 1996). The data of the patients were compared with that of 8 adult normal human subjects (3 female, 5 male) who had no known eye movement abnormalities.

2.2. Data Acquisition and Analysis

Three-dimensional position of the left eye was recorded with the magnetic field-search coil technique at 100Hz. Subjects wore a Skalar annulus containing two orthogonal coils (Skalar, Delft, Netherlands) attached to the anesthetized sclera by suction. Three orthogonal magnetic fields were produced by three pairs of coils (diameter 1.4 m), mounted in a cube-like configuration. The head of the subject was exactly in the center of the magnetic fields. Signals from all 3 fields were recorded, and the system was automatically calibrated at the beginning of the experiments (Bechert and Koenig, 1996). The eye position at the beginning or at the end of the recordings, when the subject was instructed to fixate a straight ahead target, was taken as reference position.

We use the angular position vector (actually the vector part of the eye position quaternion) for describing the eye position. The angular position vector expresses the three-dimensional orientation of the eye in terms of its rotational displacement from the reference position. As reference frame we used a head fixed, right-handed, 3-D Cartesian coordinate system determined by the field coils. This coordinate system is constructed by drawing an x-axis pointing forward in the naso-okzipital direction in the horizontal plane (torsional direction), a y-axis pointing left along the interaural line (vertical direction), and a z-axis pointing up (horizontal direction). The eye position vectors are expressed in the coordinate system according to the right-hand rule with positive values indicating leftward, downward and clockwise (as seen from the subject) rotation of the eye (i.e., when the thumb points in the direction of the vector, the fingers curl round in the direction the eye is turned); its length equals sin (a/2), where a is the amplitude of the rotation. The length of the vector is thus nearly proportional to a within the oculomotor range. Details of the quaternion representations and algorithms for computing them from search coil signals, are given in Tweed et al. (1990).

2.3. Stimuli

Subjects were seated in front of a spherical screen at a distance of 0.95 m. The head was in a comfortable upright position. Head movements were minimized by a helmet and a bite-bar attached to the helmet. After a set of calibration data was recorded the subject had to perform saccades by following a laser dot projected by a mirror galvanometer system onto the inner surface of a sphere in complete darkness. The laser could be pointed in any direction within about 30° of straight ahead. Sudden changes in laser position, with the shutter closed during the motion, provided the stimulus for the rapid gaze shifts (saccades). As indicator for the precision of LL we measured the variability of the torsional component of eye movements sampled during 40 s of random saccades by calculating the standard deviation of the distances, along the torsional axis, of all eye position vectors to the plane of best fit (nonplanarity). Statistical comparison was performed using student's t-test for unpaired samples with a significance level of $p < 0.05$.

3. RESULTS

The major consequence of LL is that eye position vectors should remain confined to a single plane (no change in torsional eye position). This notion is illustrated in Fig. 1 (top row) for a normal subject. The figure shows position vectors sampled during 40s of random saccades. To avoid clutter, vectors are not drawn as arrows but only the tips are indicated. The vectors are viewed from the front of the subject on the left, from the right side in the middle, and from above on the right. The side and top views show that the change in torsional eye position is minimal. In normal subjects, the average nonplanarity of the eye

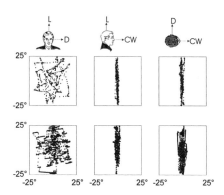

Figure 1. 2-D projections of the position vectors during random saccades in three views of a normal subject (top row) and a patient with IDCA-C. (Left column: front view; middle column: right side view; right column: top view; L=left, D=down, CW = clockwise).

position cloud was 0.82° ± 0.24° for random saccades over the same (±25°) horizontal and vertical range, with a maximum change in torsional ocular position of ±2°.

All patients had a cerebellar atrophy on MRI scan and showed severe cerebellar eye signs including gaze evoked nystagmus, reduced smooth pursuit gain, and reduced visual suppression of the vestibuloocular reflex. Eye positions during random saccades of a patient with IDCA-C (without extra-cerebellar symptoms) is shown in the bottom row of Fig. 1. This patient had in addition downbeat nystagmus (best seen in the front view on the left). Despite severe cerebellar eye signs in this patient 3-D coordination of the eye movements during random saccades was only little different from normal subjects with an average nonplanarity of 1.17°, slightly surpassing the upper normal limit of 1.06° (mean + 1 standard deviation of normals).

The average nonplanarity of all patients for random saccades is shown in Fig. 2. About half of the patients in both, the group without extracerebellar symptoms (ADCA-III and IDCA-C) and the group with extracerebellar symptoms showed pathological values with a highest value of 1.78° in a patients with ADCA-III. There was no significant difference between the two patient groups. There was also no correlation (r=0.3) between severity of the cerebellar disease and the amount of deviation from LL.

4. DISCUSSION

Why is it worthwhile to study three-dimensional eye movements and in particular Listing's law. If this law represents a neurally imposed constraint on oculomotor output, and sev-

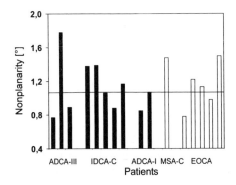

Figure 2. Nonplanarity values (average deviation from a perfect plane) for all patients. The continuous line indicates the upper normal limit.

eral evidences point in this direction, it might teach us more about the principles the brain uses to govern motor control in general. We would briefly like to recapitulate this issue.

If the brain wants to move the eyes and by that the gaze direction from one target to the other there are in three dimensions infinitely many solutions to this problem, since the torsional orientation about the line of sight in the case of a point target is not defined. This problem is called kinematic redundancy.

If the line of sight has to be moved from 30° right to 30° left, which rotation axis should the oculomotor system chose? The eyes could be moved about a pure vertical axis and would end up in the correct position. But the eyes could also be moved about a pure torsional axis, and, in fact, a rotation about any axis lying in the sagittal plane between the two positions would fulfill the task. The gaze direction would always end up in the correct position, but the difference between the different rotation axes is the final torsional orientation about the line of sight. The question is, does the brain, confronted with infinitely many solutions to a problem, decide for a certain stategy and if so will this strategy be the same under all circumstances. The answer is yes. The oculomotor system strictly adheres to a rule that defines the torsional position for each gaze direction. Under normal conditions, for saccades and pursuit the amount of torsion is fixed for all eye positions, independent of from where the eye has reached a particular position and this torsional orientation does not change. One advantage of keeping eye position vectors confined to a single plane in this way is that it permits continuous tracking of a target without buildup of ocular torsion (Tweed et al. 1992). Another advantage may be a facilitation of cooperation, allowing fixation, saccades and pursuit to follow one another in quick succession without carrying the eye position vector out of the common (Listing's) eye position plane.

In this study we attempted to quantify the amount of deviation from LL in patients with cerebellar ataxia to evaluate if the cerebellum plays a major role in the implementation of LL. To our surprise, despite severe cerebellar eye signs, only half of the patients showed a small increase in the average nonplanarity compared to normals. There was no difference between patients with or without additional extracerebellar symptoms and there was no correlation between the severity of cerebellar symptoms and the amount of deviation from LL. These results may either support the notion that LL is largely determined by passive constraints like pulleys and associated tissues (Demer et al. 1995) and that the cerebellum may only be reponsible for the fine tuning of LL, or that the assumed neural mechanism for LL resides in other structures than the cerebellum.

However, our results might have been influenced by adaptive processees in chronic lesions since in a more acute unilateral cerebellar lesion involving the cerebellar vermis, its deep nuclei, and the dorsolateral medulla Helmchen and coworkers (1997) found larger pathological deviations during and after voluntary saccades indicating more severe disturbances of 3-D eye movement coordination in the acute situation. To definitely answer the question of cerebellar involvement in 3-D eye movement coordination further studies in acute circumscribed lesions are necessary.

ACKNOWLEDGEMENTS

This study was supported by the Deutsche Forschungsgemeinschaft, SFB 307- A10. D. A. has been a visiting scientist under the EEC 'Human Capital and Mobility Program'.

REFERENCES

Bechert K, Koenig E (1996) A search coil system with automatic field stabilization, calibration, and geometric processing for eye movement recording in humans. Neuro-ophthalmology 16: 163–170

Crawford JD, Vilis T (1991) Axes of eye rotation and Listing's law during rotations of the head. J Neurophysiol 65: 407–423

Demer JL, Miller JM, Poukens V, Vinters HV, Glasgow BJ (1995) Evidence for fibromuscular pulleys of the recti extraocular muscles. Invest Ophthalmol Visual Sci 36: 1125–1136

Donders FC (1847), Beitrag zur Lehre von den Bewegungen des menschlichen Auges. In: Holländ Beitr Anat Physiol Wiss 1: 104–145

Ferman L, Collewijn H, Hansen TC, van den Berg AV (1987) Human gaze stability in the horizontal, vertical and torsional direction during voluntary head movements, evaluated with a three-dimensional scleral induction coil technique. Vis Res 27: 811–828

Fetter M, Tweed D, Misslisch H, Koenig E (1994) Three-dimensional human eye movements are organized differently for the different oculomotor subsystems. Neuro-ophthalmology 14: 147–152

Haslwanter T, Straumann D, Hepp K, Hess BJM, Henn V (1991) Smooth pursuit eye movements obey Listing's law in monkey. Exp Brain Res 87: 470–472

Helmchen C, Glasauer S, Büttner U (1997) Pathological torsional eye deviation during voluntary saccades: a violation of Lisitng's law. J Neurol Neurosurg Psychiatry 62: 253–260

Helmholtz H von (1863) Ueber die normalen Bewegungen des menschlichen Auges. Arch Ophthalmol IX (2): 153–214

Henn V, Straumann D, Hess BJM, Haslwanter T, Kawachi N (1992) Three-dimensional transformation from vestibular and visual input to oculomotor output. Ann NY Acad Sci 656: 166–180

Klockgether T, Wüllner U, Dichgans J, Grodd W, Nägele T, Petersen D, Schroth G, Schmidt O, Voigt K (1993) Clinical and imaging correlations in inherited ataxias. Adv Neurol 61: 77–96

Klockgether T, Zühlke C, Schulz JB, Bürk K, Fetter M, Dittman H, Skalej M, Dichgans J (1996) Friedreich's ataxia with retained tendon reflexes: Molecular genetics, clinical neurophysiology, and magnetic resonance imaging. Neurology 46: 118–121

Leigh RJ, Zee DS (1991) The neurology of eye movements. 2nd ed. FA Davis, Philadelphia, pp 424–428

Nakayama K (1975) Coordination of extraocular muscles. In: Lennerstrand G, Bach-y-Rita P (eds) Basic mechanisms of ocular motility and their clinical implications. Pergamon, Oxford, pp 193–207

Schnabolk C, Raphan T (1994) Modeling three-dimensional velocity-to-position transformation in oculomotor control. J Neurophysiol 71: 623–638

Tweed D, Vilis T (1990) Geometric relations of eye position and velocity vectors during saccades. Vis Res 30: 111–127

Tweed D, Cadera W, Vilis T (1990) Computing three-dimensional eye position quaternions and eye velocity from search coil signals. Vis Res 30: 97–110

Tweed D, Fetter M, Andreadaki S, Koenig E, Dichgans J (1992) Three-dimensional properties of human pursuit eye movements. Vis Res 32: 1225–1238

Tweed D, Fischer D, Misslisch H, Fetter M, Zee DS, Koenig E (1994a) Rotational kinematics of the human vestibuloocular reflex I: gain matrices. J Neurophys 72: 2467–2479

Tweed D, Fetter M, Fischer D, Misslisch H, Koenig E (1994b) Rotational kinematics of the human vestibuloocular reflex II: velocity steps. J Neurophys 72: 2480–2489

Tweed D, Misslisch H, Fetter M (1994c) Testing models of the oculomotor velocity to position transformation. J Neurophys 72: 1425–1429

Wessel K, Zeffiro T, Lou J-S, Toro C, Hallett M (1995) Regional cerebral blood flow during self-paced sequential finger opposition task in patients with cerebellar degeneration. Brain 118: 379–393

56

EFFECT OF TARGET PREDICTABILITY ON THE INITIATION OF SMOOTH PURSUIT IN HEALTHY SUBJECTS AND PATIENTS WITH CEREBELLAR LESION

C. Moschner,[1] T. J. Crawford,[2] W. Heide,[1] P. Trillenberg,[1] D. Kömpf,[1] and C. Kennard[3]

[1]Department of Neurology
Medical University of Lübeck
Lübeck, Germany
[2]Department of Psychology
Lancaster University
Lancaster, UK
[3]Department of Clinical Neuroscience
Charing Cross and Westminster Medical School
London, UK

1. INTRODUCTION

Repeated presentation of a continuously moving visual target can elicit two types of smooth eye movements that can be identified by their time of onset (Kao and Gellman 1994). One type builds up well before the target motion appears and represents an anticipatory smooth eye movement (ASEM) that is solely driven by predictive expectations derived from prior target presentations (Kowler et al. 1984; Kao and Morrow 1994, Barnes et al. 1997). ASEM are more frequent and faster during presentation of highly predictable stimuli, but they are not necessarily extinguished by making the target movement unpredictable (Kowler et al. 1981). Smooth pursuit eye movements (SP), the second type of slow eye movements, begin with a certain delay after target onset (Tychsen and Lisberger 1986, Carl and Gellman 1987). If SP is elicited by an unexpected target motion, the first 100–125 ms of the smooth eye movement (initiation phase) are directly controlled by the target motion that was perceived before SP onset (Tychsen and Lisberger 1986). This way, SP initiation operates as an open-loop system. After this, visual feedback and extraretinal input of eye and head movements provide an internal signal that controls steady-state pursuit, the so called maintenance phase of SP (Tychsen and Lisberger 1986, Carl and Gellman 1987). Although SP is predominantly controlled by visual input, pursuit maintenance during longer periods of tracking is optimised

Current Oculomotor Research, edited by Becker *et al.*
Plenum Press, New York, 1999.

by expectations of the target motion. For example, during tracking of sinusoidal stimuli, prediction of target motion significantly contributes to the adjustment of gaze velocity and phase lag (van den Berg 1988, Barnes and Asselman 1991). The same kind of predictive control seems to maintain SP during tracking of a constantly moving target that suddenly disappears for a short period of time (Boman and Hotson 1992). However, prediction of target motion not only maintains SP, it also effects pursuit initiation. Using predictable and randomised step-ramp stimuli, Kao and Morrow (1994) have recently studied the predictive control mechanisms of pursuit initiation in healthy human subjects. They have shown that target predictability modifies the timing of SP initiation, the acceleration during the initial phase of the visually-triggered SP, and the acceleration of ASEM. Our main objective was to study the impact of cerebellar dysfunction on predictive and direct visual control of SP initiation. Electrophysiological studies in monkeys and clinical studies in humans have established the crucial role of the cerebellum, especially the floccular region, in the steady-state control of SP (for further references, see Baloh et al. 1986, Blanks 1988, Keller 1989, Keller and Heinen 1991, Moschner et al. 1994, Büttner and Straube 1995). However, the cerebellum may also take part in the control of SP initiation. Recent studies have used step-ramps (Straube et al. 1997) or pure ramp stimuli (Lekwuwa et al. 1995) to study SP initiation in patients with cerebellar lesion. In response to non-predictable stimuli, cerebellar patients had significantly slower eye velocities than healthy subjects during the initiation phase of SP. There were contradictory findings regarding the effect of cerebellar lesion on the latency of SP onset. In response to non-predictable step-ramps, patients with predominant lesion of the cerebellar hemispheres showed normal latencies (Straube at al. 1997). On the other hand, Lekwuwa and colleagues (1995) noticed a significant delay of smooth pursuit onset in patients with diffuse cerebellar lesion only when non-predictable ramps were presented. When they have used a predictable ramp stimulus the latencies of patients and controls were not significantly different. Furthermore, a cerebellar defect may impair the ability to generate very fast ASEM (Lekwuwa et al. 1995, Moschner et al. 1996). Similar to Kao and Morrow (1994), we have now used repeated predictable and unpredictable step-ramp stimulation to elicit smooth eye movements in cerebellar patients and healthy control subjects. By comparing the initial eye acceleration, we have quantified possible cerebellar deficits of ASEM generation and initial SP. Furthermore, pursuit latencies were measured to clarify the cerebellar influence on the timing of pursuit initiation.

2. METHODS

2.1. Subjects

Eye movements of six patients (age 44.8 y. ± 14.9) with a cerebellar lesion and six healthy control subjects (age 48.2 y. ± 17.7) were recorded with a magnetic search-coil system. In patients, cerebellar lesion was either due to an ideopathic (n=3) or autosomal-dominant cerebellar degeneration (n=2), or to Friedreich's ataxia (n=1).Subjects were asked to track a red laser dot with optimal speed and accuracy.

2.2. Experimental Paradigms

We used a step-ramp stimulus pattern where the dot stepped in the horizontal plane from centre position to an eccentric position. This was immediately followed by a constant velocity motion of the target into the same direction (centrifugal ramp), or into the opposite direction of the step (centripetal ramp). The ramp was finished by a second step back to the centre position. Step-ramps were presented sequentially with a constant inter-trial interval of 1500ms. In the predictable condition (PRED), a sequence of seven identical centripetal ramps to the left was followed by seven similar ramps to the right. In the randomised condition (RAND), centrifugal and centripetal ramps to both sides were presented in a balanced, pseudo-randomised order. The following results exclusively refer to centripetal ramps tested with ramp velocities of 10°/s or 20°/s and step sizes of 2° or 4°, respectively.

2.3. Data Analysis

Based on the method described by Carl and Gellman (1987), we measured the acceleration of possible ASEM during an interval between 80 ms prior to and 100 ms after target onset and the time of onset of each visually triggered SP response. The response latency was determined by the time interval between the onset of the stimulus step and the onset of the SP response. SP acceleration was measured over the first 60 ms-period after the time of SP onset. Trials were rejected if a saccade occurred within this period (about 20 % of all trials), so that SP acceleration data always referred to a pre-saccadic interval of pursuit initiation.

3. RESULTS

The results revealed significant deficits of smooth pursuit initiation in the group of patients with cerebellar lesion in comparison to healthy control subjects. The following two tables summarise the results in the experiments with randomised (table 1) and predictable step-ramp stimulation (table 2).

3.1. Latency of Smooth Pursuit Onset

In the PRED condition, mean latency of SP responses was always significantly prolonged in patients compared to healthy controls (p<0.01; Mann-Whitney U-test), irrespective of the stimulus velocity. In the RAND condition, the same trend was significant in trials with the slower 10°/s-ramp velocity (p<0.01) but not with 20°/s-ramp velocity (p=0.09). This was probably due to the large inter-individual variability in the patients group (compare 1 SD values). In controls, corresponding latencies were shorter in the

Table 1. Randomised step-ramps

	Group			
	Controls		Patients	
	Stimulus velocity			
	10 °/s	20 °/s	10 °/s	20 °/s
Latency of SP initiation [ms]	155 + 9	151 + 16	201 + 27*	186 + 42
Initial acceleration of SP [°/s^2]	42 + 12	75 + 28	32 + 9	38 + 13*
Anticipatory acceleration [°/s^2]	3.3 + 1.5	3.1 + 1.6	2.3 + 0.4	2.5 + 1.2

Group mean values ± 1 SD.
* = significant difference between patients and controls (p < 0.01; Mann–Whitney U-test).

Table 2. Predictable step-ramps

	Group			
	Controls		Patients	
	Stimulus velocity			
	10 °/s	20 °/s	10 °/s	20 °/s
Latency of SP initiation [ms]	126 + 6	125 + 12	180 + 13*	185 + 19*
Initial acceleration of SP [°/s^2]	47 + 22	74 + 31	29 + 10	33 + 9*
Anticipatory acceleration [°/s^2]	3.3 + 2.7	4.1 + 1.6	2.2 + 1.0	2.5 + 0.6

Group mean values ± 1 SD.
* = significant difference between patients and controls (p < 0.01; Mann – Whitney U-test).

PRED condition compared to the RAND condition (p<0.05, Wilcoxon rank test) whereas in patients, the difference between PRED and RAND trials was insignificant.

3.2. Eye Acceleration during SP Initiation

Mean acceleration of initial SP was decreased in patients compared to controls only when the faster ramp velocity of 20°/s was presented. This decrease of initial SP acceleration in the patient group (in comparison to controls) was found under both conditions, RAND (Table 1, p<0.01; Mann-Whitney U-test) and PRED (Table 2; p< 0.01). In none of the groups did we find a significant effect of target predictability on initial SP acceleration, i.e. the peak acceleration during SP initiation was about the same in the RAND condition compared to the PRED condition. In healthy subjects, initial acceleration increased with the higher stimulus velocity. In patients, the eye acceleration did not further increase with a stimulus velocity of 20 °/s (compared to stimulus velocities of 10 °/s), irrespective whether randomised or predictable step-ramps were presented.

3.3. ASEM

The mean acceleration of anticipatory eye movements was low in both groups, controls and patients. In the PRED condition the mean anticipatory eye acceleration ranged between 2 and 8°/s^2 in controls and between 2 and 4 °/s^2 in patients. In some individuals, controls and patients, anticipatory acceleration occasionally reached 25 to 40 °/s. However, the mean initial acceleration did not differentiate between both groups. Furthermore, in both groups, the difference of mean anticipatory acceleration in the PRED condition compared to the RAND condition was insignificant.

4. DISCUSSION

4.1. ASEM

In the present study, mean ASEM acceleration remained slow in both groups, cerebellar patients and healthy controls. In healthy subjects, it did not significantly increase with faster ramp velocities of 20°/s and the difference between mean ASEM acceleration during predictable stimulation and randomised stimulation was insignificant, which is discrepant to prior observations (Kao and Morrow1994). This discrepancy was probably related to methodical differences between the two studies. For example, we have used a longer inter-trial time interval (1500 compared to 625 ms) and we gave different verbal instruction asking not only for fast but also very accurate responses. Due to the lack of fast ASEM in the control group, we could not identify a significant deficit of ASEM generation in the patients, although a tendency towards slower anticipatory eye movements was found in the patients' group (compare corresponding mean values in table 1 and 2). On the other hand, the presence of slow ASEM in patients underlines that predictive control of slow eye movement is, at least, partially preserved after a degenerative cerebellar lesion.

4.2. Timing of Smooth Pursuit Onset

Our results on smooth pursuit initiation in healthy subjects were basically consistent with previous studies that have used the step-ramp paradigm. The mean latency of SP towards an unpredictable step-ramp target motion was about 150 ms, independent of the ramp velocity (Carl and Gellman 1987, Kao and Morrow 1994). Predictable presentation of repeated step-ramps significantly shortened the latency to about 125 ms (Kao and Morrow 1994). Thus, the latency of pursuit initiation in healthy humans is not only determined by the time required to process visual information of the actual target motion. With higher levels of target predictability, the latency is reduced by predictive control mechanisms that are based on the experience of previous target motion. We have now demonstrated that cerebellar dysfunction due to a degenerative lesion disturbs the initiation of smooth pursuit in humans. When step-ramps were presented in randomised order the mean latency of SP onset was significantly delayed in patients compared to controls. This shows that optimal timing of SP initiation requires the intact function of cerebellum. Some electrophysiological studies in monkeys gave evidence that cerebellar structures involved in SP initiation may include the caudal fastigial nuclei (Fuchs et al. 1994) and/or the floccular region (Stone and Lisberger 1990). This would explain, why the timing of pursuit onset remained unchanged in patients with more lateral lesions of the cerebellar hemispheres (Straube et al. 1997). Another important finding of our study was that the timing of smooth pursuit onset in cerebellar patients was not improved by target predictability. The mean latency of SP in cerebellar patients was not significantly shorter in the PRED condition than in the RAND condition. Obviously, the predictive control mechanism that shortens pursuit onset in healthy humans during predictable stimulation are impaired in cerebellar patients; at least, it cannot compensate for the delay of SP.

4.3. Initial SP Acceleration

The acceleration of initial PS varies depending on individual factors and various target properties (Tychsen and Lisberger 1986, Carl and Gellman 1987; Kao and Morrow 1994). In healthy subjects, prediction significantly increases initial SP acceleration when ramp velocity exceeds 20–30°/s (Kao and Morrow 1994). With the slower target velocities used in this study the predictive increase of SP remained insignificant in our control subjects. In cerebellar patients, initial SP acceleration was significantly slower than in healthy subjects when the faster stimulus velocity of 20 °/s was presented. This deficit of SP acceleration was observed with predictable and unpredictable stimulation. These findings question the results of Lekwuwa and colleagues (1995) who proposed a preserved predictive input to the cerebellum that is able to compensate for decreased eye velocity during SP initiation.

4.4. Conclusions

The human cerebellum does not only control (steady-state) gaze velocity during maintenance of SP. It also takes part in the control of initial smooth pursuit acceleration and in the timing of SP initiation. Predictive control of smooth eye movements is not completely deactivated by cerebellar lesion because cerebellar patients are able to generate ASEM. However, improvement of SP initiation by prediction is ineffective in cerebellar patients, and prediction fails to compensate for decreased initial SP acceleration. Thus, the cerebellar deficit of SP initiation seems to be independent from the amount of predictive input provided to the cerebellum.

REFERENCES

Baloh RW, Yee RD, Honrubia V (1986) Late cortical cerebellar atrophy. Clinical and oculographic features. Brain 109: 159–80.

Barnes GR, Asselman PT (1991) The mechanism of prediction in human smooth pursuit eye movements. J Physiol (Lond) 439: 439–61.

Blanks RHL (1988) Cerebellum. In: Büttner-Ennever JA (ed) Neuroanatomy of the oculomotor system. Elsevier, Amsterdam, pp 225–72.

Boman D, Hotson J (1992) Predictive smooth pursuit eye movements near abrupt changes in motion direction. Vision Res 32: 675–689.

Büttner U, Straube A (1995) The effect of cerebellar midline lesions on eye movements. Neuroophthalmology 15: 75–82.

Carl JR, Gellman RS (1987) Human smooth pursuit: Stimulus dependent responses. J Neurophysiol 57: 1446–62.

Fuchs AF, Robinson FR, Straube A (1994) Participation of caudal fastigial nucleus in smooth pursuit eye movements. I. Neuronal activity. J Neurophysiol 72: 2714–28.

Kao GW, Morrow MJ (1994) The relationship of anticipatory eye movement to smooth pursuit initiation. Vision Res 34: 3027–36.

Keller EL (1988) Cerebellar involvement in smooth pursuit eye movement generation: Flocculus and vermis. In: Kennard C, Rose F (eds) Physiological aspects of clinical neuro-ophthalmology. Chapman and Hall, London, pp 341–55.

Keller EL, Heinen SJ (1991) Generation of smooth-pursuit eye movements. Neuronal mechanisms and pathways. Neurosci Res 11: 79–107.

Kowler E, Martins AJ, Pavel M (1984) The effect of expectations on slow oculomotor control. IV. Anticipatory smooth eye movements depend on prior target motions. Vision Res 24: 197–210.

Kowler E, Steinman RM. (1981) The effect of expectations on slow oculomotor control. III. Guessing unpredictable target displacements. Vision Res 21: 191–203.

Lekwuwa GU, Barnes GR, Grealy MA (1995) Effects of prediction on smooth pursuit velocity gain in cerebellar patients and controls. In: Findlay JM, Walker R, Kentridge RW (eds) Eye movement research. Mechanisms, processes, and applications. Elsevier, Amsterdam, pp 119–21.

Moschner C, Perlman S, Baloh RW (1994) Comparison of oculomotor findings in the progressive ataxia syndromes. Brain 117: 15–25.

Moschner C, Zangemeister WH, Demer JL (1996) Anticipatory smooth eye movements of high velocity triggered by large target steps: Normal performance and effect of cerebellar degeneration. Vision Res 36: 1341–9.

Straube A, Scheurer W, Eggert T (1997) Unilateral cerebellar lesions affect initiation of ipsilateral smooth eye movements in humans. Ann Neurol 42: 891–898.

Stone LS, Lisberger SG (1990). Visual response of Purkinje cells in the cerebellar flocculus during smooth-pursuit eye movements in monkeys. I. Simple spikes. J Neurophysiol 63: 1241–61.

Tychsen L, Lisberger SG (1986) Visual motion processing for the initiation of smooth-pursuit eye movements in humans. J Neurophysiol 56: 953–68.

Van den Berg, AV (1988) Human smooth pursuit during transient perturbations of predictable and unpredictable target movement. Exp Brain Res 72: 95–108.

57

OCULAR MOTOR DISORDERS ASSOCIATED WITH INBORN CHIASMAL CROSSING DEFECTS

Multi-Planar Eye Movement Recordings in See-Saw and Congenital Nystagmus

P. Apkarian,[1] L. J. Bour,[2] J. van der Steen,[1] and H. Collewijn[1]

[1]Department of Physiology
Faculty of Medicine and Health Sciences
Erasmus University Rotterdam
PO Box 1738, 3000 DR Rotterdam, The Netherlands
[2]Department of Neurology
Clinical Neurophysiology
Academic Medical Centre
Amsterdam, The Netherlands

1. INTRODUCTION

The present study briefly reviews the accompanying ocular motor function and dysfunction in two major inborn conditions of naturally occurring aberrant optic pathway projections, i.e., albinism and non-decussating retinal-fugal fibre syndrome (Apkarian et al. 1994;1995; Apkarian 1996). The latter is a rare, isolated achiasmatic condition in which nasal retinal projections and concomitant visuotopic and retinotopic mapping misroute due to the inborn and isolated absence of the optic chiasm. The achiasmatic ocular motor profile is compared with that of albinos who also present with optic pathway misrouting but in opposite form from that of the achiasmatic condition. In albinism there is a preponderance of erroneously decussating temporal retinal-fugal fibres whilst in achiasmatic syndrome there is a complete absence of decussating nasal retinal-fugal fibres. The simplified sketches of Figure 1, adapted from Polyak (1957), emphasize the normal organisation of retinal-fugal projections compared to the relative majority of contralateral projections pathognomonic to albinism and the nonextant contralateral projections characteristic of the achiasmatic condition.

Current Oculomotor Research, edited by Becker *et al.*
Plenum Press, New York, 1999.

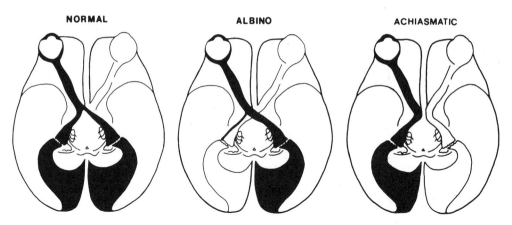

Figure 1. The simplified models, adapted from Polyak, 1957 as depicted in Apkarian et al., 1995, reflect a tangential view of the primary visual pathway projections of a normal, albino, and achiasmat. For the normal model, nasal retinal fibres project to the contralateral hemisphere whilst temporal retinal fibres project to the ipsilateral hemisphere. For the albino, temporal retinal fibres cross in error at the chiasm resulting in a preponderance of contralateral projections. For the achiasmat the absence of a chiasma precludes decussation resulting in both nasal and temporal retinal projections to the ipsilateral hemisphere and a complete absence of contralateral projections.

In either of these congenital anomalies, developmental chiasmal misrouting of the retinal-fugal fibres results in widespread visual system disorganisation that apparently and consequently stimulates the rearrangement of retinal-topic mapping of visual information throughout the visual pathways. In albinos, with a central segment of temporal retinal fibres erroneously decussating, the medial portions of the lateral geniculate layers (LGN) which represent, at least in part, the ipsilateral visual field, fall into misalignment (Guillery 1990;1996). For the achiasmats, all nasal retinal fibres fail to decussate and the entire ipsilateral hemifield is represented in the targeted LGN layers in complete mirror reversal. Of particular interest is that despite the striking chiasmal crossing errors and subsequent visual field misprojections and mismapping, both albinos and achiasmats present with normal visual fields. For the albinos, based on temporal retinal lesions or albino animal models, partial or full bi-nasal hemianopsia is expected (Elekessy et al. 1973; Guillery and Casagrande 1977). For the achiasmats, based on experimentally induced split chiasm conditions in animal models or trauma induced split chiasm conditions, bi-temporal hemianopsia is expected (Fisher et al. 1968; Traquair et al. 1935). The normal visual fields in albinos and achiasmats suggest a striking neural plasticity and functional reorganisation, at least at higher visual processing structures, which apparently allows for compensation of the resultant visuotopic rearrangements and inconsistencies.

However, one major aspect of visual processing in the two aberrant chiasmal conditions that apparently is unable to fully compensate for the inborn rearrangements of the albino and achiasmatic visual pathways concerns the ocular motor systems. Albinos and achiasmats present with ocular motor impairments including interocular misalignments as well as ocular motor instabilities (Abel 1989; Apkarian et al. 1983; Apkarian et al. 1995; Collewijn et al. 1985; Leigh and Zee 1991). For both albinos and achiasmats the ocular motor instabilities are typically present in the form of classic congenital nystagmus (Apkarian 1996; Collewijn et al. 1985; Leigh and Zee 1991). However, in addition to congenital nystagmus in the horizontal planes, the achiasmats also present with nystagmus in the

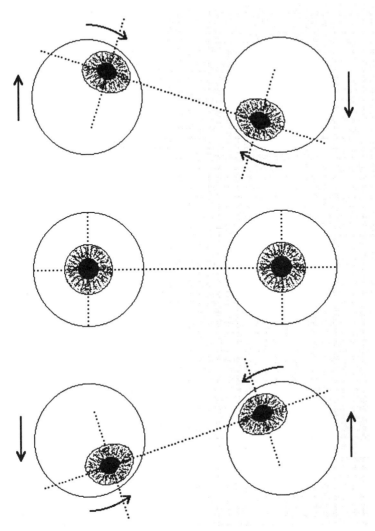

Figure 2. Simplified schematic of classic see-saw nystagmus with upward movement and intorsion of one eye and simultaneous downward movement and extorsion of the fellow eye.

vertical and torsional planes (Apkarian et al. 1994; 1995; Apkarian 1996). The latter takes the form of the rare but classic see-saw nystagmus (Maddox 1914) with upward movement and intorsion of one eye and simultaneous downward movement and extorsion of the fellow eye (see also see-saw model presented in Figure 2).

There are several unresolved issues of interest concerning ocular motor instabilities associated with the two abnormal chiasmal conditions described. First, the etiology of the accompanying ocular motor instabilities in the two chiasmal defects remains enigmatic. Secondly, see-saw nystagmus with the exception of a rare and purportedly isolated congenital form (Schmidt and Kommerell 1974; Zauberman and Magora 1969) typically accompanies various inborn or acquired disorders or accidental infarcts that affect the midline including diverse tumors (Alvord and Lofton 1988; Bataini et al. 1991; Dutton 1994; Iraci et al. 1981; MacCarty et al. 1970), demyelinating disorders (Samkoff and

Smith 1994), or degenerative diseases (Bergin and Halpern 1986). However, in contrast to see-saw nystagmus *per se*, anatomical and physiological substrates for congenital nystagmus remain perplexing (Daroff et al. 1978; Leigh and Zee 1991; Optican and Zee 1984; Yee et al. 1976). For example, distinct from albinos or achiasmats, patients with isolated idiopathic or hereditary congenital nystagmus show neither demonstrable evidence of visual pathway misrouting (Apkarian and Shallo-Hoffmann 1991) nor any other detectable pathology (Leigh and Zee 1991). Furthermore, although both albinos and achiasmats with clear evidence of aberrant visual pathways also present with classic congenital nystagmus profiles, at least in the horizontal planes, the direct relationship between misrouted primary optic pathways and accompanying ocular motor instabilities continues to prove elusive.

In describing the various profiles of see-saw and congenital nystagmus which occur in albinism and non-decussating retinal fugal fibre syndrom, the present study strives to provide empirical ocular motor descriptions that, in future, may help yield a better understanding of underlying mechanisms of ocular motor disorders associated with inborn chiasmal crossing defects as well as those associated with isolated, idiopathic or congenital nystagmus.

2. METHODS

2.1. Patient History

In the present study, the ocular motor profiles of two patients are presented. Both patients are of normal intelligence and with the exception of ocular motor related misalignments and instabilities and chiasmal misrouting, test negative for accompanying neurological and or endocrinopathic disorders. Patient ACH is a female achiasmat tested at the age of 16 years; patient ALB is a male albino tested at the age of 25 years.

Patient ACH: ACH is a dizygotic twin; extensive pedigree evaluation of the family tree registered no relatives with notable hereditary or idiopathic visual system anomalies including congenital nystagmus. Ophthalmic evaluation of ACH revealed normal fundi including well defined macular and foveal reflexes, pigmentation and retinal vasculature; irides were also normal. Optical refraction yielded spherical and cylindrical corrections of OD: S = -5.25, C = -1.5 axis 50 deg; OS: S = -6.75. Corrected Snellen acuity at 6 metre viewing distance was 0.3 (20/60) OD viewing, 0.2 (20/100) OS viewing and 0.3 (20/60) OU viewing. At near viewing (20 cm) OU acuity was 1 (20/20). An alternating esotropia of 20 to 25 prism diopters was present together with a variable hypotropia (2 to 5 deg) of the left eye with right eye fixation. The right eye is generally the preferred eye of fixation particularly in straight ahead position. When gaze angle increases ACH prefers to fixate with the eye in adduction. That is, typically the left eye will fixate a far right target while the right eye will fixate a far left target. In Figure 3, an example of the achiasmat's esotropia is depicted. Note from the first Purkinje image that the right eye is fixating the target while the left eye is misaligned.

In the horizontal planes, ACH presents with classic congenital nystagmus (Abadi and Pascal 1995; Daroff et al. 1978; Yee et al. 1976) and in the vertical and torsional planes, classic see-saw nystagmus (Daroff 1965; Druckman et al. 1966; Maddox 1914) Accompanying the ocular motor instabilities is a mild head shudder and torticollis with head tilt toward right shoulder. ACH shows no evidence of stereopsis; colour vision is normal. Visual fields as tested with either static or kinetic perimetry also are normal.

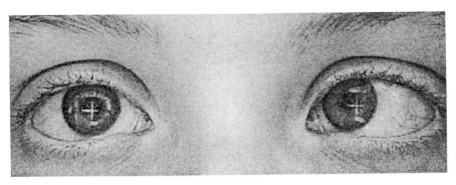

Figure 3. Interocular misalignment of ACH with alternating esotropia. Typically this patient prefers to fixate more eccentric positioned targets with the fixating eye in adduction

Patient ALB: The albino genotype for ALB is unknown but phenotype and family pedigree analysis suggests autosomal recessive, oculocutaneous albinism or OCA2. Ophthalmic evaluation of ALB revealed foveal and macular hypoplasia, peripheral fundus hypopigmentation and iris diaphany. ALB presents with blue irides, light brown hair colour and no tanning when exposed to sun light. Optical refraction yielded spherical corrections of OD: S = +10; OS: S = +11.25. Corrected Snellen acuity at 6 metre viewing distance was 0.1 (20/200) OD viewing, 0.15 (20/300) OS viewing. At near viewing (20 cm) OU acuity was 0.4 (20/50). A variable esotropia and hypertropia was present. The left eye is generally the preferred eye of fixation particularly in straight ahead gaze. When gaze angle is elevated, ALB also prefers to fixate with the left eye. In Figure 4, an example of the albino's hypertropia is depicted. Note from the first Pukinje image, the interocular misalignments.

In the horizontal planes, ALB presents with classic congenital nystagmus (Abadi and Pascal 1995; Daroff et al. 1978; Yee et al. 1976) and in the vertical planes, with an oblique component and interocular amplitude disconjugacy. ALB shows no evidence of stereopsis; colour vision is normal. Visual fields as tested with static perimetry also are normal.

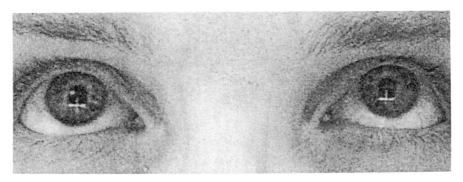

Figure 4. Interocular alignment of ALB with hypermetropia and esotropia while fixating a target positioned along the vertical meridian.

2.2. Eye Movement Recordings

Calibration and Recording: Measurement of ocular rotation in three dimensions (3D) was implemented with the dual scleral induction coil technique (Ferman et al. 1987). Raw data were digitized with a sample frequency of 500 Hz. To account for the various offsets, corrective alterations were added to the calibration procedures (see e.g., Hess et al. 1992). Calibration consisted of an *in vitro* and an *in vivo* protocol. For *in vivo* calibration, cooperation of the patient was required.

For the *in vitro* calibration, the following procedure was implemented. The straight ahead position (0 degrees) was used as the reference target. The three gain components of the direction and the torsion coil (coil vectors) were obtained by directing a gimbal system to symmetrically positioned targets with respect to the reference target. Under these conditions, offsets inherent to the dual search coil could then be determined. Measurements with the gimbal system obtained from eccentric target positions across the different meridians also were used as a calibration check. Via a rotation matrix (Robinson, 1963), sine and cosine components of direction and torsion coils were converted to 3D Fick coordinates. After Haustein (1989), Fick coordinates were converted to rotation vectors (see also Tweed et al. 1990).

For the *in vivo* calibration the subject fixated a reference target positioned at straight ahead. To obtain the corresponding 'zero fixation' position for each eye, monocular measurements were implemented. Following the experimental protocol, all successful and successful 'zero position fixations' within a given test session were marked for further offline calibration and analysis. To compensate for long-term drift and/or sudden shifts of eye movement signals (particularly those from the torsion coil) repeated fixation of the zero fixation reference target was implemented. A third-order polynomial was fit through successive 'zero-fixations' that extended over a given fixation measure. Zero-fixations were also parsed into "foveation periods" (Bedell et al. 1989; Chung and Bedell 1996; Daroff et al. 1978; Yee et al. 1976). Criteria for foveation periods included,

1. target fixation accuracy to within +/- 30 minutes in both vertical and horizontal planes,
2. eye velocity of no greater than 7.5 deg/sec in both vertical and horizontal planes. Mean velocities and standard deviations (across all trials) were calculated for foveation periods across the duration of the fixating epoch.

Stimulus: For the achiasmat, the stimulus grid consisted of targets presented in horizontal, vertical and oblique meridians from primary position to ±20 deg eccentricity; fixation targets consisted of red spots (6' radius) with black cross hairs superimposed. For the albino, the stimulus grid was slightly modified such that the targets were presented in isovergence; fixation targets consisted of red LEDs (7' radius) positioned in horizontal, vertical and oblique meridians from primary position to ±30 deg eccentricity.

3. RESULTS

3.1. Achiasmat

As depicted in Figure 5, during target fixation at straight ahead position with binocular viewing, ACH demonstrates in the horizontal planes classic congenital nystagmus characterised by unidirectional jerk left with slow eye movement foveation. Frequency of

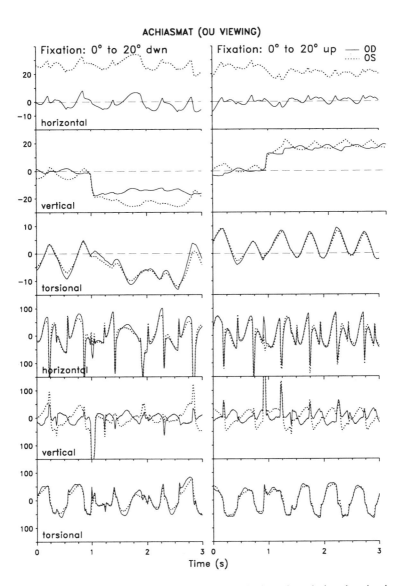

Figure 5. For achiasmat ACH, depicted from top to bottom are the horizontal, vertical, and torsional components of rotation vectors and corresponding horizontal, vertical, and torsional components of rotation vector velocities for the right eye (solid traces) and left eye (dotted traces). Target fixation of ACH under OU viewing conditions for about 1 second at straight ahead position is followed first by a 20 degree downward (leftmost column) or upward (rightmost column) saccade and then about two seconds of target fixation at 20 degrees downward or upward gaze angle. Rightward, upward, and clockwise (upper pole toward the right shoulder) rotation are plotted as positive values along the Y coordinates. Note the classic CN waveforms in the horizontal planes, striking interocular phase disconjugacy in the vertical planes, and pendular nystagmus in the torsional planes. Note also the persistent interocular esotropia and intermittent hypertropia.

the latter is about 2 Hz; amplitude varies between 5–10 degrees. Note also from the upper most traces, depicting the horizontal planes, that the right eye is fixating the target whilst the left eye is variably esotropic. In the vertical and torsional planes classic see-saw nystagmus is present and is characterized by conjugate, pendular oscillation in the torsional planes with a superimposed disjunctive vector in the vertical planes. The frequency of the vertical and torsional components of the see-saw nystagmus are similar to and in phase with the congenital nystagmus in the horizontal planes. As depicted under fixation conditions of 20 degrees eccentricity in downgaze (leftmost column), the frequency of the nystagmus appears to slightly decrease to about 1.7 Hz whereas with 20 degrees upgaze (rightmost column) the frequency increases to about 2.5 Hz. In contrast, amplitude of the see-saw nystagmus in the vertical and torsional planes appears independent of vertical gaze angle. Mean torsion also does not change significantly with vertical gaze angle. Note also that at downgaze OS is hypotropic.

3.2. Albino

As depicted in Figure 6, particularly during target fixation with both eyes at straight ahead position, ALB demonstrates in the horizontal planes classic congenital nystagmus characterised by unidirectional jerk right nystagmus with extended foveation, having a frequency of about 4.5 Hz and an amplitude between 3 and 7 degrees. In the vertical planes a small vertical component can be observed beating upwards with an amplitude of about 1–3 degrees. In addition, in phase with the horizontal and vertical nystagmus, a torsional component with an amplitude of 2 to 3 degrees also can be observed with the fast phase beating in counter clockwise direction. With 30 degrees downward gaze the frequency of the nystagmus increases to about 5.5 Hz (4th panel to the left) and in the torsional planes the amplitude of nystagmus for OD diminishes whereas the nystagmus in the comparable plane for OS appears to reverse direction (3rd and 6th panels to the left). Also with 30 degrees downward gaze, the mean torsion of OD increases by about 5 degrees whereas the mean torsion of OS decreases by about 2 to 3 degrees. The latter results in cyclovergence of about 4 degrees (3rd panel to the left). Interestingly, with 30 degrees upgaze the frequency and amplitude of the nystagmus in the horizontal and vertical planes does not significantly alter. However, the amplitude of the fast phase in the torsional planes clearly increases in amplitude (6th panel to the right). Compared to downgaze the mean torsion of OD diminishes by about 1 degree whereas the mean torsion of OS increases by the substantial amount of about 10 degrees. The latter results in cyclovergence of about minus 11 degrees (3rd panel to the right). Note also that ALB shows a variable esotropia from 10 to 15 degrees.

4. DISCUSSION AND CONCLUSIONS

As described in the result section the inborn visual pathway perturbations in non-decussating retinal fugal fibre syndrome as well as in albinism are associated with various profiles of ocular motor pathology. In general, the present study emphasizes the rather complicated eye movement profiles associated with chiasmal crossing defects. Achiasmats present with particularly complicated aberrant ocular motor profiles including vertical and horizontal interocular misalignments as well as profound ocular instabilities and dysconjugacies that extend across horizontal, vertical and torsional eye movement planes. Albinos also present with complicated interocular misalignments and ocular motor instabilities al-

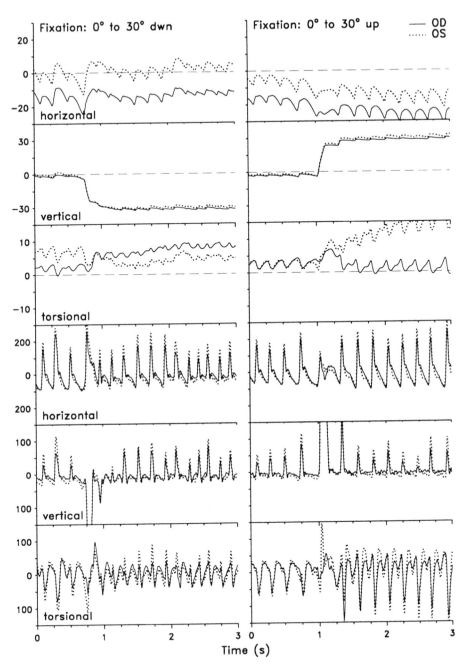

Figure 6. For albino ALB depicted from top to bottom are the horizontal, vertical, and torsional components of rotation vectors and corresponding horizontal, vertical, and torsional components of rotation vector velocities for the right eye (solid traces) and left eye (dotted traces). Target fixation of ALB under OU viewing conditions for about 1 second at straight ahead position is followed first by a 30 degree downward (leftmost column) or upward (rightmost column) saccade and then about two seconds of target fixation at 30 degrees downward or upward gaze angle. Rightward, upward, and clockwise (upper pole to the right shoulder) rotation is positive. Note the classic CN waveforms in the horizontal planes, an oblique component and amplitude disconjugacy in the vertical planes, and pendular nystagmus in the torsional planes.

beit the latter are typically in the form of irregularities within primarily the horizontal planes. However, as observed in the albino profile included in the present study, the primary classic congenital nystagmus prevalent in albinism may also be accompanied by instabilities within the vertical and torsional planes as well. In fact, there are albino studies which also report the presence of so-called micro see-saw nystagmus (Apkarian et al., 1996). Also as illustrated in the present study, detection of various vertical and torsional instabilities whether in albinos, achiasmats or idiopathic congenital nystagmats typically requires highly sensitive recording and/or observation procedures. Moreover, research and investigation into the underlying normal and abnormal anatomical structures of ocular motor anomalies is also of importance. For example, parasellar lesions including disorders that affect the interstitial nucleus of Cajal or related structures, have been documented in patients with ocular motor instabilities within particularly the torsional and vertical planes as in see-saw nystagmus (Crawford et al. 1991; Halmagyi et al. 1994; Nakada and Kwee 1992). However, until the mechanisms of normal vertical, horizontal and torsional ocular motor generation and control are fully deciphered, the link between misrouted optic pathways, idiopathic congenital nystagmus, and horizontal, vertical and torsional ocular motor instabilities remains enigmatic. Hopefully, comprehensive three dimensional ocular motor investigations, particularly developmental, may help to lead the quest towards a better understanding between normal and abnormal visual pathway ontogenesis, structure and ocular motor (dys)function.

REFERENCES

Abadi RV, Pascal E (1995) Eye movement behaviour in human albinos. In: Findlay JM, Walker R, Kentridge RW (eds) Eye Movement Research. Mechanisms, Processes and Applications. Elsevier, Amsterdam, pp 255–268

Abel LA (1989) Ocular oscillations. Congenital and acquired. Bull Soc Belge Ophtalmol 237: 163–189

Alvord EC Jr, Lofton S (1988) Gliomas of the optic nerve or chiasm. J Neurosurg 68: 85–98

Apkarian P (1996) Chiasmal crossing defects in disorders of binocular vision. Eye 10: 222–232

Apkarian P, Bour L, Barth PG (1994) A unique achiasmatic anomaly detected in non-albinos with misrouted retinal-fugal projections. Eur J Neurosci 6: 501–507

Apkarian P, Bour LJ, Barth PG, Wenniger-Prick L, Verbeeten B. Jr (1995) Non-decussating retinal-fugal fibre syndrome. An inborn achiasmatic malformation associated with visuotopic misrouting, visual evoked potential ipsilateral asymmetry and nystagmus. Brain 118: 1195–1216

Apkarian P, Bour LJ, van der Steen J, de Faber JTHN (1996) Chiasmal crossing defects in disorders of ocular motor function: three dimensional eye movement recordings in albinism and non-decussating retinal fugal fibre syndrome. Invest Ophthalmol Vis Sci 37 (suppl.): 228

Apkarian P, Shallo-Hoffmann J (1991) VEP projections in congenital nystagmus; VEP asymmetry in albinism: a comparison study. Invest Ophthalmol Vis Sci 32: 2653–2661

Apkarian P, Spekreijse H, Collewijn H (1983) Oculomotor behavior in human albinos. Doc Ophthalmol 37: 361–372

Bataini JP, Delanian S, Ponvert D (1991) Chiasmal gliomas: results of irradiation management in 57 patients and review of literature. Int J Radiation Oncology Biol Phys 21: 615–623

Bedell HE, White JM, Abplanalp PL (1989) Variability of foveations in congenital nystagmus. Clinical Vision Sci 4: 247–252

Bergin DJ, Halpern J (1986) Congenital see-saw nystagmus associated with retinitis pigmentosa. Ann Ophthalmol 18: 346–349

Chung STL, Bedell HE (1996) Velocity criteria for "foveation periods" determined from image motions simulating congenital nystagmus. Optometry & Vision Sci 73: 92–103

Collewijn H, Apkarian P, Spekreijse H (1985) The oculomotor behaviour of human albinos. Brain 108: 1–28

Crawford JD, Cadera W, Vilis T (1991) Generation of torsional and vertical eye position signals by the interstitial nucleus of Cajal. Science 252: 1551–1553

Daroff RB (1965) See-saw nystagmus. Neurology 15: 874–877

Daroff RB, Troost BT, Dell'Osso LF (1978) Nystagmus and related ocular oscillations. In: Glaser JS (ed) Neuro-ophthalmology. Harper and Row, Hagerstown, pp 219–240.

Druckman R, Ellis P, Kleinfeld J, Waldman M (1966) Seesaw nystagmus. Arch Ophthalmol 76: 668–675

Dutton JJ (1994) Gliomas of the anterior visual pathway. Survey of Ophthalmol 38: 427–452

Elekessy EI, Campion JE, Henry GH (1973) Differences between the visual fields of Siamese and common cats. Vision Res 13: 2533–2543

Ferman L, Collewijn H, Jansen TC, van den Berg AV (1987) Human gaze stability in the horizontal, vertical and torsional direction during voluntary head movements, evaluated with a three-dimensional scleral induction coil technique. Vision Res 27: 811–828

Fisher NF, Jampolsky A, Scott AB (1968) Traumatic bitemporal hemianopsia. Part I. Diagnosis of macular splitting. Amer J Ophthalmol 65: 237–242

Guillery RW (1990) Normal and abnormal visual field maps in albinos: central effects of non-matching maps. Ophthalmic Paediat & Genetics 3: 177–183

Guillery RW (1996) Why do albinos and other hypopigmented mutants lack normal binocular vision, and what else is abnormal in their central visual pathways? Eye 10: 217–221

Guillery RW, Casagrande VA (1977) Studies of the modifiability of the visual pathways in Midwestern Siamese cats. J. Comp Neurol 174: 15–46

Halmagyi GM, Aw ST, Dehaene I, Curthoys IS, Todd MJ (1994) Jerk-waveform see-saw nystagmus due to unilateral meso-diencephalic lesion. Brain 117: 789–803

Haustein W (1989) Considerations on Listing's law and the primary position by means of a matrix description of eye position control. Biol. Cybern 60: 411–420

Hess BJM, van Opstal AJ, Straumann D, Hepp K (1992) Calibration of three-dimensional eye position using search coil signals in rhesus monkey. Vision Res 32: 1647–1654

Iraci G, Gerosa M, Tomazzoli L, Pardatscher K, Fiore DL, Javicoli R, Secchi AG (1981) Gliomas of the optic nerve and chiasm. A clinical review. Child's Brain 8: 326–349

Leigh RJ, Zee DS (1991) The Neurology of Eye Movements. Edition 2. FA Davis Co, Philadelphia

MacCarty CS, Boyd AS Jr, Childs DS Jr (1970) Tumors of the optic nerve and optic chiasm. J. Neurosurg 33: 439–444

Maddox EE (1914) See-saw nystagmus with bitemporal hemianopia. Proc Royal Soc Med 7: 12–13

Nakada T, Kwee IL (1992) Role of visuo-vestibular interaction in pathological ocular oscillation: new model and control system analysis. Medical Hypotheses 38: 261–269

Optican LM, Zee DS (1984) A hypothetical explanation of congenital nystagmus. Biol Cybern 50: 119–134

Polyak S (1957) The vertebrate visual system. University of Chicago Press, Chicago

Robinson DA (1963) A method of measuring eye movement using a scleral search coil in a magnetic field. IEEE Transactions on Biomedical Electronics BME-10: 137–145

Samkoff LM, Smith CR (1994) See-saw nystagmus in a patient with clinically definite MS. Eur Neurol 34: 228–229

Schmidt D, Kommerell G (1974) Congenitaler Schaukelnystagmus (Seesaw Nystagmus). Graefes Archs Klin Exp Ophthal 191: 265–272

Traquair HM, Dott NM, Russell WR (1935) Traumatic lesions of the optic chiasma. Brain 58: 398–411

Tweed, D, Cadera W, Vilis T (1990) Computing three-dimensional eye position quaternions and eye velocity from search coil signals. Vision Res 30: 97–110

Yee RD, Wong EK, Baloh RW, Honrubia V (1976) A study of congenital nystagmus: waveforms. Neurology 26: 326–333

Zauberman H, Magora A (1969) Congenital "see-saw" movement. A rare anomaly of ocular motility. Br J Ophthal 53: 418–421

58

CONTROL OF PURPOSIVE SACCADIC EYE MOVEMENTS AND VISUAL FIXATION IN CHILDREN WITH ATTENTION-DEFICIT HYPERACTIVITY DISORDER

Douglas P. Munoz, Karen A. Hampton, Kim D. Moore, and Jenny E. Goldring

MRC Group in Sensory-Motor Neuroscience
Department of Physiology, Queen's University
Kingston, Ontario, K7L 3N6 Canada

1. INTRODUCTION

Attention-deficit hyperactivity disorder (ADHD) is a common disabling disease affecting approximately 5% of children (Barkley 1990; Silver 1992). ADHD is characterized by the symptoms of impulsivity, hyperactivity, and inattention and these core symptoms persist into adulthood. The diagnosis of ADHD remains difficult because it usually involves the subjective evaluation of a child's behavior by parents, teachers, and physicians. At present, the etiology of ADHD remains unknown. A frontostriatal deficit as been hypothesized for the following reasons. First, ADHD subjects lack inhibitory control and often act impulsively (Chelune et al. 1986; Grodzinsky and Diamond 1992), which is similar to other frontal lobe disorders. Second, regional blood flow and glucose metabolic studies have revealed frontal and/or striatal abnormalities in ADHD subjects (Lou et al. 1984, 1989; Zametkin et al. 1990). Third, neuroimaging studies have shown altered architecture in the frontal lobes, caudate nucleus and rostrum of the corpus callosum (Giedd et al. 1994; Castellanos et al. 1996a). A dopamine disorder has also been proposed (Levy 1991) for the following reasons. First, the action of methylphenidate, the main pharmacotherapy for ADHD, is to block dopamine reuptake. Second, there is evidence for abnormal levels of catecholamine metabolites in the CSF of ADHD subjects (Castellanos et al. 1996b).

Saccades are rapid eye movements that shift the line of sight rapidly from one target of interest to another. Between saccades the eyes remain fixed on a target while the visual system performs a detailed analysis of the visual image. Several brain areas have been implicated in the control of saccadic eye movements (Wurtz and Goldberg 1989;

Current Oculomotor Research, edited by Becker *et al.*
Plenum Press, New York, 1999.

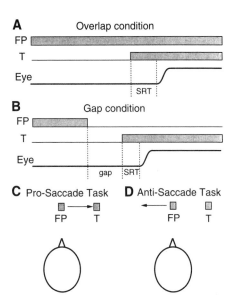

Figure 1. Schematic showing the different behavioral paradigms used. In the overlap condition (*A*), the central fixation point (FP) remained illuminated when an eccentric target (T) appeared. In the gap condition (*B*), the FP disappeared 200 ms before the appearance of the eccentric T. The gap duration was either kept constant at 200 ms or varied randomly from 0–800 ms. Within a block of trials, subjects were instructed to either look from the FP to the T (*C*: Pro-saccade Task) or from the FP to the opposite side of the vertical meridian of the T (*D*: Anti-saccade Task). SRT: saccadic reaction time.

Leigh and Zee 1991) including regions of frontal cortex and the basal ganglia (e.g., caudate nucleus) that have also been implicated in ADHD. We therefore hypothesize that children with ADHD may have some deficits in controlling visual fixation, suppressing unwanted reflexive saccades, and generating voluntary purposive saccades. To test this hypothesis, we recorded eye movements from children diagnosed with ADHD and age-matched controls recruited to perform the tasks illustrated in Fig. 1. In a pro-saccade task (Fig. 1C), the subject is required to look from a central fixation point (FP) to an eccentric target (T). In an anti-saccade task (Fig. 1D), the subject is required to suppress the reflexive saccade to the eccentric target and instead generate a voluntary saccade to the opposite side (Hallett 1978). One aim of this study is to determine whether ADHD children have difficulties performing the anti-saccade task. Saccadic reaction times (SRTs) in the pro- and anti-saccade tasks are dependent upon the state of fixation at the time of target appearance. SRTs are increased when the initial fixation point remains illuminated during the appearance of the new saccade target (overlap task; Fig. 1A), and reduced when the initial fixation point disappears some time prior to target appearance (gap task; Fig. 1B) (Saslow 1967; Fischer and Weber 1993; Munoz and Corneil 1995). If ADHD children have difficulties engaging and disengaging visual fixation, then they may not show the same distributions in SRTs in the gap and overlap conditions. SRTs can sometimes be reduced to a minimum of about 100 ms (Fischer and Weber 1993). It has been suggested that subjects generating an abundance of these short-latency *express saccades*, especially in the overlap condition may have some underlying pathology affecting the saccadic system (Biscaldi et al. 1996).

2. METHODS

All experimental procedures were reviewed and approved by the Queen's University Human Research Ethics Board. Children between the ages of 6 and 17 years were recruited from the greater Kingston area. All subjects were informed of the nature of the study and consented to participate. Parents provided informed consent for minors. Participants in the study were reimbursed $10.00 per recording session. All subjects reported no known visual disorders other than refractive errors. Subjects were able to wear their prescription lenses during the recording sessions. Our subject pool consisted of 64 control children and 49 children diagnosed with ADHD. The mean age of each group was 10.4 years. The ADHD children were studied on days when they did not take their prescribed drug treatment methylphenidate (off-meds) and on separate days when they did take their medication (on-meds). We therefore describe results from 3 experimental groups: control, ADHD off-meds, and ADHD on-meds.

Subjects were seated upright in a dental chair equipped with a head rest which could be adjusted for height so that they faced the center of a translucent visual screen, 100 cm away. The experiments were performed in darkness and silence except for the controlled presentation of visual stimuli that consisted of red light emitting diodes (LEDs; CIE x = 0.73, CIE y = 0.26). One LED (2.0 cd/m^2) was back projected onto the center of the translucent screen and served as a central fixation point (FP) to start all trials. Eccentric target LEDs (5.0 cd/m^2) were mounted into small boxes on portable stands that were positioned 20° to the left and right of the central FP. Between trials the screen was diffusely illuminated (1.0 cd/m^2) with background slides to reduce dark adaptation and boredom. Each recording session lasted not more than 40 minutes and there were breaks between blocks of trials during which participants were provided with snacks and drinks to maintain alertness.

In the pro-saccade task (Fig. 1C), children were instructed to look from the FP to an eccentric target that appeared randomly either 20° to the left or right. Each trial began when the background illumination was turned off. After a 250 ms period of darkness, the FP appeared. After 1000 ms one of two events occurred. In the overlap condition (Fig. 1A), the FP remained illuminated while the eccentric target appeared. In the gap condition (Fig. 1B), the FP disappeared and, after a gap period of 200 ms, the eccentric target appeared. The target remained illuminated for 1000 ms, after which all LEDs were turned off and the background illumination came on to signify the end of the trial. Target location (20° right or left) and fixation condition (gap or overlap) were randomly interleaved within a block of trials.

In the anti-saccade task (Fig. 1D), the presentation of stimuli was identical to that described above. Children were instructed to look at the FP but then, after the appearance of the eccentric target, they were asked to look to the opposite side of the vertical meridian. Once again target location (20° right or left) and fixation conditions (gap or overlap) were randomly interleaved within a block of trials.

In a separate experiment design to study fixation stability, children performed pro-saccades in the gap condition only. In this separate experiment, the FP was illuminated for 1500 ms and the gap period was varied randomly between one of five intervals: 0 ms, 200 ms, 400 ms, 600 ms, or 800 ms. The target then appeared randomly either 20° right or left. Thus, in this experiment, the children knew they had to make an eye movement, but they did not know where or when the target would appear. We measured the number of intrusive saccades generated by each subject during the final 1000 ms of fixation upon the visible FP and during the gap period.

Horizontal eye movements were measured using DC electrooculography (EOG). Ag-AgCl skin electrodes were placed on the outer canthus between each eye and the temple to record horizontal eye position. A ground electrode was placed just above the eyebrows in the center of the forehead. The EOG signal was amplified and low pass filtered with a Grass P18 amplifier rated for human use. To minimize EOG drift, subjects wore the electrodes for approximately 10 minutes before the onset of calibration and recording.

The experimental paradigms, visual displays, and storage of eye movement data were under the control of a 486 computer running a real-time data acquisition system. Horizontal eye position was digitized at a rate of 500 Hz. Digitized data were stored on a hard disk, and subsequent off-line analysis was performed on a Sun Sparc 2 workstation. Horizontal eye velocity was computed from the position traces by applying software differentiation (finite impulse response filter). The onset and termination of each saccade was determined when eye velocity respectively increased or decreased beyond 30°/s. Saccades were scored as correct if the first movement after target appearance was in the correct direction (i.e., toward the target in the pro-saccade task; away from the target in the anti-saccade task). Saccades were scored as incorrect if the first saccade after target appearance was in the wrong direction (i.e., away from the target in the pro-saccade task; toward the target in the anti-saccade task). Saccadic reaction time (SRT) was measured from the time of target onset to the onset of the first saccade. Mean SRTs were computed from trials with reaction latencies between 90 ms and 1000 ms after target appearance. Movements were classified as anticipatory and were excluded from analysis if they were initiated less than 90 ms after target appearance. This anticipatory cutoff was obtained from viewing SRT distributions for correct and incorrect movements in the pro-saccade task. Saccades that were initiated less than 90 ms after target appearance were correct about 50% of the time, whereas saccades initiated more than 90 ms after target appearance were correct more than 95% of the time. SRTs of up to 1000ms were included so as not to miss responses of slower subject groups.

From the data of each subject, we computed the following values: the mean SRT for correct trials; the coefficient of variation of SRT for correct trials ((CV = standard deviation / mean) * 100); the percentage of express saccades (latency: 90 - 140 ms) (Fischer et al. 1993); and the percentage of direction errors (saccades away from the target in the pro-saccade task; saccades toward the target in the anti-saccade task).

3. RESULTS

Three separate experiments are described. In the first experiment the subjects performed the pro-saccade task in overlap and gap conditions with the gap duration fixed at 200 ms. In the second experiment, stimulus conditions remained identical but subjects were asked to generate anti-saccades. In the third experiment, subjects were run in the pro-saccade task only with gap condition and the gap was varied randomly from 0 - 800 ms in 200 ms increments to study fixation instability.

3.1. Pro-Saccade Task

Figure 2A illustrates the mean SRTs obtained in the pro-gap and pro-overlap conditions for the 3 experimental groups: control, ADHD off-meds, and ADHD on-meds. Mean SRT for all groups was significantly increased in the overlap condition compared to the gap condition. Note that mean SRT did not vary between groups except in the overlap

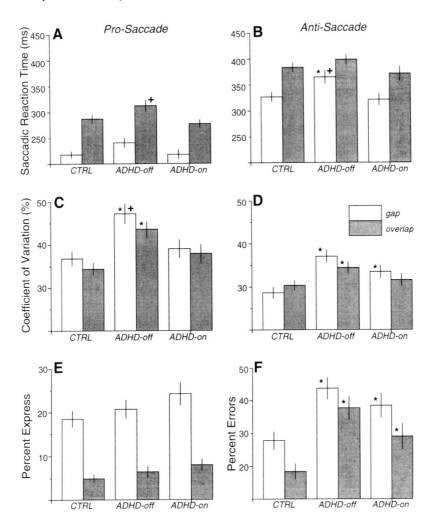

Figure 2. Quantification of parameters in the gap (empty bars) and overlap (filled bars) conditions of pro-saccade (**A,C,E**) and anti-saccade (**B,D,F**) tasks. Values represent mean (± SEM) from control and ADHD off-meds and on-meds children. **A,B**. Mean saccadic reaction times for correct responses. **C,D**. Coefficient of variation (standard deviation of SRT/mean SRT x 100%). **E**. Percentage of express saccades (SRT = 90 – 140 ms) in the pro-saccade task. **F**. Percentage of errors (i.e., reflexive pro-saccades) generated in the anti-saccade task. * denotes values significantly different from control (t-test, p < 0.01). + denotes significant differences between ADHD off-meds and ADHD on-meds groups. Gap duration was fixed at 200 ms.

condition, when the mean SRT for the ADHD off-meds group was significantly elevated relative to the ADHD on-meds group (t-test, p < 0.01).

Although mean SRTs did not vary much between groups, there were systematic differences in intra-subject variance among the 3 groups (Fig. 2C). The coefficient of variance (CV) for the ADHD off-meds group was significantly greater than the control group in both the gap and overlap conditions (t-test, p < 0.01). The CV for the ADHD off-meds group was also greater than the ADHD on-meds group in the gap condition (t-test, p < 0.01).

It has been reported that abnormal numbers of express saccades may reflect some underlying pathology in the saccadic system (Biscaldi et al. 1996). Figure 2E shows the percentage of express saccades (SRT between 90 - 140 ms) for the 3 groups in the gap and overlap conditions. All groups generated more express saccades in the gap, compared to overlap conditions but there were no significant differences between the groups in the percentage of express saccades elicited.

3.2. Anti-Saccade Task

The mean SRTs for correct anti-saccades were greater than the mean SRTs for pro-saccades as described previously (Fischer and Weber 1992). Figure 2B illustrates the mean SRTs obtained in the anti-gap and anti-overlap conditions for the 3 groups of subjects. Note that mean SRT did not vary between groups except in the gap condition, when the mean SRT for the ADHD off-meds group was significantly elevated relative to both the control and ADHD on-meds groups (t-test, $p < 0.01$).

Figure 2D illustrates the intra-subject variance for the 3 groups of subjects in the anti-saccade task. Once again, the amount of intra-subject variance, expressed as the CV, was elevated in the ADHD off-meds group. The CV in both the anti-gap and anti-overlap condition was significantly greater than the CV for the control group (t-tes, $p < 0.01$). In addition, the CV in the anti-gap condition for the ADHD on-meds group was significantly greater than that of the control group.

Direction errors in the anti-saccade task have been associated with pathology of the frontal lobes (Guitton et al. 1985). Figure 2F summarizes the percentage of direction errors generated by children in the 3 subject groups. All groups generated more errors in the gap condition as compared to the overlap condition. Of importance here, the percentage of direction errors generated by the ADHD off-meds group was the highest of the 3 experimental groups. Both the ADHD off-meds and ADHD on-meds groups generated significantly more direction errors than the control group (t-test, $p < 0.01$).

3.3. FIXATION INSTABILITY

To measure fixation instability, each subject performed blocks of pro-gap trials with random duration gap periods ($0 - 800$ ms). For each subject we counted the number of intrusive saccades that subjects made in the final 1000 ms of instructed fixation upon the visible FP and during the gap period. We then computed the rate of instability for each subject for these two epochs. Figure 3 plots the mean rate of intrusive saccades during these two intervals for the 3 experimental groups. For control children, the intrusive saccade rate was 0.24 saccades/s during fixation of the FP and 0.22 saccades/s during the gap period. For the ADHD children off-meds, this rate was significantly elevated (t-test, $p < 0.01$) to 0.54 and 0.50 saccades/s during visible fixation and the gap period, respectively. The rates obtained on days when ADHD children took medication were 0.45 and 0.42 saccades/s, respectively, which were also significantly greater than control (t-test, $p < 0.01$).

4. DISCUSSION

We have demonstrated that the ability to accurately control visual fixation and suppress unwanted saccades is impaired in children with ADHD. Specifically, ADHD chil-

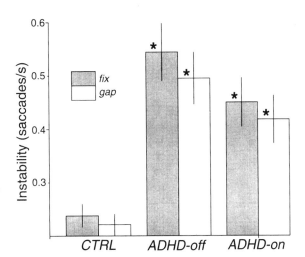

Figure 3. Quantification of mean fixation instability for control and ADHD off-meds and on-meds children. Instability was measured as the rate of generation of saccades $\geq$ 2° in amplitude during instructed fixation of the visible FP (filled bars) or during the randomized gap period (empty bars). * denotes values significantly different from control (t-test, p < 0.0005)

dren had: 1) greater intra-subject variance in SRTs (Fig. 2C,D); 2) more direction errors in the anti-saccade task (Fig. 2F); and 3) greater fixation instability (Fig. 3). In addition, we found that task performance of many ADHD children improved during medication with methylphenidate. Our results confirm and extend previous reports in the literature that have described deficits in eye movement control in children with ADHD. Previous studies have described difficulties in suppressing intrusive saccades during either visual fixation (Shapira et al. 1980; Paus 1992) or during smooth pursuit eye movements (Bala et al. 1981; Blysma and Pivik 1989). Ross and colleagues (1994) studied ADHD children in a delayed memory-guided saccade task and found that ADHD children were significantly impaired in their ability to delay a saccade to a flashed visual stimulus. Rothlind and colleagues (1991) studied ADHD children in an anti-saccade task and noted differences between ADHD children and age-matched control subjects in terms of direction errors but these differences failed to reach significance. However, each subject only performed 10 trials in each condition, whereas we collected between 40–60 trials in each condition from each subject.

The greater intra-subject variance and increased frequency of intrusive saccades among ADHD subjects is indicative of their symptoms of inattention. Such results would be predicted if the subjects had reduced abilities to stay on task. This could manifest itself as poor fixation control and would result in saccades being triggered at inappropriate times. It is important to note that treatment with methylphenidate reduced these impairments among many ADHD children. The increased frequency of direction errors in the anti-saccade task among ADHD children represents a measure of their impulsivity. Accurate completion of this task requires suppression of pro-saccades to the stimulus, and then generation of a voluntary saccade to the opposite side. ADHD children had no difficulties with the latter. Their main deficit in the anti-saccade task was the inability to suppress reflexive pro-saccades to the stimulus. Once again, treatment with methylphenidate reduced error rates in many children.

Despite the reduced fixation stability in ADHD children, there was no significant increase in the frequency of express saccades. This observation suggests that the primary mechanisms for controlling visual fixation and generating express saccades may be somewhat separate. This is consistent with the recent hypothesis that express saccades result from advanced preparation of saccadic motor programs (Paré and Munoz 1996; Dorris et al. 1997), rather than reduction in fixation-related activity (Munoz and Wurtz 1992).

Our results suggest that eye movement testing may provide useful insight into the diagnosis of ADHD and the effectiveness of prescribed drug therapies. In addition, the fixation instability and excessive direction errors in the anti-saccade task are consistent with a frontostriatal dysfunction hypothesis producing the symptoms of ADHD. Indeed, neurological patients with lesions of the dorsolateral frontal cortex have difficulties suppressing reflexive pro-saccades in the anti-saccade task (Guitton et al. 1985). Future work may elucidate the precise locus of dysfunction in ADHD subjects.

REFERENCES

Bala SP, Cohen B, Morris AG, Atkin A, Gittelman R, Kates W (1981) Saccades of hyperactive and normal boys during ocular pursuit. Develop Med Child Neurol 23: 323–336.

Barkley RA (1990) Attention deficit hyperactivity disorder: a handbook for diagnosis and treatment. Guildford Press, New York.

Biscaldi M, Fischer B, Stuhr V (1996) Human express-saccade makers are impaired at suppressing visually-evoked saccades. J Neurophsyiol 76: 199–214.

Bylsma FW, Pivik RT (1989) The effects of background illumination and stimulant medication on smooth pursuit eye movements of hyperactive children. J Abnormal Child Psych 17: 73–90.

Castellanos FX, Giedd JN, Marsh WL, Hamburger SD, Vaituzis AC, Dickstein DP, Sarfatti SE, Vauss YC, Snell JW, Rajapakse JC, Rapoport JL (1996a) Quantitative brain magnetic resonance imaging in attention-deficit hyperactivity disorder. Arch Gen Psychiatry 53: 607–616.

Castellanos FX, Elia J, Kruesi MJP, Marsh WL, Gulotta CS, Potter, WZ, Ritchie GF, Hamburger SD, Rapoport JL (1996b) Cerebrospinal fluid homovanillic acid predicts behavioral response to stimulants in 45 boys with attention deficit/ hyperactivity disorder. Neuropsychopharm 14: 125–137.

Chelune GJ, Ferguson W, Koon R, Dickey TO (1986) Frontal lobe disinhibition in attention deficit disorder. Child Psychiat Human Dev 16: 221–234.

Dorris MC, Paré M, Munoz DP (1997) Neuronal activity in monkey superior colliculus related to the initiation of saccadic eye movements. J Neurosci 17: 8566–8579.

Fischer B, Weber H (1992) Characteristics of "anti" saccades in man. Exp Brain Res 89: 415–424.

Fischer B, Weber H (1993) Express saccades and visual attention. Behav Brain Sci 16: 553–610.

Fischer B, Weber H, Biscaldi M, Aiple F, Otto P, Stuhr V (1993) Separate populations of visually guided saccades in humans: reaction times and amplitudes. Exp Brain Res 92: 528–541.

Giedd JN, Castellanos FX, Casey BJ, Kozuch P, King AC, Hamburger SD, Rapoport JL (1994) Quantitative morphology of the corpus callosum in attention deficit hyperactivity disorder. Am J Psychiatry 151: 665–669.

Grodzinsky GM, Diamond R (1992) Frontal lobe functioning in boys with attention-deficit hyperactivity disorder. Dev Neuropsych 8: 427–445.

Guitton D, Buchtel H, Douglas R (1985) Frontal lobe lesions in man cause difficulties in suppressing reflexive saccades and in generating goal-directed saccades Exp Brain Res 58: 455–472.

Hallett P (1978) Primary and secondary sacades to goals defined by instructions. Vision Res 18: 1279–1296.

Leigh RJ, Zee DS (1991) The neurology of eye movements. FA Davis, Philadelphia.

Levy F (1991) The dopamine theory of attention deficit hyperactivity disorder (ADHD). Australian NZ J Psychiatry 25: 277–283.

Lou HC, Henriksen L, Bruhn P (1984) Focal cerebral hypoperfusion in children with dysphasia and/or attention deficit disorder. Arch Neurol 41: 825–829.

Lou HC, Henriksen L, Bruhn P, Borner H, Nielsen JB (1989) Striatal dysfunction in attention deficit and hyperkinetic disorder. Arch Neurol 46: 48–52.

Munoz DP, Corneil BD (1995) Evidence for interactions between target selection and visual fixation for saccade generation in humans. Exp Brain Res 103: 168–173.

Munoz DP, Wurtz RH (1992) Role of the rostral superior colliculus in active visual fixation and execution of express saccades. J Neurophysiol 67: 1000–1002.

Paré M, Munoz DP (1996) Saccadic reaction time in the monkey: advanced preparation of oculomotor programs is primarily responsible for express saccade occurrence. J Neurophysiol 76: 3666–3681.

Paus T (1992) Impaired voluntary suppression of reflexive saccades in attention-deficit hyperactivity disordered boys. Thalamus 8: 1–23.

Ross RG, Hommer D, Breiger D, Varley C, Radant A (1994) Eye movement task related to frontal lobe functioning in children with attention deficit disorder. J Am Acad Child Adolesc Psychiatry 33: 869–874.

Rothlind JC, Posner MI, Schaughency EA (1991) Lateralized control of eye movements in attention deficit hyperactivity disorder. J Cog Neurosci 3: 377–381.

Saslow MG (1967) Effects of component displacement-step stimuli upon latency of saccadic eye movements J Opt Soc Am 57: 1024–1029.

Shapira YA, Jones MH, Sherman SP (1980) Abnormal eye movements in hyperkinetic children with learning disability. Neuropadiatrie 11: 36–44.

Silver LB (1992) Attention-deficit hyperactivity disorder. A clinical guide to diagnosis and treatment. American Psychiatric Press, Washington.

Wurtz RH, Goldberg ME (1989) The neurobiology of saccadic eye movements. Elsevier, Amsterdam

Zametkin AJ, Nordahl TE, Gross M, King C, Semple WE, Rumset J, Hamburger S, Cohen RM (1990) Cerebral glucose metabolism in adults with hyperactivity of childhood onset. N Engl J Med 323: 1361–1366.

59

A COMPARISON OF EYE MOVEMENTS IN FAMILIES WITH MULTIPLE OCCURRENCE OF SCHIZOPHRENIA AND NORMAL FAMILIES

Rebekka Lencer, Katja Krecker, Carsten P. Malchow, Achim Nolte, and Volker Arolt

Klinik für Psychiatrie
Medizinische Universität zu Lübeck
D-23538 Lübeck, Germany

1. INTRODUCTION

Why are psychiatrists interested in eye movements? Since the discovery of Diefendorf and Dodge in 1908 and the findings of Holzman and colleagues in 1974 it has been suggested that eye tracking dysfunction (ETD) may serve as a biological marker for schizophrenia in genetic linkage studies (Levinson et al. 1991). Already in those earlier studies a higher prevalence of ETD was found in both schizophrenic patients (50–86%) and their relatives (45%) when compared to normal subjects. ETD as a measurable indicator for vulnerability to schizophrenia may help to identify those individuals who carry the genetic trait without suffering from the disease (Grove et al. 1992).

In this article we present the results of eye movement studies obtained in a genetic epidemiological study. Using ETD as a phenotypic marker we found a significant linkage of ETD to markers on the short arm of chromosome 6 (6p21–23) in families with multiple occurrence of schizophrenia (so-called multiplex families, Arolt et al. 1996).

Although schizophrenic patients show lower gain values (ratio of eye to target velocity) and higher saccade rates (predominantly catch-up saccades) than normal individuals (Abel at al. 1991; Radant and Hommer 1992), not much is known about the neurophysiological mechanisms underlying eye tracking dysfunction in schizophrenic patients. Are these saccades, especially catch-up saccades, generated to compensate for periods of low eye velocity or do they, like anticipatory saccades, interrupt normal smooth pursuit eye movements due to pathological disinhibitions in higher cerebral structures such as the frontal eye field (FEF) (Levin 1984)? Recent results suggest that 1); a defect occurs in matching eye velocity to target velocity which results in low gain and 2); the resulting position errors are compensated for by implementing catch-up saccades towards the moving target (Radant and Hommer 1992). Such saccades have been shown to be in-

Current Oculomotor Research, edited by Becker *et al.*
Plenum Press, New York, 1999.

accurate (i.e. hypometric) in schizophrenic patients (Schoepf et al. 1995), indicating a dysfunction that may be located in the medial superior temporal visual area (MST). Schoepf et al. also reported a deficit in smooth pursuit maintenance while smooth pursuit initiation and saccadic task latencies remained within normal ranges.

Abnormalities in saccadic eye movements have often been observed in schizophrenic patients. Some groups have shown hypometria in visually guided saccades (Cegalis et al. 1982; Schmid-Burgk et al. 1982; Schmid-Burgk et al. 1983; Mackert and Flechtner 1989, Moser et al. 1990). Schizophrenic patients performed at higher error rates with antisaccadic tasks (Fukushima et al. 1988; Matsue et al. 1994; Sereno and Holzman 1995, Crawford et al. 1995). Saccade latencies appeared normal in most studies (Iacono et al. 1993; Levin et al. 1981), but Mackert et al. (1989) found increased latencies during a reflexive saccadic task. Few studies have examined saccadic eye movement abnormalities amongst schizophrenic patients and their relatives and none have made comparisons with normal families without psychotic disorders. Schreiber et al. (1995) demonstrated increased rates of hypometric saccades in both schizophrenic patients and their first degree relatives compared to a control group. Clementz et al. (1994) reported increased antisaccade error rates in schizophrenic patients and their first degree relatives but no significant results concerning hypometria.

The genetic epidemiological study mentioned above (Arolt et al 1996) provided us with the opportunity to conduct a detailed analysis on both smooth pursuit and reflexive saccadic task performance not only in schizophrenic patients but also in their family members and in members of families without any history of psychotic disorders (normal families).

2. MATERIALS AND METHODS

2.1. Subjects

Eye movements were recorded from 8 multiplex families (67 members) and another 9 normal families (80 members) of German ethnic origin. Individuals had to have 1); no neurological disease, 2); no significant history of head trauma, 3); normal or corrected to normal vision and 4); no history of substance abuse or CNS-active medication involving lithium, clozapine or benzodiazepines since such agents can affect oculomotor performance. Subjects were divided into 4 groups:

1. The group consisting of all members of the normal families (mean age 37.03 ± 14.5 (SD) years),
2. Multiplex family members who were diagnosed as schizophrenic (N = 19, mean age = 34.43 ± 11.08 (SD) years),
3. The 1°-relatives of such schizophrenic patients (N = 27, mean age = 47.48 ± 14.13 (SD) years),
4. All non-1°-relatives (2° up to 5°-relatives) of those schizophrenic patients (N = 21, mean age = 50.86 ± 22.57 (SD) years).

2.2. Assessment of Eye Movements

Eye movements were recorded by using a high resolution infra-red technique at a sampling rate of 200 Hz. The stimulus was displayed by an array of light emitting diodes.

For the smooth pursuit task, a triangle wave stimulus at a constant velocity of 30°/s (±15° from the centre, ramp movements started from the left) was used. For investigating saccadic eye movements, subjects had to track 30 target steps within 30 seconds. These steps were randomized with respect to their duration, amplitude (range 3°-18°) and direction. Calibration steps of 10° to the left and right of the central point were presented at the beginning and end of all tasks.

2.3. Data Analysis

Smooth pursuit velocity gain (average smooth eye velocity/ target velocity) was calculated after the original data had been desaccaded. Saccades were considered to have occurred when both movement amplitudes exceeded 0.5° and velocity changes exceeded 40°/s (compared to the mean velocity of 50–25ms prior to the event). Gains were only calculated for each half cycle of target movement and not for the whole trial. After a preliminary cycle, the 30°/s trial consisted of 9 rightward and 9 leftward half cycles of target movements. Rates and amplitudes of the total number of saccades (TS) were also determined and saccades were classified either as catch-up saccades (CUS, saccades starting behind the target and moving in its direction), back-up saccades (BUS, saccades opposite in direction to the target which bring the eye back to the target), anticipatory saccades (AS, saccades moving in the direction and ahead of the target) or square wave jerks (SWJ, opposite directed paired saccades with an intersaccadic interval of 50–500 msec).

During the saccadic tasks, eye movements were analyzed to assess hypometria, hypermetria, misdirected saccades and initial saccadic response latencies.

2.4. Statistics

For an appropriate analysis of the multidimensional nature of this study, and for considering the influence of age (as a covariate) on oculomotor performance, a multivariate analysis of variance (MANOVA) was performed. Univariate analysis of variance (ANOVA) was used whenever the MANOVA test indicated significant differences. All data presented in this study were corrected for age by means of regression analysis.

3. RESULTS

3.1. Smooth Pursuit Maintenance

Figure 1 shows the single gain values for each half cycle of target movement at 30°/s. Gain values from the different groups were significantly different from one another (F=15.04, P<0.001, D.F.=3). As expected, the normal families yielded the highest gain levels followed in order by the non 1°-relatives, the 1°-relatives and lastly, the schizophrenics. Furthermore, direction and target cycle were revealed as significantl main effects (target direction: F=3.27, p=0.001, D.F.=8; target cycle: F=15.30, P<0.001, D.F.=1; group x target cycle: F=2.02, P=0.003, D.F.=24; group x target direction: F=3.74, P=0.013, D.F.=3). It is obvious from Figure 1 that amongst normal families, unlike the other groups, the differences between individual gain values over the whole course of one trial were negligible. Directional asymmetries of smooth pursuit maintenance with higher gains in rightward as compared to leftward pursuit appeared amongst the schizophrenic patients, their 1° and non-1° relatives. In the schizophrenic patients, gain decreased con-

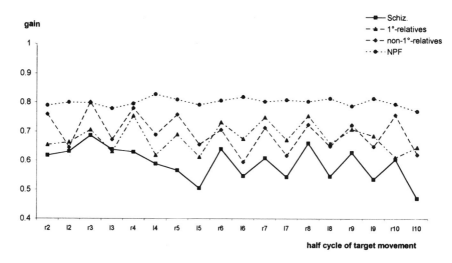

Figure 1. Gain values for each target movement to the right (r2, r3,..., r10) and to the left (l2, l3,..., l10) at 30°/s for normal family members (NPF), schizophrenic patients (Schiz.), their 1° and non-1° relatives.

sistently from the third rightward (r3) to the fifth leftward (l5) target movement until the same pattern was achieved as was seen in both groups of relatives.

3.2. Saccades and Saccade Subtypes which Occurred during Smooth Pursuit

Following analysis of saccade subtypes we found statistically significant differences in TS-, CUS- and AS-rates amongst the four different groups (TS-rates: F=9.53, P<0.01; CUS-rates: F=3.23, P=0.02 and AS-rates: F=6.12, P<0.01). Rates were generally higher in the schizophrenic patients than they were in the normal families. In both groups of rela-

Table 1. Rates and amplitudes of different saccade categories during smooth pursuit of a 30°/s target in normal family members (NPF), schizophrenic patients (Schiz.), their 1° (1°-rel.), and non-1° relatives (non-1°-rel.)

Saccade rates (n/s)	NPF	Non-1°relatives	1°-relatives	Schizophrenic pat.
TS [*,†]	2.45	2.86	2.82	3.10
CUS[*]	2.10	1.99	1.99	2.60
BUS	0.05	0.20	0.10	0.03
AS[*]	0.25	0.64	0.68	0.46
SWJ	0.10	0.03	0.04	0.02
Saccade amplitudes (°)				
TS	3.73	3.75	3.91	4.03
CUS	3.65	3.16	3.42	3.63
BUS	2.14	2.84	2.40	2.18
AS[*]	5.04	7.98	7.46	6.63
SWJ	3.92	3.18	5.73	4.58

* indicates statistically significant (p<0.01) differences amongst the groups
† total saccades

tives, TS-rates were higher than those of normal families and lower than those of schizophrenic patients, whereas CUS-rates were as low as they were in the normal families. AS-rates in both groups of relatives were as high as those of schizophrenics and tended to be highest amongst the 1° relatives.

Significant differences amongst the groups concerning the amplitudes of each saccade category were only revealed for AS-amplitudes (F= 5.74, P<0.01) which were larger in both groups of relatives compared to manifest schizophrenics and members of normal families.

3.3. Saccade Task

Frequencies of hypometric saccades were significantly higher in both schizophrenics and their relatives compared to members of normal families. Schizophrenic patients and their relatives also exhibited higher rates of misdirected saccades. Latencies of initial saccadic responses were increased in both schizophrenic patients and their relatives while in normal families they remained unchanged.

4. DISCUSSION

A large overall reduction in gain could be shown in schizophrenic patients when compared to healthy subjects. Additionally, a directional asymmetry in smooth pursuit maintenance with higher gain values for rightward as compared to leftward target movements was observed. This gain reduction was accompanied by an excess of catch-up saccades and, to a lower extent, of anticipatory saccades. Essentially the same deficit in smooth pursuit maintenance was found in both groups of relatives. Anticipatory saccades with large amplitudes were the predominant types observed. With predictable stimuli, for which the turnarounds of the target are known to the subject, anticipatory saccades may occur whenever the predictive component of the smooth pursuit system fails to compensate for the slowness of the visually guided component. This strategy, which originates from the saccadic system and which is accompanied by a decrease in gain, appears to have been utilized particularly by the two groups of relatives. In general, smooth pursuit maintenance is driven by extraretinal signals that include predictive mechanisms (Jürgens et al 1987). In schizophrenic patients, this predictive component may compensate to a certain extent for the very minor visually guided component of the smooth pursuit system (Trillenberg et al 1997). Our results suggest that at higher velocities, i.e. target velocities at the high end of the range that can be followed optimally by the smooth pursuit system, this predictive component was not sufficiently compensated for. With predictable stimuli, an ipsiversive directional deficit in smooth pursuit maintenance (frequently interrupted by catch-up saccades) has been observed in patients with lesions in the FEF system (Heide et al 1996). This would indicate a motor disorder in schizophrenic patients. However, a directional smooth pursuit maintenance deficit may also be caused by lesions within the MST. Considering that catch-up saccades towards the moving target were found to be hypometric in schizophrenic patients but not in patients with lesions of the FEF, support is provided for the idea that the defect may be located within the MST.

There were no differences amongst the groups concerning the amplitudes of both catch-up and back-up saccades: this indicates that the threshold at which a compensatory saccade appeared to correct for a positional error was not augmented either in the schizophrenic patients or their relatives.

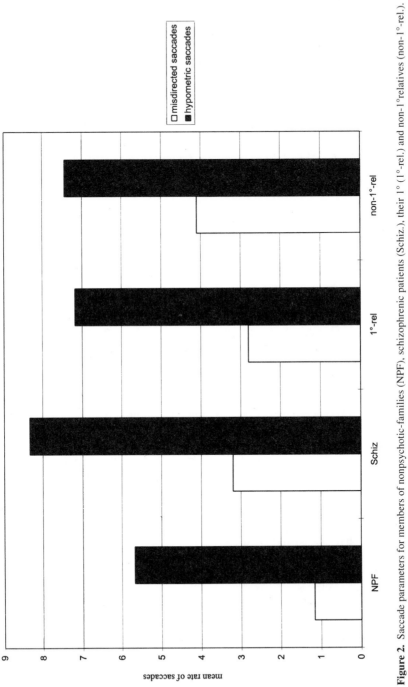

Figure 2. Saccade parameters for members of nonpsychotic-families (NPF), schizophrenic patients (Schiz.), their 1° (1°-rel.) and non-1°relatives (non-1°-rel.).

The accuracy of saccadic eye movements was similarly impaired in both schizophrenic patients and their relatives compared to members of nonpsychotic families. Increased rates of both hypometric and misdirected saccades were found in those groups. Reduced saccadic eye movement accuracy might act as an indicator for predisposition to schizophrenia. Such a view agrees with the findings of Schreiber et al. (1995) who reported impaired saccadic eye movements in both schizophrenic patients and their first-degree relatives.

5. CONCLUSION

Our findings confirm the hypothesis that the genetic vulnerability to schizophrenia is associated with deficits in both smooth pursuit maintenance and saccadic hypometria. In both schizophrenic patients and their relatives we found leftward pursuit to be more impaired than rightward pursuit. Functional brain imaging strategies are needed for localizing the structural lesions in the main cortical centers involved in oculomotor control in schizophrenic patients and their relatives.

REFERENCES

Abel LA, Friedman L, Jesberger JA, Malki A, Meltzer HY (1991): Quantitative assessment of smooth pursuit gain and catch-up saccades in schizophrenia and affective disorders. *Biol Psychiatry* 29:1063–1072.

Arolt V, Lencer R, Nolte A, Müller-Myhsok B, Purmann S, Schürmann M, et al (1996): Eye tracking dysfunction is a putative phenotypic susceptibility marker of schizophrenia and maps to a locus on chromosome 6p in families with multiple occurrence of schizophrenia. *Am J Med Gen* 67:564–579.

Cegalis JA, Sweeny JA, Dellis EM (1982): Refixation saccades and attention in schizophrenia. *J Psychiatry Res* 7: 189–98

Clementz BA, McDowell JE, Zisock S (1994): Saccadic system functioning among schizophrenic patients and their first degree relatives. *J Abnormal Psychology* 103:277–87

Crawford TJ, Haeger B, Kennard C, Reveley MA, Henderson L (1995): Saccadic abnormalities in psychotic patients. *Psychol Med* 25:461–483

Diefendorf AR, Dodge R (1908). An experimental study of the ocular reactions on the insane from photographic records. *Brain* 31:451–489.

Fukushima J, Fukushima K, Chiba T, Tanaka S, Yamashita I, Kato M (1988): Disturbances of voluntary control of saccadic eye movements in schizophrenic patients. *Biol Psychiatry* 23:670–77

Grove WM, Clementz BA, Iacono WG, Katsanis J (1992): Smooth pursuit ocular motor dysfunction in schizophrenia: Evidence for a major gene. *Am J Psychiatry* 149:1362–1368.

Heide W, Kurzidim K, Kömpf D (1996): Deficits of smooth pursuit eye movements after frontal and parietal lesions. *Brain* 119:1951–1969.

Holzman PS, Proctor LR, Levy DL, Yasillo NJ, Meltzer HY, Hurt SW (1974). Eye-tracking dysfunction in schizophrenic patients and their relatives. *Arch Gen Psychiatry* 31:143–151.

Iacono WG, Tuason VB, Johnson RA (1993): Dissociation of smooth pursuit and saccadic eye tracking in remitted schizophrenics. *Arch Gen Psychiatry* 38:991–96

Jürgens R, Kornhuber AW, Becker W (1987): Prediction and strategy in human smooth pursuit eye movements. In: Lüer G, Lass U, Shallo-Hoffmann J, editors. *Eye movement research. Physiological and psychological aspects.* Göttingen: CJ Hogrefe, pp 55–75.

Levin S, Holzman PS, Rothenberg SJ, Lipton RB (1981): Saccadic eye movements in psychotic patients. *Psychiatry Res* 5:47–58

Levin S (1984): Frontal lobe dysfunctions in schizophrenia- I. eye movement impairments. *J Psychiatr Res* 18:27–55.

Levinson DF, Mowry BJ (1991): Defining the schizophrenia spectrum: Issues for genetic linkage studies. *Schizophr Bull* 17:491–514.

Mackert A, Flechtner M (1989): Saccadic reaction times in acute and remitted schizophrenics. *Euro Arch Psychiatry Neurol Sci* 239:33–38.

Mackert A, Flechtner M, Frick K (1989): Reaktionszeiten und visopatiale Aufmerksamkeitsstörung bei Schizophrenen mit Negativsymptomatik. *Fortschr Neurol Psychiat* 57:535–43

Matsue Y, Saito H, Osakabe K (1994): Smooth pursuit eye movement and voluntary control of saccades in the antisaccade task in schizophrenic patients. *Jpn J Psychiatry Neurol* 48:13–22

Moser A, Kömpf D, Arolt V, Resch T (1990): Quantitative analysis of eye movements in schizophrenia. *Neuroophthalmology* 10:73–80

Radant AD, Hommer DW (1992): A quantitative analysis of saccades and smooth pursuit during visual pursuit tracking. A comparison of schizophrenics with normals and substance abusing controls. *Schizophr Res* 6:225–235.

Schmid-Burgk W, Becker W, Jürgens R, Kornhuber HH (1983): Saccadic eye movements in psychiatric patients. *Neuropsychobiology* 10:193–98

Schmid-Burgk W, Becker W, Diekmann V, Jürgens R, Kornhuber HH (1982): Disturbed smooth pursuit and saccadic eye movement in schizophrenia. *Arch Psychiat Nervenkr* 323:381–89

Schreiber H, Rothmeier J, Becker W, Jürgens R, Born J, Stolz-Born H, Westphal KP, Kornhuber HH (1995): Comparative assessment of saccadic eye movements, psychomotor and cognitive performance in schizophrenics, their first-degree relatives and control subjects. *Acta Psychiatr Scand* 91:195–201

Schoepf D, Heide W, Arolt V, Junghanns K, Kömpf D (1995): Deficits of smooth pursuit initiation in schizophrenic patients. *Soc Neurosci* 21:922.

Sereno AB, Holzman PS (1995): Antisaccades and smooth pursuit eye movements in schizophrenics. *Biol Psychiatry* 37:394–401

Trillenberg P, Heide W, Junghanns K, Blankenburg M, Arolt V, Kömpf D (accepted 10/1997): Target anticipation and impairment of smooth pursuit eye movements in schizophrenia. *Exp Brain Res.*, in press

60

EYE-HEAD COORDINATION IN PATIENTS WITH CHRONIC LOSS OF VESTIBULAR FUNCTION

C. Maurer,[1] T. Mergner,[1] W. Becker,[2] and R. Jürgens[2]

[1]Department of Neurology
University of Freiburg, Germany
[2]Department of Neurology
Universität Ulm, Germany

1. INTRODUCTION

In healthy subjects sacccadic gaze shifts of more than 20° or so are achieved by moving both the head and the eyes. The coordination between head and eyes during such gaze shifts depends critically on vestibular information. A vestibulo-saccadic reflex (VSR) is thought to reduce the eye-in-head saccade in proportion to current head displacement (Laurutis and Robinson 1986), and following the saccade the vestibulo-ocular reflex (VOR) stabilises gaze if the head movement is still going on and visual mechanisms (smooth pursuit) are not yet effective. In monkey it has been shown that acute bilateral loss of vestibular function after labyrinthectomy causes overshoot and postsaccadic instability (Bizzi et al. 1972, Morasso et al. 1973, Dichgans et al. 1973). However, during the weeks and months following labyrinthectomy, these authors observed a conspicuous remittance of the deficits which they attributed to several compensatory mechanisms, noticeably a cervico-ocular reflex. The same is true for humans with chronic loss of vestibular function. These patients are able to use head movements for large gaze shifts and, in doing so, produce apparently normal gaze saccades without the overshoot or postsaccadic gaze instability one would expect to result from the lack of vestibular signals. There are few quantitative analyses of patients' behaviour, though. The most detailed study, to our knowledge, is that of Kasei and Zee (1978). However the small number of patients in this study (3) and their different, apparently idiosyncratic, compensatory mechanisms make it difficult to discern a general pattern. Therefore, in the present study we set out to determine the average behaviour of patients with chronic loss of vestibular function during large gaze shifts and to compare it to that of normal subjects. We will show that patients exhibit consistent traits which suggest the existence of common compensatory mechanisms. We will summarise the results of both normal subjects (Ns) and

Current Oculomotor Research, edited by Becker *et al.*
Plenum Press, New York, 1999.

patients (Ps) in terms of descriptive models which provide a framework for discussing the conceivable basis of these mechanisms.

2. METHODS

Six patients (age: 23–27 yrs) and two control groups of six normal adult subjects each (age: 20–30 yrs) participated in the study. All patients suffered from chronic bilateral vestibular loss since early childhood (complete absence of postrotatory and caloric responses). Controls were free of known neurological diseases. All subjects were naive with regard to the purpose of the experiment.

Subjects were seated at the centre of a horizontal perimeter (radius, 1.8 m) carrying a row of red light emitting diodes (LEDs), spaced 5° over a range of 120° (from 60° left to 60° right), which served as targets. There were three experimental conditions: (1) *Head-fixed*. Ss were presented with a random sequence of centrifugal and centripetal steps of up to 30°, and of midline crossing steps of up to 60°. They were instructed to "accurately fixate the light spot, follow it as rapidly as possible when it jumps, and keep the head motionless in its primary position" (there was no mechanical head restraint or support). (2) *Head-free*. The target stepped by up to 60° (centrifugal or centripetal) or 120° (midline crossing). Ss were told that in tracking the target, they were free to also move their heads if they liked. The head position achieved at the completion of given gaze reaction then was maintained till the following reaction. (3) *Preadjusted-head*. Ss were presented with a green and a red LED. They were instructed to orient their heads towards the green LED, but to fixate their gaze at the red one. By choosing different positions for the red and the green LED, initial head position was dissociated from the initial eye and gaze positions by an offset of controlled magnitude. Three offset values were used (random alternation): +30° (H<E, head closer to target than gaze), 0° (H=E, head aligned with gaze), and -30° (H>E, head further away from target than gaze). After the initial adjustment of eye and head positions, saccadic gaze shifts were elicited by stepping the red LED and extinguishing the green one. Control subjects for conditions (1) and (2) came from the first group, those for condition (3) from the second one, whereas patients were the same in all 3 conditions.

Subjects wore a lightweight plastic helmet which was coupled via a torsionally rigid, but otherwise flexible hose to a precision potentiometer recording angular head position. Eye movements (in orbit) were recorded by conventional DC-electrooculography (EOG). Eye, head and gaze position (sum of eye and head signals) as well as corresponding velocity readings (obtained by electronic differentiation) were sampled at 400 Hz, displayed on a computer screen, and stored in memory. EOG was calibrated by having Ss fixate at the centre LED while slowly rotating their heads to either side by about 30° at a frequency of less than 0.25 Hz. EOG gain then was adjusted until the gaze signal became flat, indicating that the EOG signal had the same magnitude as the potentiometer signal recording head movement.

The recorded signals were analysed off-line using an interactive computer program. The program noted for each detected eye-in-head saccade, gaze saccade and head movement the position and velocity of eye, head and gaze during several characteristic instants, e.g. start of movement, time of peak velocity, or end of movement. The resulting data set provides a fairly complete description of eye, head, and gaze behaviour (cf. Fig. 1). In a further step, the data were corrected for EOG offset and drift of EOG gain between calibration epochs.

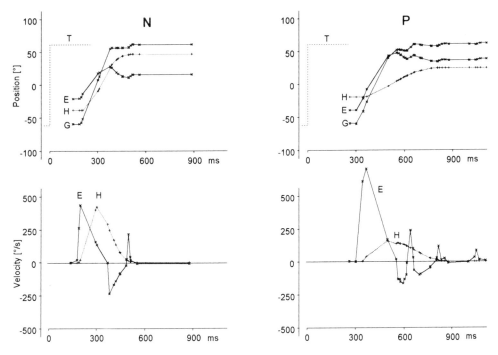

Figure 1. Response of a control subject (N) and a patient (P) to a midline crossing target step of 120°; traces reconstructed from selected sampling points. T, target; E, eye; H, head; G, gaze (=E+H). Position profiles in upper, velocity in lower panels.

3. RESULTS

Figures 1 shows typical responses (reconstructed from the sampled "characteristic points") to large target steps (120°) from a normal subject (N) and a patient (P). Qualitatively the responses are fairly similar suggesting a very effective compensation for the lack of vestibular signals in P. P's response is hypometric, and not hypermetric as it would be with acute labyrinthectomy, and there is a (small) reverse gaze drift after the saccade, whereas in the uncompensated state gaze would continue to move onward with the head for at least 100 ms (latency of pursuit system). However, a more quantitative approach to Fig. 1 reveals several differences between P and N which are representative for the average of patients and controls. Clearly, P's head movement is smaller and, by the same token, both his eye-in-head movement and the final orbital eccentricity of the eye, is larger than in N. Moreover, the delay of head movement onset (head lag) upon the start of the eye and the gaze saccade is larger and the reaction as a whole starts later than in N. Finally, postsaccadic gaze is not as stable as in N and there are more secondary saccades.

3.1. Contributions of Eye and Head to Gaze Shifts

An analysis of the contributions of the eyes and of the head to the saccadic gaze shift proper and to the maintenance of gaze position after the saccade is shown in Fig 2.

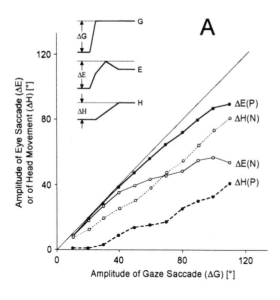

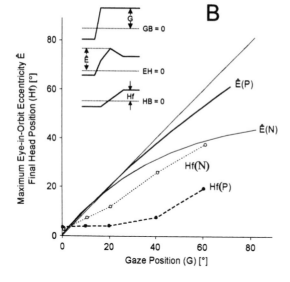

Figure 2. Comparison of eye and head contributions to gaze shifts in controls (N) and patients (P). See text and key to symbols in insets.

Panel A depicts the amplitude of the eye-in-head saccade, ΔE, and of the head movement, ΔH (see inset for definitions) as a function of the gaze amplitude. In controls (N), eye amplitude (light curve, open circles) equals gaze amplitude up to gaze shifts of about 40° and then levels off to reach an asymptotic maximum of about 50°. In other words, with saccades up to 40° the head contributes little to gaze displacement, whereas larger gaze saccades contain a head component of increasing magnitude. On the other hand, in patients (P) eye amplitude (bold, filled circles) is almost identical to gaze amplitude up to gaze shifts of 70° and reaches an asymptotic maximum of 90°. Thus, in patients the head contributes but to very large saccadic gaze shifts. Correspondingly, patients' total head movement amplitude (ΔH; dashed bold curve, filled circles) is much smaller than that observed in controls (light dashed, open circles), and frequently patients do not move the head at all when the required gaze shift is small. The difference between patients and controls is also well illustrated in panel B which considers peak orbital eye eccentricity at the end of gaze saccades ($\hat{E}$, continuous curves) and final head vs. trunk eccentricity (H_f, dashed) as a function of final gaze eccentricity during fixation (=target position). Whereas in controls $\hat{E}$ is restricted to an oculomotor range of ±40°, in patients this range is expanded to at least ±60°. The expansion is a prerequisite for the patients' strategy to make small and late head movements which contribute virtually nothing to the gaze saccade itself but serve only to reduce eye eccentricity during the subsequent gaze fixation. Finally, a comparison of the curves $H_f(N)$ and $H_f(P)$ demonstrates that patients are much more reluctant to assume an eccentric head position than controls are; for gaze positions up to ±40° they stay with their heads close to the primary position. The course of the $\Delta H(P)$ curve in panel A is direct consequence of this behaviour (if one accounts for the fact that it averages centrifugal, midline crossing and centripetal reactions, and that during a given reaction the head starts from where it stopped after completion of the preceding one).

3.2. Accuracy

The mean accuracy of patient's gaze saccades was slightly better than that of controls. In controls, the mean error of the main saccade increased from 1° with target steps of 10° to 6° with 80°-steps (undershoot errors), whereas in patients the corresponding values were 0.7° and 3.4°. However, the frequency distribution of patients' errors was broader and, consequently, comprised more instances of overshoot than that of the normal subjects. Interestingly, these differences do not seem to be related to the occurrence of head movements; the same differences between patients and controls were seen in gaze shifts that were not accompanied by head movements and particularly also in the head fixed condition.

3.3. Reaction Times

On average, patients started their gaze saccades after a longer latency than controls (mean difference 40 ms); again, also this difference between Ps and Ns cannot be attributed to "complications" by a concurrent head movement because it occurred also in the head fixed condition. Finally, a striking difference between Ps and Ns concerns the lag of the head movement with respect to the eye saccade which was by about 70 ms longer in patients.

3.4. Postsaccadic Stability

To investigate the stability of the line of gaze immediately after a saccade, we measured the eye velocity occurring 40 ms after the end of the primary gaze saccade (average across a 20 ms-epoch) and related it to the concurrent head velocity. For normal subjects this relationship indicated a virtually perfect stabilisation (slope of regression line, 0.997; coefficient of determination, 0.95). On the other hand, the linear regression describing patients' data yielded a slope of 0.91 and an offset of 11°/s, the coefficient of determination being 0.86. Thus, on average, patients' gaze drifts back at a rate of 11°/s if there is no head movement after the saccade. Interestingly, this observation also holds for the head fixed condition. This reverse drift decreases with the occurrence of sizeable postsaccadic head velocities, that is with large gaze shifts, and turns into a slight onward drift with the largest head velocities observed in patients (~150°/s). Thus, in terms of its average, gaze stability is remarkably good in patients, but individual trials exhibit a wide range of reverse or onward drifts.

3.5. Preadjusted Head Condition

The results presented so far seemed to suggest that patients achieve apparently normal gaze shifts (with regard to accuracy and postsaccadic stability) by (i) avoiding to make significant head movement *during* the eye saccade and by (ii) increasing their oculomotor range correspondingly. However, when we forced them to make sizeable *concurrent* head movements by controlling their head position at the outset of a response (-30° offset in preadjusted head condition), no significant deterioration of performance was observed. With such an initial offset the head contributed 25° to the saccadic gaze displacement of patients when the target stepped by 60°, as opposed to 5° in the normal head free condition. Without compensation for the lack of vestibular signals, one would expect an overshoot of more than 20° in this situation. Yet, patient's primary gaze saccades clearly undershot the target as did those of the control subjects. Negative offsets of initial head position sometimes give rise to 'arrested' eye-in-head saccades (Becker and Jürgens 1992) because the eye, being already close to the limit of its motor range at the start of the movement, may 'run' into this limit during the movement if the concurrent head movement is not large enough. Gaze shift then is carried on exclusively by the head until a compensatory, reverse eye movement is initiated upon approaching the desired target position. In this situation it becomes particularly important to know the exact amount of head movement because otherwise there is no means to decide whether the head has indeed brought gaze close to the target. Hence, in patients targeting accuracy should be particularly vulnerable to imperfections of the mechanisms compensating for the loss of vestibular function. Again however, no conclusive difference was observed between patients and controls. It is true, though, that our normal subjects made only a small number of such reactions (2.5%) whereas they were more frequent in patients (35%) so that a comparison is actually difficult.

Finally, in both patients and controls the analysis of the reaction times obtained with the preadjusted head condition revealed a dependence of the eye motor command centres upon the 'status' of the head motor system. Indeed, the latency of the eye saccade increases with negative offsets of initial head position (head further away from target than eye), by about 50 ms (Ns) and 30 ms (Ps), respectively. As a result, the lag of the head upon the eye vanishes in normal subjects, or even turns into a lead, and is reduced in patients. Functionally, the eye behaves as though it was waiting for the head movement in order to avoid an early arrest in the orbit.

4. DISCUSSION AND MODEL DESCRIPTION

Patients with chronic loss of vestibular function adapt to this state mainly by avoiding, or reducing and delaying, head movements during the saccadic displacement of their eyes. Such a strategy removes the necessity to continuously adjust the saccadic motor command to current head displacement, hence it does not matter for the gaze amplitude whether information on head movement is available or not. By the same token, if a certain amount of head movement is desirable in order to avoid excessive orbital eye eccentricities during gaze fixation, their late and slow commencement gives the smooth pursuit system a good chance to stabilise gaze in space without the necessity to recruit substitutes of

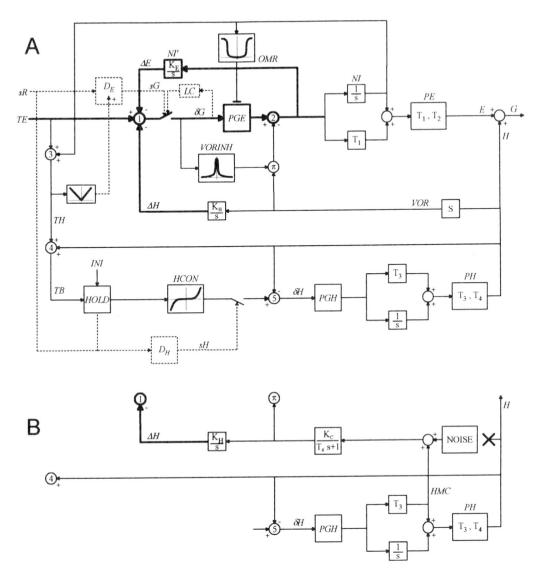

Figure 3. Descriptive model of eye-head coordination in normal subjects (A) and patients (B). Bold lines emphasise the local feedback scheme controlling the oculomotor pulse generator. *LC*, latch of local feedback circuit (Robinson 1975). *PE*, eye plant with time constants T_1=0.2 s, T_2=0.01s. *PH*, head plant with time constants T_3=0.2 s, T_3=0.1 s. See text for other symbols and full description. Note that B only shows those parts where the topology has been changed to model patients' behaviour; for other changes see text.

the VOR. However there is not only strategy but, as an indispensable prerequisite, also true plasticity as a result of which patients' oculomotor range is considerably expanded. It is puzzling, though, why the "small head movement strategy" is adopted at all since patients perform quite well if forced to make large head movements and since the same imperfections (larger variability of both accuracy and postsaccadic drift than in normal subjects) occur whether the head is moved or not. At any rate, the ability to produce fairly normal gaze saccades with considerable head contribution suggests that, in the course of adaptation, substitutes for the unavailable vestibular head movement signals have developed. The present data do not allow to pinpoint with any certainty at a single most likely source for these substitute signals, and it is beyond the scope of this report to discuss all conceivable mechanisms in detail. Instead, in the following we present a model (Fig. 3) which describes eye-head-coordination in normal subjects and which shows how a copy of efferent head motor activity (which, clearly, is but one of several conceivable mechanisms) could substitute for the vestibular afferents.

The model in Fig. 3A, which describes the behaviour of normal subjects, has been derived from schemes previously suggested by Laurutis and Robinson (1986), Guitton and Volle (1987), and Pelisson et al. (1988). The motor command for the eye-in-head saccade is generated by eye pulse generator *PGE* situated in the forward pathway of a local feedback circuit. The circuit responds to the target vs. eye offset *TE* which is identical to the desired gaze displacement. At summing junction 1, the currently achieved displacements of the eye in the head (ΔE) and of the head relative to the trunk (ΔH, identical to head vs. space) are subtracted from *TE* leaving the current gaze error δG which drives *PGE*. For the operational characteristics of *PGE* a simplified law, *PGE* output = min($25 \bullet \delta G$, 500), has been assumed. ΔE is obtained by feedback of the *PGE* activity through the resettable integrator *NI'* which acts as a model of the neural integrator *NI* on the output side. Similarly, ΔH is obtained by integrating the vestibular signal of head velocity (pathway *VOR* $\rightarrow \Delta H$; note that the vestibular transfer function (s) has been idealised by omitting its time constant of ~ 20 sec). The vestibulo-saccadic reflex mediated by ΔH is only active during saccades; during fixation, the vestibular velocity signal is channelled, through multiplicative stage π and summing junction 4, into the common final pathway ("classical" VOR). π acts as a gate which is controlled by current gaze error via the operation characteristics *VORINH*. It switches the VOR on for fixation, and off during all saccades except very small ones. To account for the eye-in-head arrest occurring at the limits of the oculomotor range, *PGE* activity is reduced, and finally inhibited, if current eye position approaches and eventually reaches these limits (inhibitory pathway through element *OMR*; in our simulations we have modelled this *PGE* inhibition by multiplication with a signal complementary to the characteristics sketched in *OMR*, that is a signal which is unity inside the oculomotor range, and zero outside). Others have placed the neural limitation of the eye movement range ahead of the pulse generator (Guitton and Volle 1987). However we wished to avoid the double transformation first of *TE* into a signal of target vs. head (*TH*) and then of *TH* into desired eye-in-head displacement which such an arrangement would require.

Yet, at least the transformation *TE*→*TH* (summing junction 3) appears to be unavoidable because the head contribution to gaze displacement depends on where the target is with respect to the head. Finally, because we assume that the head motor circuitry eventually codes head-on-body position, *TH* must be further transformed (summing junction 4) into *TB*, the target vs. body offset. The degree to which the head responds to this offset is determined by the non-linear characteristic *HCON* which is an empirical fit of the curves H_f in Fig. 2B (controls: TB-20arctan[TB/40], patients TB-40arctan[TB/40]). With the decision to start a reaction (*sR*) the desired head vs. body position is stored in *HOLD* and acts as the set value for a head motor circuit. For this circuit also a local feedback scheme has been assumed, with parameters adjusted to approximate the observed head movement trajectories. For the present purpose this assumption is sufficient although, in reality, head motor control may be considerably more complex (e.g. Zangemeister et al 1981). The head pulse generator (*PGH*) produces the activity min($20 \bullet \max(\delta G - 5°)$, 300); the 5°-dead zone has been introduced to prevent the circuit from ringing. Input *INI* allows the head to

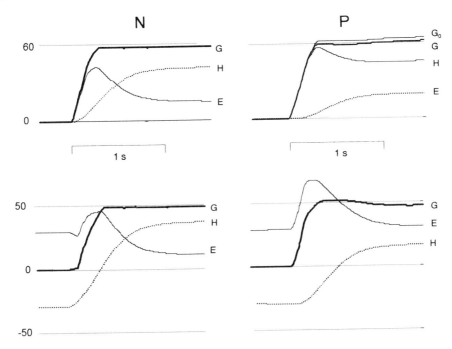

Figure 4. Simulated responses of normal subjects (N) and patients (P) to centrifugal target steps of 60° (head free condition, top panels) and 50° with an initial head offset of −30° (preadjusted head condition, lower). G, gaze; G_0, gaze when there is no substitute for VOR; E, eye; H, head. (Note: small "steps" in postsaccadic traces are digitising artefacts and actually represent drift and not saccades.)

be initially adjusted to arbitrary positions, independent of the currently fixated target (as in the preadjusted head condition).

Our scheme does not address the question how and where the decision to start a saccadic gaze response is elaborated. It assumes the occurrence of a start signal (*sR*) contingent on the arrival of the *TE* step. D_H is a delay which represents the lag of the head relative to the eye. As we have mentioned, with large target to head distances this lag decreases because the latency of the eye increases. This observation is modelled by delay D_E which rises as signal *TH* increases.

Fig. 4 N shows simulated responses of normal subjects in the head free condition (top) and the preadjusted head condition for the case of a -30° initial head offset (bottom). K_E and K_H have been set to a value of 1.05 so that gaze saccades exhibit a small undershoot. Owing to a delay D_H of 40 ms, the head movement starts only while the saccade is already in progress in the conventional head free condition, whereas it is about synchronous to the eye when initial head offset is away from the target (bottom). In the latter situation also a brief eye arrest is evident (however, we recall that this pattern was rare in controls).

To simulate the performance of patients, the parameters of the following elements of Fig. 3A were changed: Width of the oculomotor range (±60° instead of ±40°), delay D_H (110 ms instead of 40 ms), feedback gains K_E and K_H (1.0 instead of 1.05) and the head contribution characteristic *HCON* (detailed already above). Furthermore, as a substitute of the interrupted vestibular pathway, in panel B the possibility is considered that a copy of the phasic component of the head motor command (*HMC*) couples into the oculomotor circuitry. To create a realistic image of the concurrent head velocity, this copy must be modified to account for the dynamics of the head plant (*PH*). To this end it is fed through a model of the head dynamics which mimics time constant T_4 of *PH* (transfer function $K_C/(T_4s+1)$, Kc=1). It is also suggested that *HMC* is plagued by a low frequency noise which causes the larger scatter of both the saccadic end points (by affecting ΔH) and the postsaccadic drift (by affecting the pathway for gaze stabilisation through multiplicative gate π) in patients. It is unclear whether this noise actually is a property inherent to *HMC* or a product of the deafferented vestibular complex which, at its efferent end, is still tightly connected to the oculomotor circuitry. At any rate, with the topology of Fig. 3 B it would indeed also affect saccades made with the head fixed, in conformity with our observations. Finally, the local feedback for the head motor circuitry was left unchanged on the assumption that it is mainly governed by proprioceptive feedback (cervicocollic reflex). Fig. 4 P shows gaze saccades of patients simulated with these modifications. The simulated trajectories reproduce the delayed and small head contribution which is typical of patients in the head free situation but also the occurrence of large head movements when the reaction starts with a negative head offset (top). Furthermore it will be noted that the saccades land slightly off target and that following the saccade gaze is drifting. To illustrate how little the VOR substitute is challenged with patients' strategy to make small and late head movements, the thinly outlined gaze curve (G_0, Fig. 4 P) simulates the effect of a complete absence of the VOR substitute. ($K_C=0$). Finally, in the preadjusted head condition (bottom) the eye is arrested in the orbit and the saccade is brought to its end by the head movement, without negative consequence for its accuracy.

ACKNOWLEDGMENT

This work was supported by DFG Me 715.

REFERENCES

Becker W, Jürgens R (1992) Gaze saccades to visual targets: Does head movement change the metrics? In: Berthoz A, Graf W, Vidal PP (eds) Head-neck sensory-motor system. Oxford University Press, New York, pp 427–433

Bizzi E, Kalil RE, Morasso P (1972) Two modes of active eye-head coordination in monkeys. Brain Res 40:45–48.

Dichgans J, Bizzi E, Morasso P, Taglisaco V (1973) Mechanisms underlying recovery of eye-head coordination following bilateral labyrinthectomy in monkeys. Exp Brain Res 18: 548–562

Guitton D, Volle M (1987) Gaze control in humans: eye-head coordination during orienting movements to targets within and beyond the oculomotor range. J Neurophysiol 58: 427–459.

Kasai T, Zee DS (1978) Eye-head coordination in labyrinthine-defective human beings. Brain Res 144: 123–141

Laurutis VP, Robinson DA (1986) The vestibulo-ocular reflex during human saccadic eye movements. J Physiol (Lond) 373: 209–233

Morasso P, Bizzi E, Dichgans J (1973) Adjustment of saccade characteristics during head movements. Exp Brain Res 16: 492–500

Pelisson D, Pablanc C, Urquizar C (1988) Vestibuloocular reflex inhibition and gaze saccade characteristics during eye-head orientation in humans. J Neurophysiol 59: 997–1013

Robinson DA (1975) Oculomotor control signals. In: Lennerstrand G, Bach-y-Rita P (eds) Basic mechanisms of ocular motility and their clinical implications. Pergamon, Oxford, pp 337–374

Zangemeister WH, Lehman S, Stark L (1981) Simulation of head movement trajectories: model and fit to main sequence. Biol Cybern 41: 19–32

61

SUBCLINICAL SACCADIC ADDUCTION SLOWING IN PATIENTS WITH MONOSYMPTOMATIC UNILATERAL OPTIC NEURITIS PREDICTS THE DEVELOPMENT OF MULTIPLE SCLEROSIS

E. Tsironi,[1] D. Anastasopoulos,[2] Th. Mergner,[3] and K. Psilas[1]

[1]Department of Ophthalmology
[2]Department of Neurology
University of Ioannina
Box 1186, 45100 Ioannina, Greece.
[3]Department of Neurology
University of Freiburg, Neurozentrum
Breisacher Str. 64
79106 Freiburg, Germany

Many patients with acute unilateral optic neuritis (ON) develop later multiple sclerosis (MS), the risk varying widely between 35% and 75% (McDonald 1983). Many MS and ON patients are subject to abnormalities of eye movements (Reulen et al 1983). Saccadic disturbances are the commonest among them, which in many cases cannot easily be detected clinically (Meienberg et al 1986). Using electro-oculography, it was concluded that the ratio of abduction vs. adduction peak velocities represents a sensitive index of subclinical abnormality (Ventre et al 1991). However, the pathological significance of subtle abnormalities revealed by quantitative testing of eye movements remains unclear.

In this study, using infrared oculography as recording technique, we addressed the question whether subclinical internuclear ophthalmoplegia (INO) is able to provide additional paraclinical evidence in patients with clearcut monosymptomatic demyelination, such as ON. More specifically, by defining lower normal limits of conjugacy of visually-guided saccades and by documenting the subsequent development of clinically definite multiple sclerosis (CDMS) during a 2.2 year average follow-up period we were able to determine the significance of this abnormality as pathological finding.

Twenty-two consecutive patients (aged 35.3 ±10.3 yrs; mean ±S.D.) presenting with acute unilateral isolated ON and 21 age-matched controls (35.4 ±11.9 yrs) gave their in-

Current Oculomotor Research, edited by Becker *et al.*
Plenum Press, New York, 1999.

formed consent to the study. Eye movement measurements were carried out a few days after the onset of symptoms. The patients were re-evaluated every 6 months and whenever new neurologic symptoms developed. CDMS was diagnosed when new neurologic symptoms, other than new ON, emerged.

Subjects sat on a Barany chair at the centre of a 1.6 m radius cylindrical screen. Their heads were stabilized by means of a dental bite-board. A laser spot, subtending 0.2° of visual angle, was projected onto the screen and horizontally rotated by means of a mirror galvanometer. The spot was initially presented for 1500 ms as a fixation point located straight ahead with respect to the subject. It was then extinguished and, following an interval of 100 ms, it reappeared in a lateral eccentric location (4°, 8°, and 16° on either the right or left side) as target for centrifugal saccades. Timing and target location were randomized. Each subject performed 10 trials for each of the six target locations.

Eye movements were recorded using an infrared corneal reflection device (IRIS, Skalar Medical, Delft, The Netherlands). The analysis of the saccade amplitude and maximum velocity was performed separately for each eye and separately for abducting and adducting saccades by means of an interactive computer program (Anastasopoulos et al 1996). The dependency of the peak velocity (PV) on amplitude was evaluated by fitting a curve to the maximum velocity/ amplitude data according to the exponential law of the type:

$$PV = PV_{MAX} * [1\text{-}exp(\text{-}A/A_{63})]$$

Peak velocity for 4°, 8°, 12° and 15° were calculated for each normal subject from the exponential fit of abductive and adductive saccades, separately for each eye. The data were treated by a 2 X 2 X 4 factorial ANOVA, with Eye (left vs. right), Direction (abduction vs. adduction) and Amplitude (4°, 8°, 12° and 15°) as the within-subject repeated measures factors. Abduction maximum velocities were clearly higher than adduction velocities (F = 13.8, p =0.0014). Furthermore, the interaction of Direction and Amplitude proved significant (F = 10.7, p = 0.0001) reflecting the fact that the bigger the amplitude, the faster the abduction, as compared to the adduction .

As the difference between abduction and adduction PV proved more variable (coefficient of variation between 0.9 and 6.9) than their ratio (range between 0.06–0.11 respectively), we used the latter parameter (versional disconjugacy index, VDI, Ventre et al 1991) to define the lower normal limits of eye yoking. 2 X 4 factorial ANOVA of the VDI, with Gaze (left vs. right) and Amplitude (4°, 8°, 12° and 15°) as the within-subject repeated measures factors revealed a highly statistical significance for the factor Amplitude (F = 8.8, p = 0.0001), confirming that the abduction is even faster for big saccades (Fig. 1).

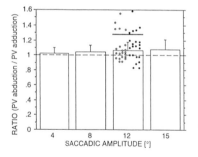

Figure 1. Comparison of ratio values of peak velocities for abducting and adducting saccades (VDI), separately for 4°, 8°, 12° and 15° saccadic amplitude (data of normal group). On average, abduction is faster than adduction, the difference increasing with amplitude. Patients' VDI data is plotted separately for rightward and leftward gaze shifts (filled and open circles, respectively) only for the 12Æ amplitude (upper normal limit, horizontal thick line).

Table 1. Overall comparison of PV and VDI between control and patient groups (mean values ±S.D.). PV values are given separately for abduction and adduction (amplitude, 12°). There was no difference between the two groups.

	Abduction PV (°/ s)	Adduction PV (°/ s)	VDI
Controls	378 ±56	358 ±53	1.06 ± 0.11
Patients	374 ±75	343 ±59	1.10 ± 0.17

In order to remain well within the range of the actual measured amplitudes, only the VDI for saccades of 12° was used to set lower normal limits of conjugacy. On the whole, there was no statistically significant difference between the patient and control groups for both PV and VDI (Table 1). In 9 patients this index was greater than 1.28 (mean +2SD) and they were thus considered as having subclinical INO (Fig. 1, filled and open circles, one patient on both sides). Seven of these patients and only 4 out of 13 patients falling within the normal conjugacy limits developed CDMS during the follow-up period (Fisher's exact p-value = 0.04).

The results of this study show that measurement of abducting vs adducting saccadic peak velocity at presentation with clinically isolated ON may prove to be useful in detecting patients who are likely to subsequently develop MS. The detection of subclinical abducting vs adducting saccadic slowing proved predictive of later development of demyelinating disease and not a mere statistical measure.

REFERENCES

Anastasopoulos D, Kimmig H, Mergner T, Psilas K (1996). Abnormalities of ocular motility in myotonic dystrophy. Brain 119: 1923–1932.

McDonald WI (1983). The significance of optic neuritis. Trans Ophthalmol Soc UK 103: 230–246.

Meienberg O, Müri R, Rabineau PA (1986). Clinical and oculographic examinations of saccadic eye movements in the diagnosis of multiple sclerosis. Arch Neurol 43: 438–443.

Reulen JP, Sanders EA, Hogenhuis LA (1983). Eye movement disorders in multiple sclerosis and optic neuritis. Brain 106: 121–140.

Ventre J, Vighetto A, Bailly G, Prablanc C (1991). Saccadic metrics in multiple sclerosis: versional velocity disconjugacy as the best clue? J Neurol Sci 101: 144–149.

62

SACCADIC TRACKING IN SCHIZOPHRENIA

Incidence of Hypometria and Intrusions Influenced by Visual Background and Pace of Stepping?

R. Jürgens,[1] W. Becker,[1] H. Schreiber,[2] B. Fegert,[1] and S. Klausmann[1]

[1]Section of Neurophysiology
[2]Department of Neurology
University of Ulm, Germany

1. INTRODUCTION

Schizophrenic patients and their relatives exhibit a genetically increased probability of impaired smooth pursuit eye movements (Levy et al. 1993). It is less clear whether also saccadic eye movements are affected. Abnormalities such as hypometric tracking of target steps or saccadic intrusions during fixation have been reported by some groups (e.g., Cegalis et al. 1982; Mather and Putchat 1983) and denied by others (e.g., Yee et al. 1987). A number of studies considering both patients and their first degree relatives, which were carried out by our group either in a hospital environment or at the patients' or their relatives' homes, demonstrated an increased rate of hypometric saccades (gain < 0.75) of up to 35% as compared to about half that rate (18%) in controls (Schreiber et al. 1995, 1997). However, a hypometria incidence of 18% in controls is much higher than what is observed in a standard laboratory environment (complete darkness except visual targets), and a recent examination of juveniles at risk of schizophrenia conducted by our group under such laboratory conditions revealed no significant increase of hypometria. We therefore asked whether differences in background structure or target step timing could be responsible for these discrepancies. We argued that there might be particular experimental sets in which the saccadic tracking system is challenged to a degree where it would operate at the limits of its capability in normal subjects and would disclose otherwise unnoticeable impairments in patients.

2. METHODS

24 normal adult subjects (Ss; paid students) tracked sequences of 130 random horizontal steps of a target (red LED) of 5–60 deg amplitude. Ss were to refixate the target as

Current Oculomotor Research, edited by Becker *et al.*
Plenum Press, New York, 1999.

447

fast and accurately as possible after a step and to precisely maintain fixation between steps. There were 4 different conditions: "Normal" tracking (NOR) in complete darkness with inter-step intervals varying randomly from 2 to 4 s. The possible influence of a visible background similar to those encountered in patients' homes was studied by dimly illuminating a coloured curtain. The curtain was at the same viewing distance as the target array (170 cm), filled 180 x 70 deg of the visual field, and displayed a regular pattern of filled circles with 1 deg diameter and a spacing of 1.5 deg (condition COL). In a 3rd condition (GRN) the background was created by permanently lighting green LEDs 2 cm beneath each locus at which the (red) target could appear. Finally, in the 4th condition (RAP) the intervals were shortened to 0.75 - 1.5 s while the target stepped again in total darkness, as in NOR. The order of these four conditions was systematically varied. Eye movements were recorded by DC EOG, and saccades were interactively analysed off-line after careful recalibration of the EOG.

3. RESULTS

Figure 1 compares the incidence of hypometric saccades in the various paradigms. Condition COL caused a clear increase of the frequency of hypometria, but only for steps exceeding 40 deg; with 60-deg steps, the mean frequency of hypometric saccades attained 9% in this condition, with individual frequencies varying from 0 − 38 %. In contrast, with the row of green LEDs (GRN) accuracy deteriorated dramatically in *all* Ss and for *all* step sizes exceeding 10 deg. Correspondingly, for steps of 60 deg, the average number of correction saccades per response changed from 1.2 in NOR to 1.7 in COL and 2.9 in GRN. Finally, the accelerated pace of target presentation (RAP) did not influence response accuracy, neither in terms of the frequency of hypometric responses nor of the mean postsaccadic error, although it forced a decrease of the average reaction time from 220 to 202 ms.

We also investigated saccades detracting the eye from the target while it was supposed to fixate (intrusions). As a global measure of the frequency and magnitude of intrusions, the absolute values of their amplitudes were summed up for each S and experimental paradigm. Again, there were clear idiosyncrasies as can be seen from Figure 2; while in many of our Ss the amount of intrusions remained almost unchanged in condition COL as compared to NOR, there was a subgroup of 9 Ss in which the cumulated intrusion amplitude rose from 16 deg in NOR to 100 deg in COL (note: the cumulated duration of the fixation periods was identical for NOR and COL: 310 s). Many Ss (among them all but one of the above 9) exhibited also a facilitation of intrusive saccades in condi-

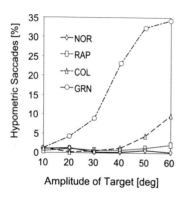

Figure 1. Percentage of hypometric saccades (saccadic amplitude 25%-75% of target amplitude) as a function of target amplitude with different experimental conditions (see METHODS for abbreviations).

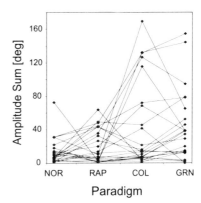

Figure 2. Amount of saccadic intrusions expressed by sum of amplitudes per session. Thin lines connect cumulative amplitudes of single Ss across the four paradigms. Note: In condition GRN, owing to the large number of saccadic corrections, the average amount of time available for intrusions was shorter than in NOR (by about 11%).

tion RED. Interestingly, Ss making many intrusions also required more corrective saccades to acquire the target (correlation coefficient between number of intrusions and number of corrections: r=0.55).

4. CONCLUSIONS

Whereas the huge increase of hypometria in condition GRN (Fig. 1) may simply be explained by the lack of red-green distinction in peripheral vision, the increased frequency of hypometria and intrusions obtained with the dimly illuminated background in condition COL points to a destabilising effect of structured visual backgrounds upon saccadic tracking. However, the effects reported here for normal adults are too small to quantitatively account for the results obtained by Schreiber et al. (1995, 1997) in normals and patients who were investigated at the subjects' homes or in hospitals. It is, none the less, conceivable that the effect of the visual background could be exploited to better unravel specific impairments of psychiatric patients such as vulnerability against distractors. Finally, it is surprising that the accelerated pace used in condition RAP is inconsequential for saccadic accuracy and even improves saccadic tracking in terms of the reaction time, at least in the normal subjects considered here. Possibly, the short fixation intervals reduced the chance that subjects were already engaged in covert shifts of attention when the next target step occurred.

REFERENCES

Cegalis JA, Sweeney JA, Dellis EM (1982) Refixation saccades and attention in schizophrenia. J Psychiat Res 7: 189–198.

Levy DL, Holzman PS, Matthysse S, Mendell NR (1993) Eye tracking dysfunction and schizophrenia: A critical perspective. Schizophr Bull 19: 461–536

Mather JA, Putchat C (1983) Motor control of schizophrenics. I: Oculomotor control of schizophrenics: A deficit in sensory processing, not strictly in motor control. J Psychiat Res, 17: 343–359.

Schreiber H, Rothmeier J, Becker W, Jürgens R, Born J, Stolz-Born, G, Westphal KP and Kornhuber HH (1995) Comparative assessment of saccadic eye movements, psychomotor and cognitive performance in schizophrenics, their first-degree relatives and control Ss. Acta Psychiatr Scand 91: 195–201

Schreiber H, Stolz-Born G, Born J, Rothmeier J, Rothenberger A, Jürgens R, Becker W, Kornhuber HH (1997) Visually-guided saccadic eye movements in adolescents at genetic risk for schizophrenia. Schizophrenia Research 25: 97–109

Yee RD, Baloh RW, Marder SR, Levy DL, Skala SM, Honrubia V (1987) Eye movements in schizophrenia. Investigative Ophthalmology and Visual Science, 28: 366–374.

63

ASYMMETRIC GAP EFFECT ON SMOOTH PURSUIT LATENCY IN A SCHIZOPHRENIC SUBJECT

Paul C. Knox[1] and Douglas Blackwood[2]

[1]Vision Sciences
Glasgow Caledonian University
Cowcaddens Rd, Glasgow G4 0BA
[2]Psychiatry
Royal Edinburgh Hospital
Edinburgh EH10 5HF

The underlying neuropathology in schizophrenia is still poorly understood and several approaches have been adopted to investigate it at a behavioural level. Studies of oculomotor performance in schizophrenia have proved particularly useful. It is clear that in schizophrenia several intriguing oculomotor deficits are manifest. In particular, smooth ocular pursuit (SP) is known to be disrupted; Holzman et al (1973) reported that SP in schizophrenics was disrupted by the intrusion of numerous small saccades giving a "cogwheel" appearance to eye position records. It has been suggested that this deficit might serve as a biological marker for the neuropathology which gives rise to schizophrenia. The development of new behavioural paradigms have provided new tools for investigating oculomotor control in schizophrenia, and perhaps better tasks for probing the SP deficit.

There has been considerable interest in the effect of the gap paradigm on saccade latency in schizophrenia. In general, schizophrenic subjects exhibit a higher frequency of express saccades in both gap and non-gap tasks than non-schizophrenic subjects and this is most pronounced when targets are presented in the right visual field (Matsue et al. 1994). This might reflect the attentional asymmetry which is a major feature of the psychopathology of schizophrenia (eg Carter et al. 1996). Recently the "gap" protocol has been applied to SP, and a "gap" effect on SP latency observed. SP latency is reduced in gap, as opposed to non-gap trials (Knox 1996, Krauzlis and Miles 1996). Given that in schizophrenic subjects there is an SP deficit, that the gap effect on saccade latency is modified, and that this is most marked in those subjects with SP dysfunction, we wished to investigate the gap effect on SP latency in a schizophrenic subject and compared it with that observed in normal subjects.

Current Oculomotor Research, edited by Becker *et al.*
Plenum Press, New York, 1999.

One subject (PH), a right handed, male, 30-year old diagnosed with chronic schizophrenia at 24, was tested. He had responded well to oral antipsychotic medication, and at
the time of testing had been free from oral medication for six months. He sat 57cm from a
visual display, which he viewed with his left eye. In each trial a square (0.3°) was presented for 1s in the middle of the display; this was extinguished and a pursuit target
moved at 8°/s from 4° to the right or left, through the centre and continued until disap-
pearing off the edge of the display. Four conditions were randomly presented in runs of
100 or 96 trials. In two the target moved to the right and in two it moved to the left. In one
condition there was no temporal gap between fixation target extinction and pursuit target
illumination (normal trials), while in the other three there was a gap of 100ms, 200ms or
400ms (gap trials). The subject was exposed to a total of 1176 trials over three sessions.
Left eye position was digitised at 1kHz and stored on disc for analysis. SP latency was
measured for each trial; data from trials where SP was not preceded by a period of steady
fixation or interrupted by blinks were discarded (305/1176 trials). Data from three normal
subjects (see Knox 1996), performing the same tasks in identical circumstances was
pooled and is presented for comparison.

PH was able to perform the tasks, there were no gross abnormalities in the eye position records. The distributions of pursuit latency were broadly similar for leftward and

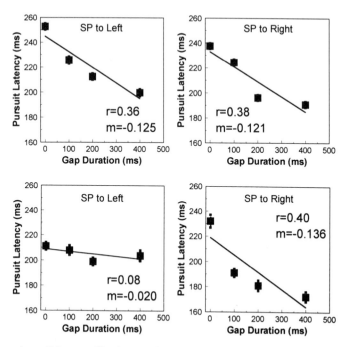

Figure 1. Comparison of the gap effect in normal subjects (a: top panels) and subject PH (b: bottom panels).
Mean±sem pursuit latency is plotted against gap duration for each condition. In a, the group mean for three normal
subjects is shown. Linear regression lines also plotted. All regressions were highly statistically significant
(p<<0.01) except that for PH, SP to left. r values, and the slope of the regression line (m) are shown. Note that in
normal subjects there is a gap duration dependent reduction in SP latency, whereas for PH there is little evidence
of a gap effect for SP to the left, and a normal or enhanced gap effect for SP to the right.

rightward pursuit with relatively few responses that might be interpreted as being clearly anticipatory (latency<100ms). There was little evidence of gaps inducing a shift from a unimodal to a bi- or even trimodal distribution. Figure 1 shows plots of mean SP latency against gap duration for pooled normal subject data (Figure 1a) and for PH (Figure 1b). SP latency in trials with no gap between the disappearance of the fixation target and the appearance of the pursuit target (leftward 211±3ms, rightward 232±5ms, mean±sem) was similar to, if lower than, that observed in normal subjects (leftward 253±2ms, rightward 237±2ms). For PH there was a large gap-duration dependent reduction in latency for rightward pursuit (eg 400ms gap, 172±4ms, reduction of 26% from 0ms gap trials in PH; 191±2ms, reduction of 20% in Normals), there was barely any effect with leftward pursuit (lowest latency at 200ms gap, 199±3ms, reduction of 6% compared with 0ms gap trials). Having found the asymmetry in the gap effect on pursuit in PH, we checked the latency of saccades which accompanied SP in the step-ramp tasks employed in these experiments. There was a significant gap effect on saccade latency both for targets appearing on the left and the right, although the magnitude of the effect was smaller for saccades to the right. At least for targets appearing on the right, there were also further significant reductions in saccade latency as gap duration increased.

In these experiments, in our schizophrenic subject PH, there was a gap effect on *pursuit latency* for targets appearing on the left and moving to the right, but little gap effect for targets appearing on the right and moving to the left. In normal subjects there is no large systematic asymmetry in the gap effect on SP latency. There was a gap effect on *saccade latency* for saccades both to the left and right. It is unlikely that the SP asymmetry observed is attributable simply to deficits in visual motion processing or the output of brainstem motor pathways; the subject reported no difficulty in seeing and following all targets and the absolute values of pursuit latency are broadly comparable with non-schizophrenic subjects performing the same tasks. Asymmetrical responses to visual targets is a consistent finding in work on schizophrenia. Clementz (1996) and Matsue et al (1994) reported a higher frequency of express saccades (to stationary targets) in schizophrenic subjects, an effect which was most pronounced for targets presented in the right visual field in subjects who also exhibited a smooth pursuit deficit. Perceptual and attentional asymmetries have also been reported in schizophrenia (eg Carter et al. 1996) and these could underlie the asymmetry in express saccade production. Further work is necessary to establish the reliability of the asymmetry in the gap effect on SP we have observed and to investigate the relationship between the pursuit system and attentional mechanisms in subjects with and without schizophrenia.

REFERENCES

Carter CS, Robertson LC, Nordahl TE, Chaderjian M, Oshora-Celaya L (1996) Perceptual and attentional asymmetries in schizophrenia: further evidence for a left hemisphere deficit Psychiatry Res 62:111–119

Clementz BA (1996) The ability to produce express saccades as a function of gap interval among schizophrenia patients. Exp Brain Res 111:121–130

Holzman, PS, Proctor LR, Hughes DW (1973) Eye tracking patterns in schizophrenia. Science 181:179–180

Knox, P. C. (1996) The effect of the gap paradigm on the latency of human smooth pursuit eye movement. NeuroReport 7:3027–3030

Krauzlis RJ, Miles FA (1996) Release of fixation for pursuit and saccades in humans: evidence for shared inputs acting on different neural substrates. J Neurophysiology 76:2822–2833.

Matsue Y, Osakabe K, Saito H, Goto Y, Ueno T, Matsuoka, H, Chiba H, Fuse Y, Sato M, (1994) Smooth pursuit eye movements and express saccades in schizophrenic patients. Schizophrenia Research 12:121–130

64

EYE-HAND COORDINATION IN PATIENTS WITH PARKINSON'S DISEASE, WILSON'S DISEASE, CEREBELLAR LESIONS, AND PARIETAL LESIONS

A. Roll,[1] W. Wolf,[1] and H. Hefter[2]

[1]Universität der Bundeswehr München
München, Germany
[2]Neurologische Klinik
Heinrich-Heine-Universität
Düsseldorf, Germany

1. INTRODUCTION

Coordinated eye and hand movements are successfully involved in many activities of human behavior. In order to execute concurrent or consecutive voluntary movements efficiently temporal and spatial coupling of the corresponding motor processes are required. A possibility to investigate interferences between both movements is the dual task methodology. Interference effects of eye and hand movements have been shown in experiments with aimed hand movements to randomized targets. Performing combined eye and hand reactions in dual task experiments, Warabi et al. (1986) have shown delayed saccadic reaction times (SRT), and Prablanc et al. (1979) reported delayed manual reaction times (MRT) compared to those in single task experiment. The reported interference effects support the hypothesis of neural processes shared by both motor systems. The kind of control processes and the involvement of distinct cerebral areas are partly known only.

The aim of the study is to compare (i) the SRT and MRT in single task experiments and (ii) the temporal relation of both reactions in dual task experiments. We were interested in the ability to coordinate eye and finger reactions in iso- and contra-directed experiments. Patient groups with deficits in brain areas which are assumed to be involved in temporal control and coordination of movements are investigated.

2. MATERIAL AND METHODS

Each trial began with the appearance of a central LED which served as fixation point. After a randomized time the fixation point was switched off and a target (LED) pre-

Current Oculomotor Research, edited by Becker *et al.*
Plenum Press, New York, 1999.

sented either 8° left or right from the fixation point was presented. Horizontal saccadic eye movements were recorded with an infrared recording system (SKALAR IRIS). Isometric finger reactions consist of pressing the forefinger within a splint to the left or right and were measured with a force measurement. In the two single task conditions, subjects had to respond by either horizontal saccade (Spro) or finger reaction (Mpro) to the target direction as fast as possible. In the three dual task conditions both reactions were required, in which the eye and finger reactions could be iso-directed (both reactions to target direction, Spro/Mpro) or contra-directed (one reaction to and the other opposite to target direction, Spro/Manti and Santi/Mpro). Each individual performed 10–15 training trials guided by the experimenter to ensure that the task was understood correctly. Reaction times (RT) below 100 ms were excluded as anticipatory reactions. Groups of patients with mild to moderate Parkinson's disease, Wilson's disease, cerebellar lesions and parietal lesions are compared to corresponding specifically age-matched control groups. Medication of patients was interrupted the day before measurement device. Both patients and control subjects had normal (or corrected to normal) vision, and they were naive with respect to the aim of the study.

3. RESULTS AND DISCUSSION

Median SRT and MRT of patient and control groups are shown in Figure 1. The left two columns of plots compare directly the RTs between patient and control groups of all experiments. The right two columns show SRT and MRT separately for each group and allow a comparison of temporal relation between eye and hand reactions easily. Statistical significance was calculated by the u-test and is given within plots (n.s. = not significant, * for $P<0.05$, ** for $P<0.01$, *** for $P<0.001$).

The MRTs are significantly larger in all patient groups compared to their corresponding control groups, but there are differences in the increase of MRT between patient groups. The differences of SRTs between patient and control groups show more variability. SRTs of patient groups are partly not different at all, but some are significantly larger or slower than SRTs of the control groups.

The Parkinson group shows no deficits with reflexive prosaccades but much larger SRT if making a voluntary antisaccade. In dual task performances there is a typical temporal order with the eyes starting before the hand begins to move (Abrams et al. 1990). We have found this temporal order in the Parkinson and control group, too, but in the experiment Santi/Mpro Parkinson patients reacted with the opposite temporal order (hand starts before the saccade) in more than 50 % of trials. Patients seem to change their strategy and prefer to begin with the manual proreaction before executing the more difficult antisaccade. In the Wilson group, there is a tendency of changing the temporal order in this experiment, too. This patient group is the only one which shows an increase in SRT with respect to the performance of the control group in all experiments even in prosaccades in the single task experiment. Patients with cerebellar lesions and with parietal lesions have no significant differences of prosaccades in the single task condition but more deficits in dual task conditions than the other two patient groups. Comparing SRT in single task and in the iso-directed dual task experiment shows that an additional hand reaction produces a larger prolongation of SRT in the cerebellar and the parietal patient group than in the corresponding control groups. These two patient groups show significantly shorter SRT in experiment Spro/Manti than control groups but a large difference between SRT and MRT. In experiment Santi/Mpro, patients with cerebellar lesions show larger SRT than the control

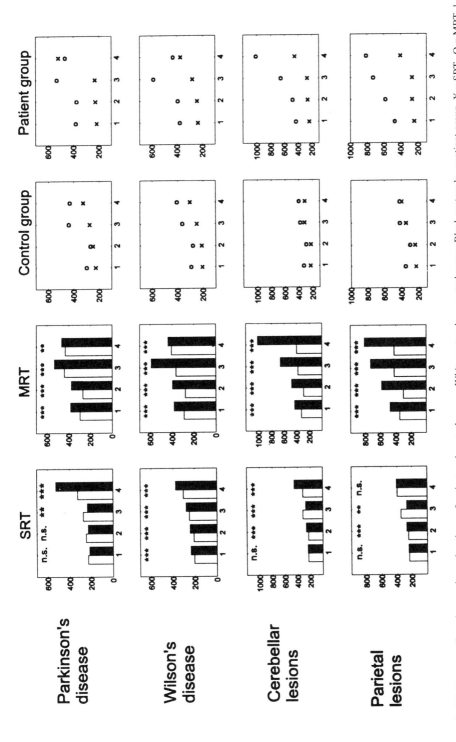

Figure 1. Median saccadic and manual reaction times of patient and control groups. White rectangle = control group. Black rectangle = patient group. X = SRT . O = MRT. 1 = single task experiment. 2 = Spro/Mpro. 3 = Spro/Manti. 4 = Santi/Mpro.

group and very large differences between RTs of both reactions. Patients with parietal lesions show no significant difference of SRT in comparison to the control group in this experiment but also a large difference between SRT and MRT, too.

These findings show that all patient groups have deficits in the coordination of eye and hand reactions in dual task experiments and reacted in a more sequential way than the control groups, but each of the four patient groups shows a different pattern in size and distribution of SRT and MRT differences compared to the corresponding control group. Further analysis of saccade amplitudes, RTs of corrective saccades, number of saccades, kind and proportion of errors and dependence of these parameters on the temporal order of saccades and hand reactions should characterize the differences between the patient groups more exactly. The specific impairments associated with the different brain deficits of the investigated patient groups in a given task may contribute to understand the involvement of different brain areas in the control of coordination of eye and hand movements.

REFERENCES

Abrams RA, Meyer DE, Kornblum S (1990) Eye-Hand Coordination: Oculomotor Control in Rapid Aimed Limb Movements. J Exp Psychol Hum Percept Perform 16(2): 248–267

Prablanc C, Echaillier J F, Komilis E, Jeannerod M (1979) Optimal Response of Eye and Hand Motor Systems in Pointing at a Visual Target, I. Spatio-Temporal Characteristics of Eye and Hand Movements and Their Relationships when Varying the Amount of Visual Information. Biol Cybern 53: 113–124

Warabi T, Noda H, Kato T (1986) Effect of aging on sensorimotor functions of eye and hand movements. Exp Neurol 92: 686–697

65

A SIMPLE APPROACH TO VIDEO-BASED 3D EYE MOVEMENT MEASUREMENT

Sven Steddin and Alexander Weiß

Department of Neurology
Ludwig-Maximilians University
Klinikum Großhadern
Munich, Germany

1. INTRODUCTION

Measurement of 3D eye movements by image processing of video data has recently been the subject of several publications. On the basis of the applied architecture, existing systems can be divided into three basic groups: I.) Images of the eyes are stored on video tapes prior to analysis (Clarke et al. 1991). This requires expensive time-base corrected analog video recorders, which often greatly decrease the quality of the image data due to noise. II.) Images are analysed online without storage of the video data (Steddin and Brandt 1995); thus, there is a risk of losing data, if the online detection of the pupil temporarily fails, or if torsion is not calculated properly. III.) More reliable semi-realtime systems detect the pupil online, and store only those parts of the image which are relevant for offline calculation of the eye's torsion (Moore et al. 1991). This method has resulted in sampling rates of only a few frames per second due to the time-consuming online calculation of pupil position and eye torsion.

Recently, the introduction of the PCI-bus (Peripheral Component Interconnect bus) technology made possible realtime storage of uncompressed digital video data directly on hard disk, making expensive and image degrading analog video recorders obsolete. Processing of the stored data is done offline. Each frame can be accessed directly, and sequences of the video can be replayed in realtime or even faster.

2. HARD DISK RECORDING OF IMAGES OF THE EYE

We developed a video eye movement recording system (VEMRS) based on this new PCI-bus technology which incorporates all of its special features mentioned above. Eye movement analysis of video data is done interactively after a recording session.

Current Oculomotor Research, edited by Becker *et al.*
Plenum Press, New York, 1999.

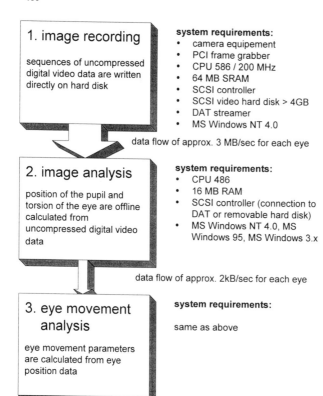

1. image recording

sequences of uncompressed digital video data are written directly on hard disk

system requirements:
- camera equipement
- PCI frame grabber
- CPU 586 / 200 MHz
- 64 MB SRAM
- SCSI controller
- SCSI video hard disk > 4GB
- DAT streamer
- MS Windows NT 4.0

data flow of approx. 3 MB/sec for each eye

2. image analysis

position of the pupil and torsion of the eye are offline calculated from uncompressed digital video data

system requirements:
- CPU 486
- 16 MB RAM
- SCSI controller (connection to DAT or removable hard disk)
- MS Windows NT 4.0, MS Windows 95, MS Windows 3.x

data flow of approx. 2kB/sec for each eye

3. eye movement analysis

eye movement parameters are calculated from eye position data

system requirements:

same as above

Figure 1. Different stages of eye movement analysis in a video eye movement recording system (VEMRS): 1) image recording: hard disk recording of video; 2) image analysis: image processing for calculation of eye position; 3) analysis of eye movement data (slow phase vel., etc.). All steps can be done either on a single computer or distributed over several computers.

For well-known reasons (Moore at al. 1996), 3D analysis is actually restricted to a range of ±10° in the horizontal and vertical directions. Eye position is given in Fick coordinates. Pupil diameter and pupil area are given in pixels and square pixels. Data conform to the Matlab format and can be processed by any other program.

Equipped with two 8 GByte hard disks, the VEMRS records 60 minutes of video data of the right and left eye (~2.25 MB/s/eye). Offline analysis is done at 10 frames/s on a Pentium Pro (200 MHz), thus resulting in 3 hours of unattended processing time for each hard disk.

Special hardware makes possible the use of rapid scan cameras (70 Hz non-interlaced frame rate), the concomitant registration of analog and digital input channels, and the measurement of head and limb movements with an ultrasonic motion analysis system (zebris Medizintechnik GmbH, Tuebingen).

Digital video hard disk recording has various advantages, e.g. images are not contaminated by noise as in analog recording on video recorders. Thus, detection of the pupil and analysis of ocular torsion are more reliable. Furthermore, hard disk recording gives random access to any frame within a video sequence. Time-consuming winding operations of video recorders are thus obsolete. Repeated replaying of video sequences results in no reduction of image quality unlike with video recorders.

We decided to analyse the video data offline. Therefore, all parameters required for automatic detection of the pupil and for measurement of ocular torsion can be fitted interactively to an optimum. Contrary to online systems, incorrect detections can be fixed and reevaluated. During offline analysis results can be compared to the original image data, thus allowing effective control of detection.

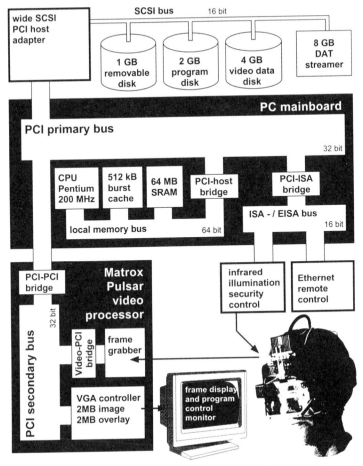

Figure 2. Hardware setup of the video eye movement recording system (VEMRS).

Currently, the hardware required for building a binocular version of the VEMRS system costs less than $20000. Future improvements of computer hardware (e.g. hard disk capacity, speed of CPU, lower prices) will increase the performance of the VEMRS and the analysis software, thus making its use less expensive.

REFERENCES

Clarke AH, Teiwes W, Scherer H. (1991) Video-oculography - An alternative method for measurement of three-dimensional eye movements. In: Schmid R, Zambarbieri D (eds) Oculomotor control and cognitive processes. Elsevier, Amsterdam, pp 431–443

Moore ST, Curthoys IS, McCoy SG. (1991) VTM - An image-processing system for measuring ocular torsion. Computer Methods and Programs in Biomedicine 35: 219–30

Moore ST, Haslwanter T, Curthoys IS, Smith ST. (1996) A geometric basis for measurement of three-dimensional eye position using image processing. Vision Res. 36: 445–59

Steddin S, Brandt T. (1995) Rapid scan video-oculography (RASVOG) for measurement of rapid eye movements. J. Neurol 242, Suppl 2: 64

66

IMPROVED THREE-DIMENSIONAL EYE MOVEMENT MEASUREMENT USING SMART VISION SENSORS

A. H. Clarke, D. Schücker, and W. Krzok

Vestibular Research Lab
Department of Otorhinolaryngology
Freie Universität Berlin

1. INTRODUCTION

State-of-the-art imaging technology, based on video sensors, permits accurate three-dimensional measurement of eye movement (horizontal, vertical, torsional). The non-invasive nature of such imaging techniques is particularly attractive for use in the clinic, where due consideration must be given to patient comfort, and in those experimental situations where operating conditions preclude the use of more invasive techniques such as scleral search coils.

However, a number of drawbacks arise with those video-oculography systems which adhere to standard video conventions. The major disadvantage is the restriction of the image sampling rate (typically 30 Hz). As a workaround, some manufacturers also provide increased sampling rates (i.e. 60 Hz, in some cases multiples up to 240 Hz), by simply decimating the number of horizontal lines included in each frame. A further disadvantage of video-based systems is the necessary digitisation of the analogue video signal before any image processing can be performed. While modern framegrabber devices provide on-line video digitisation, the delay of 33 ms for frame acquisition can be restrictive in such applications where the response, or latency time of the eye position measurement is crucial (e.g. graphic, or virtual environment rendering, or eye-guided processes). Furthermore, storage and processing after full frame acquisition can lead to bottleneck situations.

A new approach is described here that rests on the premise that any series of images of the moving eye is of necessity largely redundant, i.e the content of the image remains theoretically constant. Thus, with conventional digitising and processing of video images, the majority of pixel operations, although necessary for the technology employed, introduce only a loss of processing time. This is reflected, in the fact that for each image typically 400,000 pixels are digitised and stored; whereas after final processing, only three

Current Oculomotor Research, edited by Becker *et al.*
Plenum Press, New York, 1999.

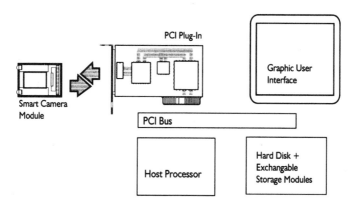

Figure 1. Illustration of smart vision eye tracker system. The sensor chip is packaged with the lens and lighting diodes; this module is attached to a head-mounted, free-field-of-view assemblyor to a light-occluding mask. Data from the chip are transferred via parallel bus to a DSP board, where final processing is performed.

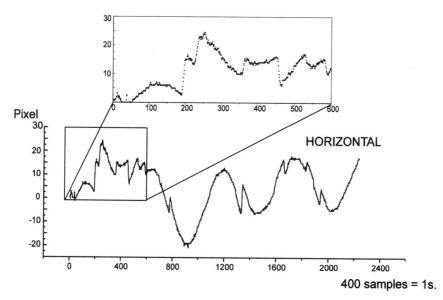

Figure 2. Example of online eye tracking at 400 /s using smart sensors. Eye movement pattern elicited by oscillation of the head (i.e. vestibulo-ocular reflex). Note the complex pattern of slow and rapid phases. The blow-up demonstrates the adequate acquisition, which is achieved with a sampling rate of 400 /s.

data values (corresponding to the three orthogonal components of eye position) are extracted. The recently introduced techniques for image compression (e.g. JPEG) also illustrate the substantial reduction in data capacity when the image redundancy is reduced.

2. DIGITAL CAMERA SOLUTIONS

Recently, a number of digital cameras have become available, which provide solutions to these problems. In particular, the most recent CMOS devices, which include on-chip analog-to-digital conversion free the user from the video timing conventions, and permit direct pixel addressing of the areas-of-interest.

Of particular interest for high-speed object tracking are the more complex devices, known as smart vision sensors, which incorporate sensor array, A/D conversion, storage registers and pixel-parallel processors (Clarke, 1994). With such devices, the entire image acquisition and pre-processing tasks can be performed on-chip, without any transfer to a framegrabber or external processor. Thus, only non-redundant information is subsequently transferred to the host computer. This approach also eliminates errors due to analogue video processing or VTR fluctuations, resulting in improved image registration. This novel technology combines the advantages of video techniques with image sampling rates of beyond two hundred per second.

With the current lab system priority is given during online image acquisition to achieving high sampling rate and preprocessing the image pixels. In essence, this involves compressing the image data for efficient transmission and storage. With this technique, the limiting factor is the maximum permissible irradiation to the eye by the infrared light source, rather than the performance of the processing circuitry. Since all relevant pixel data are stored, the user is free to define the algorithm for subsequent processing.

While the simpler approaches (e.g. pupil centroid) can be rejected for their artefact susceptibility, it appears that the more adequate "circle approximation" techniques for the pupil perimeter (e.g. Barbur et al, 1988) must also be rejected in favour of ellipse-fitting (Pilu et al, 1996) which represents a better approximation to the pupil form of most eyes, and allows for compensation of any geometric distortion during eye rotation (Moore et al, 1994).

Besides the problem of pupil form, the greatest souces of error are image artefacts caused by shadowing, reflections from tear fluid, pupil occlusion. To overcome this, an algorithm based on the generalised Hough transform has been implemented (Hough, 1962), which has proved extremely robust against such artefacts.

For 3D tracking, the torsional eye position calculated using the polar correlation algorithm (Hatamian & Anderson, 1983). The parallel processing features of the smart sensor are being exploited here to develop robust preprocessing algorithms to improve the grey level images of the iris under low lighting levels.

REFERENCES

Clarke AH, 1994 Image processing techniques for the measurement of eye movement. In Ygge J, Lennerstrand G (Eds), Eye Movements in Reading. Elsevier, Oxford, NY pp 21–38.

Barbur J, Thomson WD, Forsyth PM (1987) A new system for the simultaneous measurement of pupil size and two-dimensional eye movements. Clin Vision Sci 2: 131–142.

Hatamian M, Anderson DJ (1983) Design considerations for a realtime ocular counterroll instrument. IEEE Trans Biomed Engg BME-13: 65–70.

Hough PVC (1962) Metods and means for recognising complex patterns. US Patent 3069654.

Moore ST, Haslwanter T, Curthoys IS, Smith ST (1994) A geometric basis for measurement of three dimensional eye position using image processing. (submitted to Vision Res).

Pilu M, Fitzgibbon A, Fisher R (1996) Ellipse-specific direct least-square fitting. IEEE Int Conf Image Proc, Lausanne.

CONTRIBUTORS

Dr. A. Accardo
Universita die Trieste
via Valerio 19
I-34100 Trieste
Italy
accardo@gnbts.univ.trieste.it
via Dr. Parissutti;

Robert Althoff
Neuroscience Program and College of
   Medicine
University of Illinois
2424 Beckman Institute 405 N. Mathews
   MC-251
Urbana, IL 61801
U.S.A.
ralthoff@s.psych.uiuc.edu
Tel. ++1 217 244 4458; Fax ++1 217 244
   8371

Dr. Dimitrios Anastasopoulos
Department of Neurology
University of Ioannina
Panepistimoupolis Ioanninon
GR-45110 Ioannina, Greece
danastas@cc.uoi.gr
Tel. ++30 651 78265; Fax++30 651 78265

Dr. Dora Angelaki
Dept. of Surgery (Otolaryngology)
University of Mississippi Medical Center
2500 North State Str.
Jackson MS 39216, USA
dea@fiona.umsmed.edu
Tel. ++1 601 9845090; Fax ++1 601
   9845107

Dr. Patricia Apkarian
Dept. of Physiology, School of Medicine
   and Health Sciences
Erasmus University Rotterdam
P.O. Box 1783
3000 DR Rotterdam
The Netherlands
apkarian@fys1.fgg.eur.nl
Tel. ++31 10 408 7568; Fax++31 10 408
   7594

Dr. Graham Barnes
Institute of Neurology
MRC Human Movement and Balance Unit
23, Queen Square
WC1N 3BG London
Great Britain
g.barnes@ion.ucl.ac.uk
Tel. ++44 171 8373611 ext 3069; Fax

Mrs. Cécile Beauvillain
Laboratoire de Psychologie Expérimentale
   URA 316 CNRS
Université René Descartes
28 rue Serpente
F 75006 Paris, France
beauvi@idf.ext.jussieu.fr
Tel. ++33 1 40 51 9871; Fax++33 1 40 51
   9871

Wihelm Becker
Sektion Neurophysiologie
University of Ulm
Albert Einstein Allee 47
D-89081 Ulm
Germany

Dr. Giampaolo Biral
Dipartimento di Scienze Biomediche
Università di Modena
Via Campi 287
I 41100 Modena
Italy
rferrari@unimo.it
Tel. ++39 59 428213; Fax ++39 59 428236

Dr. Monica Biscaldi
AG-Hirnforschung
Institut fuer Biophysik
Hansastr. 9
D-79104 Freiburg, Deutschland
biscaldi@sun2.ruf.uni-freiburg.de
Tel. ++49 761 203 9539; Fax ++49 761
203 9540

Dr. Jean Blouin
Fac. Sciences du Sport
UMR CNRS Mouvement et Perception
   Univ. de la Méditerrannée
163, ave. de Luminy
F 3288 Marseille
France
blouin@laps.univ-mrs.fr
Tel. ++33 4 9117 2277; Fax ++33 4 9117
2252

Dr. Lo Bour
Department of Neurolopgy / Clinical
   Neurophysiology
University of Amsterdam Medical Centre
Meibergdreef 9
D 1106 A2 Amsterdam
The Netherlands
bour@amc.uva.nl
Tel. ++31 250 663515; Fax ++31 250
669187

Dr. med. Stephan A. Brandt
Neurologische Klinik
Charité, Humboldt Universität Berlin
Schumannstr. 20/21
D-10117 Berlin
Deutschland
sbrandt@neuro.charite.hu-berlin.de
Tel. ++49 30 2802 2648; Fax ++49 30
2802 5047

Prof. Ulrich Buettner
Neurologische Klinik
Ludwig-Maximilians- Universität
Klinikum Großhadern
D-81377 München
Germany
ubuettner@brain.nefo.med.uni-muenchen.
   de
Tel. ++49 89 7095 2560; Fax ++49 89
7095 8883

Prof. Jean Buettner-Ennever
Institute of Anatomy,
Ludwig-Maximilian University
Pettenkoferstr. 11,
D - 80336 München, Germany
Buettner@anat.med.uni-muenchen.de
Tel. ++49 89 5160 4880; Fax ++49 89
5160 4857

Dr. Yue Chen
Department of Psychology
Harvard University
33 Kirkland St. / WJH782
Cambridge MA O2139, USA
ychen@wjh.harvard.edu
Tel. ++1 617 495 3884; Fax ++1 617 495
3764

Dr. Andrew H Clarke
Klinikum Benjamin Franklin
Vestibular Research Lab ENT Clinic
Hindenburgdamm 30
D - 12200 Berlin, FRG
clarke@zedat.fu-berlin.de
Tel. ++49 30 8445 2434; Fax ++49 30 834
2116

PD Dr.-Ing. Heiner Deubel
Ludwig-Maximilians-Universitaet
   Muenchen
Institut fuer Psychologie
Leopoldstr. 13
D - 80802 München
Germany
DEUBEL@MIP.PAED.UNI-MUENCHEN.
   DE
Tel. ++49 89 2180 5282; Fax ++49 89
2180 5282

Mr. Jochen Ditterich
Center for Sensorimotor Research, Dept.
  of Neurology
Ludwig-Maximilians-University Munich
Marchioninistr. 23
D 81377 Munich
Germany
ditterich@gnf99m.nefo.med.uni-muenchen.
  de
Tel. ++49 89 70906 134; Fax ++49 89
  70906 101

Dr. Karine Dore
Laboratoire de Psychologie Expérimentale
28, rue Serpente, F 75006 Paris
France
kdore@idf.ext.jussieu.fr
Tel. ++33 1 4051 9874; Fax ++33 1 4051
  7085

Dr. Andrew Eadie
Physical Sciences
Glasgow Caledonian University
Cowcaddens Road
G4 0BA Glasgow
United Kingdom
asea@gcal.ac.uk
Tel. ++44 141331 3657; Fax ++44 141331
  3653

Prof. Yoshinobu Ebisawa
Faculty of Engineering
Shizuoka University
3-5-1 Johoku, 432-8561 Hamamatsu
Japan
ebisawa@sys.eng.shizuoka.ac.jp
Tel. ++81 53 478 1244; Fax ++81 53 478
  1244

Prof. dr. Casper J. Erkelens
Helmholtz Instituut
Research Group Physics of Man
Utrecht Unuversity, P.O.Box 80.000
350 8 TA Utrecht
 The Netherlands
c.j.erkelens@fys.ruu.nl
Tel. ++31 30 253 2832; Fax ++31 30
  2522664

Dr. Stefan Everling
Department of Physiology
Queen's University
K7L 3N6 Kingston, Ontario, Canada
stefan@ss2.biomed.QueensU.CA
Tel. 001 613 545 6360; Fax 001 613 545
  6340

PD Dr. Michael Fetter
Department of Neurology
Eberhard-Karls University
Hoppe-Seyler-Str. 3
D 72076 Tübingen, Germany
michael.fetter@uni-tuebingen.de
Tel. ++49 7071 29 80445; Fax++49 7071
  29 6507

Prof. Dr. Burkhart Fischer B
Arbeitsgruppe Hirnforschung
University Freiburg
Hansa-Str. 9a
D-79104 Freiburg, Germany
bfischer@uni-freiburg.de
Tel. ++49 761 203 9536; Fax ++49 761
  203 9540

Dr. Stefan Glasauer
Klinikum Großhadern -NRO
Zentrum für Sensormotorik
Marchoninistr. 23
D-81377 München, Germany
sglasauer@nefo.med.uni-muenchen.de
Tel. ++49 89 70906 139; Fax ++49 89
  70906 101

Dr. Michael E. Goldberg
Laboratory of Sensorimotor Research
NEI
49 Convent Drive
Bethesda MD 20892-4435, USA
meg@lsr.nei.nih.gov

Dr. Brooke Hallowell
School of Hearing and Speech Sciences
Ohio University
208, Lindley Hall, Athens OH 45701, USA
HALLOWELL@ouvaxa.cats.ohiou.edu
Tel. ++1 740 593 1356; Fax ++1 740 593
  0287

PD Dr. Wolfgang Heide
Klinik für Neurologie
Medizinische Universität zu Lübeck
Ratzeburger Allee 160
D 23562 Lübeck
Germany
heide@medinf.mu-luebeck.de
Tel. ++49 451 5003472; Fax ++49 451
  5002489

Prof. Dieter Heller
Department of Psychology
Technical University of Aachen
Jaegerstr. 17
D-52056 Aachen
Germany
diheller@psycho.rwth-aachen.de
Tel. ++49 241 806012; Fax ++49 241
  8888318

Mr. Jörg Hofmeister
Department of Psychology
University of Dundee
DD1 4HN Dundee
United Kingdom
JHOFMEIS@psycho.rwth-aachen.de
Tel. ++49 1382 344629
Fax++49 1382 229993

Dr. K. Holmqvist
Department of Cognitive Science
Lund University
Kungshuset
 Lundagaerd
S - 222 22 Lund
Sweden
kenneth.holmqvist@fil.lu.se
Tel. ++46 70 5579 265
Fax ++46 46 222 4817

Dr. Jana Holsanova
Department of Cognitive Science
Lund University
Kungshuset, Lundagaerd
S - 222 22 Lund
Sweden
Jana.Holsanova@fil.lu.se
Tel. ++46 46 222 97 58; Fax ++46 46 222
  4817

Dr. Uwe Ilg
Sektion für Visuelle Sensomotorik
Neurologische Universitätsklinik
Hoppe-Seyler-Str. 3
D 72076 Tübingen, Germany
uwe.ilg@uni-tuebingen.de; Tel. ++49 7071
  2980432; Fax ++49 7071 295724

Dr. Isabelle Israel
CNRS - College de France
Lab. de Physiol.de la Perception et de
  l'Action
11 place Marcelin Berthelot
75005 Paris, France
isi@ccr.jussieu.fr; Tel. ++33 144 271 288;
  Fax ++33 144 271 382

Dr. Jim Ivins
Psychology
University of Sheffield
Western Bank, S102 TP Sheffield, England
J.P.IVINS@SHEF-AC-UK
Tel. ++44 114 222 6515; Fax ++44 114
  222 6515

Dr. Reinhart Jürgens
Sektion Neurophysiologie
Universität Ulm
Albert-Einstein-Allee 47
D 89081 Ulm, Germany
reinhart.juergens@medizin.uni-ulm.de
Tel. ++49 731 502 5500; Fax++49 731 502
  5501

ZK Zoi Kapoula
Laboratoire de Physiologie de la
  Perception et de l'Action
CNRS-Collège de France
11, place Marcelin Berthelot
F 75231 Paris, France
zk@ccr.jussieu.fr; Tel. ++33 1 4427 1635;
  Fax ++33 1 4427 1382

Prof Alan Kennedy
University of Dundee
Psychology Department
DD1 4HN Dundee, Scotland (UK)
A.KENNEDY@dundee.ac.uk
Tel. ++44 1382 223181; Fax ++44 1382
  22993

Dr. Hubert Kimmig
Neurologische Universitätsklinik
Universität Freiburg
Breisacher Str. 64
D-79106 Freiburg
Deutschland
kimmig@sun1.ruf.uni-freiburg.de
Tel. ++49 761 270 5306; Fax ++49 761
270 5390

Dr. Paul Charles Knox
Vision Sciences
Glasgow Caledonian University
Cowcaddens Road
G4 0BA Glasgow
United Kingdom
P.C.Knox@gcal.ac.uk
Tel. ++44 141 331 3695
Fax ++44 141 331 3387

Dr. C. Krischer
KFA, IBI
ROTDORNWEG 5
52428 Juelich
Deutschland
okrischer@aol.com
Tel. ++49 2461 50932; Fax ++49 2461
910506

Dr. Markus Lappe
Allgemeine Zoologie und Neurobiologie
Ruhr Universität Bochum
Universitätsstr. 150
D 44780 Bochum
Germany
lappe@jeannie.neurobiologie
.ruhr-uni-bochum.de
Tel. ++49 234 700 4369; Fax ++49 234
709 4278

Dr. Cyril Latimer
University of Sidney
Department of Psychology
NSW 2006 Sydney
Australia
cyril@psych.su.oz.au
Tel. ++61 2 9351 2481; Fax. ++61 2 9351
2481

Dr. Rebekka Lencer
Klinik für Psychiatrie
Nedizinische Universität zu Lübeck
Ratzeburger Alle 160
D 23568 Lübeck, Germany
106624.1705@compuserve.com
Tel. ++49 451 500 2441; Fax ++49 451
500 2603

Mr. Michael MacAskill
Department of Medicine
Christchurch School of Medicine
P.O.Box 4345
Christchurch, New Zealand
m.macaskill@cheerful.com
Tel. ++64 3 3640 640 ext 88; Fax ++64 3
3640 640 935

Dr. Christoph Maurer
Neurologische Klinik
Universität Freiburg
Breisacher Strasse 64
D 79106 Freiburg, Germany
Maurer@nz11.ukl.uni-freiburg.de

McHenry
Department of Surgery
University of Mississippi
Jackson, Mississippi
Tel. ++1 601 984 5090; Fax++1 601 984
5090

Thomas Mergner
Neorological University Clinic
University of Freiburg
Breisacher Strasse 64
D-79106 Freiburg
Germany

Mr. Carsten Moschner
Klinik für Neurologie
Medizinische Universität zu Lübeck
Ratzeburger Allee 160
23538 Lübeck, Deutschland
moschner@medinf.mu-luebeck.de
Tel.++49 51 500 6050; Fax++49 51 500
4944

PD Dr. René Mueri
Department of Neurology
Inselspital
CH 3010 Bern
Switzerland
rene.mueri@insel.ch
Tel. ++41 31 632 2111; Fax ++41 31 632
9679

Prof. Douglas Munoz
Department of Physiology
Queen's University
K7L 3N6 Kingston, Ontario, Canada
doug@biomed.queensu.ca
Tel. ++1 613 545 2111; Fax++1 613 545
6840

Nasios
Department of Neurology
University of Ioannina
Panepistimioupolis Ioannina
GR-45110 Ioannina
Greece

Mr. Ulrich Nies
Institute of Psychology
Technical University of Aachen
Jägerstr. 17
52056 Aachen
Germany
ULRINIES@psycho.rwth-aachen.de
Tel. ++49 241 803992; Fax ++49 241 8888
318

Mr. Ingo Paprotta
Department of Experimental Psychology
Ludwig-Maximilians-Universität München
Leopold Strasse 13
d 80802 München, Germany
paprotta@psy.uni-muenchen.de
via Deubel;

Dr. Paolo Perisutti
Dpt. Chirurgico-occulista
Istituto Infanzia
via dell' Istria 56/1
I-34137 Trieste
Italy
Tel. ++40 3785 395; Fax ++40 660 919

Dr. Ralph Radach
Institute of Psychology
RWTH Aachen
Jaegerstr. 17
D-52056 Aachen, Germany
raradach@psycho.rwth-aachen.de
Tel. ++49 241 803993; Fax++49 241 8888
318

Dr. Eyal Reingold
Department: Psychology
University of Toronto
100 St. George Street
M5S 3G3 Toronto, Ontario, Canada
reingold@psych.toronto.edu
Tel. ++1 905 629 2036; Fax ++1 905 629
0337

Mrs. Anke Roll
Mathematik und Datenverarbeitung
Universität der Bundeswehr München
Werner-Heisenberg-Weg 39
D-85577 Neubiberg, Germany
anke.roll@unibw-muenchen.de
Tel. ++49 89 6004 3605; Fax++49 89 6004
3613

Mr. Walter Schroyens
Laboratory of Experimental Psychology
University of Leuven
Tiensestraat 102
B-3000 Leuven, Belgium
Walter.Schroyens@psy.kuleuven.ac.be

Dr. Georg Schweigart
Neurophysiologie (Gebäude MA4)
Ruhr-Universität Bochum
Universitätsstraße
44780 Bochum, Deutschland
georg@neurop.ruhr-uni-bochu.de

Mrs. Astrid Spantekow
University of Bremen
Brain Research Institute
P.O. Box 33 04 40
D - 28334 Bremen, Germany
spanteko@zfn.uni-bremen.de
Tel. ++49 4121 218 2438; Fax ++49 4121
218 4932

Mr. Sven Steddin
Zebris Medizintechnik
Wilhelmstr. 134
D-72074 Tübingen
Deutschland
steddin@zebris.de
Tel. ++49 7071 27003; Fax ++49 7071
  27005

Mrs. Mariko Takeda
Wakayama University
Dept. Psychology Faculty of Education
930 Sakaedani
640-8510 Wakayama
Japan
85688691@people.or.jp
Tel. ++81 75 711 2723
 FaxTel. ++81 75 711 2723

Tsironi
Department of Opthamology
University of Ioannina
GR-45110 Ioannina
Greece

Prof. Jan A.M. van Gisbergen
231 Medical Physics & Biophysics
University of Nijmegen
Geert Grooteplein 21
6525 EZ Nijmegen
The Netherlands
vangisbergen@mbfys.kun.nl
Tel. ++31 24361 4247
 Fax ++31 24 354

PhD Jocelyne Ventre-Dominey
Vision et Motricité
INSERM U94
16 av. Doyen Lépine
69500 Bron, France
ventre-dominey@lyon151.inserm.fr
Tel. ++33 4 72913410; Fax ++33 4
  72913401

Mrs. Martien Wampers
Laboratory of Experimental Psychology
University of Leuven
Tiensestraat 102
B 3000 Leuven, Belgium
Martien.Wampers@psy.kuleuven.ac.be
Tel. ++32 16 32 59 65; Fax ++32 16 32 60
  99

Prof. Dr. Takahiro Yamanoi
Div. Electronics and Information Eng.,
  Fac. Eng.
Hokkai Gakuen University
S26, W11, Central ward
O64 Sapporo, Japan
yamanoi@eli.hokkai-s-u.ac.jp
Tel. ++81 11 841 1161 ext. 866; Fax Tel.
  ++81 11 551 2951

Prof. Wolfgang Zangemeister
Neurologische Klinik
Universität Hamburg
Martinistr. 52
D 20251 Hamburg, Germany
zangemeister@uke.uni-hamburg.de
Tel. ++49 40 4717 2607; Fax ++49 40
  4717 5088

INDEX